Artificial Intelligence to Analyze Psychophysical and Human Lifestyle

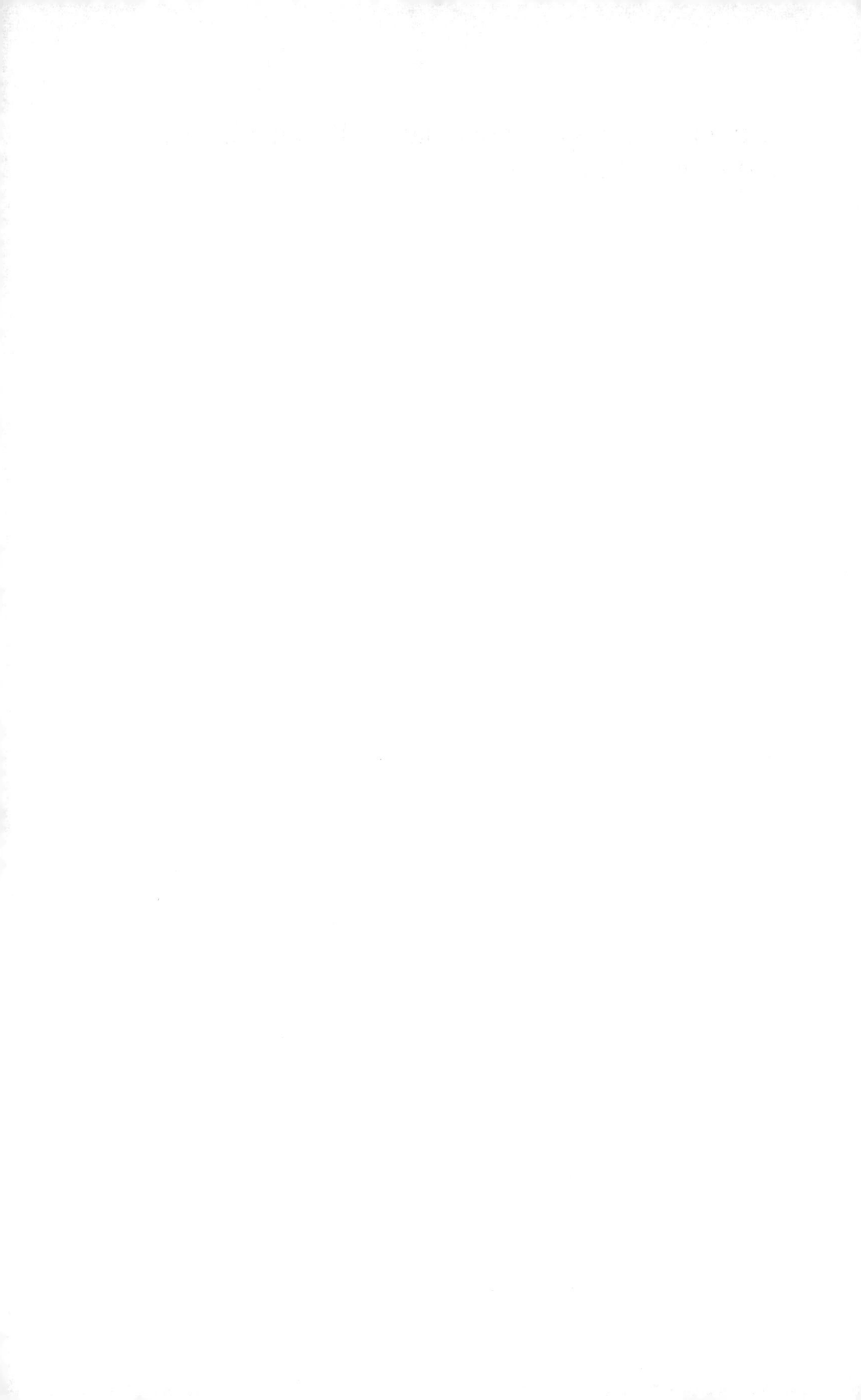

Gunjan Chhabra · Sunil Kumar · Sunil Gupta ·
Pooja Nagpal

Artificial Intelligence to Analyze Psychophysical and Human Lifestyle

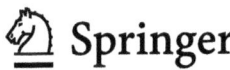

Gunjan Chhabra
Department of Computer Science
and Engineering
Graphic Era Hill University
Dehradun, Uttarakhand, India

Sunil Gupta
School of Computer Science
University of Petroleum and Energy Studies
Dehradun, Uttarakhand, India

Sunil Kumar
Department of Computer Science
and Engineering, Amity School
of Engineering and Technology
Amity University Madhya Pradesh
Gwalior, Madhya Pradesh, India

Pooja Nagpal
School of Engineering and Technology
K. R. Mangalam University
Gurgaon, Haryana, India

ISBN 978-981-99-3038-8   ISBN 978-981-99-3039-5 (eBook)
https://doi.org/10.1007/978-981-99-3039-5

This Springer imprint is published by the registered company Springer Nature Singapore Pte Ltd.
The registered company address is: 152 Beach Road, #21-01/04 Gateway East, Singapore 189721,
Singapore

Contents

Chapter 1
The Interaction and Convergence of the Internet of Things and Artificial Intelligence

1.1 Introduction

Several projections and expert papers have been written about the convergence of the Internet of Things (IoT) and artificial intelligence (AI). There has been increased emphasis for quite some time on how each functions, along with why "the IoT requires AI," across a broad range of business domains [1–5]. The fast rise of various types of AI throughout all stages of the IoT paradigm is difficult to maintain [6]. The use of machine learning (ML) in conjunction with big data as a combined effect to unleash the possible future and innovative possibilities in the IoT is now ranked highly in forecasts for 2017 [7, 8], with the change to new features listed as essential stages "to feed ML engines and even more, AI demands" [9].

As mentioned by Chowanda [10], IoT and linked systems boost AI adoption since smart management is obligated to produce a sense of the massive amounts of data created by sensing devices [11, 12]. Perhaps an overview of different instances in which it is now a reality would make it more tangible [13]. Before beginning, two points should be made. First, both technologies are overarching words, not specific domains [14, 15]. Behind the facades of IoT and AI, it's not difficult to see what they have in common: knowledge converted into data which are transformed into intelligence and changed into choices for shared objectives over several use instances. Humans will also look a little further into how AI affects the emerging methods and stages in hybrid IoT and industrial IoT (IIoT) scenarios [16, 17].

Second, it is vital to recall that the (series of) domains open to technology innovation and Industry 4.0, as illustrated in the third stage of Industry 4.0, don't exist in perfect isolation. Consider some prominent intelligent automations (or rather technology areas): digitized duplication, mixed reality, clouds, big data, and robots [18, 19]. It is rather evident that they all interact with one another, such as AI and IIoT. And this manifests in the growth of wireless networks and, in the context of business models, in the growing importance of AI algorithms and their strengths, and their assistance to augmented and virtual duplicates in the realm of Industry 4.0 technologies [20].

G. Chhabra et al., *Artificial Intelligence to Analyze Psychophysical and Human Lifestyle*, https://doi.org/10.1007/978-981-99-3039-5_1

1.1.1   AI and IoT: A Vision

When one considers the fundamental and essential levels, the integration of the IoT and AI should come as no surprise [21]. For many years, various versions of AI have been used to analyze information, locate information, and convert data into meaningful information, with a concentration on the increase of unstructured information. Consider integrated data governance, or even records capture [22]—where AI is nothing new—or help support applications that accumulate different types of information from various sources in different configurations and offer them to a unified communications representative, end-to-end communication, and deep insight, conceivably with the logic of AI. And consider text analytics when wireless transmission is included in the computation [23].

Even from the perspective of the challenging job of storing information on various servers, there are AI providers that offer, for example, the protection of private information and adherence to the General Data Protection Regulation (GDPR) [24]—which is to be responsible for compliance and private details regarding subject protection queries or requirements from authorities, so that the customer understands where private details are placed [25] and what the reasons are for legitimately analyzing data. The integration of AI and the IoT may be considered "new" and is likely to attract greater attention soon, for these reasons:

- The reality is that the IoT and AI are indeed fairly recent in many businesses and organizations, although they are not so in many others [26].
- The many requirements for the IoT and AI to function together over several application scenarios and real implementations, with some use cases and goals (e.g., preventative and anticipatory management rather than reactive management), are only applicable to medium-scale enterprises.
- A possible misconception about IIoT behavior, as well as the related domains and goals of platforms found in, for example, smart manufacturing and "Industry 4.0."
- The distinctions around how the IoT and AI are now employed together and in more enduring ways in which more "sophisticated" types of AI and ML integrate with a growing emphasis on a "fully independent" intellect [27].
- With the evolution in the IoT industry, particularly in the IIoT, there is an increasing, yet reasonable, emphasis on Intelligence IoT development and infrastructure.
- A lack of understanding of the method and the Application Programming Interface (API) industry—to which we would advise readers to look at the progression in knowledge operations in wireless communication, which is more difficult with startups [28].
- The reality is that the IoT has been primarily implemented in industrial applications within a wider definition, with unique benefits, but less within the purview of servicing, data modeling, and integrated operational processes in industries such as supply chain management, exploration and production, healthcare products, housing developments, aerospace, protection, infrastructure, and medical

services, in which the IIoT and data analysis have enabled organizations to realize the returns.

- A possibly too developed recognition of learning operations and the IIoT (and frequently for innovations) not only makes the impact on the client side counts the most but also drastically transforms corporate entrepreneurial operations.
- Too much emphasis is placed on diverse sets of technology rather than actual instances of how they are employed in practice, frequently with aims and advantages that may genuinely save a life.
- The never-ending natural need to comprehend objects by assigning them labels, even if they encompass various dependent facts, instead of understanding holistically and interconnecting dots on a profound level. Fast progression throughout all stages makes it extremely difficult to stay current.

The substance of these primary reasons is followed by various instances of the IIoT and AI being used nowadays.

1.1.2   The Core of the IoT and AI

The IoT is mainly a device to connect sensor systems, controllers, and wireless communications that use hardware resources, applications, and modern architecture strategies to collect information from a wide range of potential equipment for a diverse range of applications, goals, advancements, and inventions. The components and integrated devices (e.g., sensing devices) that empower catching a wide range of "ailment and situational state" information, and converting that information inside the diverse work environment [29], contain IoT access points, IoT devices, IoT modern communications, equipment, and software, where accumulation and assessment occur, as well as their real implementation, which is founded upon it, possible architectures such as sensor networks, and so on.

The foundation of the IoT is collecting information from interconnected devices and using that information for a meaningful cause, such as authenticating customers and network devices to perform desired actions depending on the processed and visible information. So, from the standpoint of "real" equipment (devices, actuators, etc.), the IoT operates in two ways: from information to organized process (which might also be an investigation or any other kind of human activity [30]); and "additional" information [31].

1.2   The IoT with AI: A Perspective of Industry 4.0

Industry operations and smart communications, as defined in development mechanisms such as smart manufacturing and supply chain 4.0, mainly connect the software industry and operational logistics, the IoT and digital forensics, "deep" statistical methods, and a shift toward quasi-automated and communication devices. This is a steady transition from automation to independence at the object level in the IIoT and even beyond: smart cities, remote monitoring, exploration, production activities, robots, and so on [32]. As we will see, the IoT and AI are already being employed in this field for a variety of applications, although it takes time and is a question of integrating user regulation with timely actions at the appropriate stages.

Let's examine some of the many application scenarios and domains where AI and the IoT are already being utilized in tandem in different stages and domains. The network architecture is composed of numerous levels, and AI is progressively being implemented in all categories, from enabled AI in the IoT to AI in infrastructures, such as cloud computation or network virtualization [33], as well as the associated technology, equipment, and communication systems. Integrated AI will be especially important here, as the purpose of both IoT technology and cloud technology is to analyze the information near its deployment.

1.2.1 The Role of AI and the IoT in Infrastructure Design

AI is coming to the forefront of providing services at differing stages. In organizational management, system development, in which self-directed decision-making in that network is addressed, intellectual ability is progressing farther into that line of work, farthest from the aspect where all the information is stored and analyzed, allowing us to understand how the facility works [34].

Within the large scale of supportive enhancement, the cumulative use of AI and the IIoT extends much further, with inferential enhancement and predictive modeling with planned maintenance of essential building resources being among the important instances, and ML being used to notify a facility controller that concerns are about to take place inside particular building locations or technical devices. AI and the IoT are on track to become the foundations of the developing software concept of facility optimization. From a construction standpoint, it is worth noting that AI and the IoT are rapidly being employed in an "integrated" manner in modern living spaces (smart buildings and workplaces).

1.2.2 The Role of AI and the IoT in eHealth

Healthcare is a vast field, in that AI and the IIoT are being used in combination in various medical organizations. The IoT is already playing a significant role in healthcare. The same is true for AI where it is gaining importance in medical facilities such as hospitals (e.g., computer-aided diagnostics).

Hospital-linked healthcare data, hospital instruments, and both infrastructure and healthcare resources are looking for a home. AI and the IoT already collaborate in terms of: interconnectivity and information transfer between medical centers; and empowering hospital technicians to have an obvious, clear, and precise view of the situation inside a facility in real-time and to act on it with an emphasis on physicians, healthcare coverage, the expense of health coverage (both for patient populations and services), and the quality of healthcare, evaluated on the bases of patient care and "health promotion" [35].

Medical facilities have service delay issues, which is where AI and the IoT enter preventative analysis and the time management arena. Furthermore, AI and the IoT are being utilized to enhance health operations for those who interact with doctors. There are a few instances of the IIoT and ML in medicine, but the majority of them are in practice. The simultaneous use of AI and the IoT in the digital economy of the medical industry will only rise with real-time health systems (RTHSs), the rising use of automation in treatment, intelligent beds in smarter hospitals, virtual healthcare, and so on.

Researchers have looked at some of the illustrations of consulting firm studies from 2020, such as the rising use of robotic systems for the delivery of a drug (there is more than enough autonomous navigation in clinics), the transition from passive to engaged customer participation, and authentic improvements with AI using information from smart technology, to name a few. Finally, analysts predict that, by 2022, 80% of smart healthcare will gather GPS information, healthcare IoT device information, and include AI to detect trends, saving approximately 30% of physicians' time.

1.2.3   Robotic Systems and Automated Systems: AI and the IoT in Industry 4.0 and Beyond

There are various recognized instances where companies have a formal convergence/integration between ML and IIoT. And there is much more to be said on the level of scientific facets, such as the difficulties of attempting to bring AI to the authority, where users observe an area before actually summarizing some hybrid utilization instances. We're not focusing on the application of AI and the IoT in production as a whole because it's a wide topic with overlapping numerous sectors, as we've discussed, but instead on bots and robotic systems (functional bots) that are often hybrid-industry instances [36].

Robotic systems (and robots) currently employ deep learning (DL), the IIoT and AI, computer vision, and the detection of trends, motion, etc.; for instance, utilizing computer vision techniques, depending on their particular roles. Given the numerous factors to consider when installing automated systems, advanced manufacturing robotic systems feature a plethora of sensing devices, smart systems, and have AI on board (the utilized materials, the standard interface, factory approval, preventing unsafe motions, etc.). DL is already being used in conjunction with computer vision systems to allow robotic systems and bots to perform comparable jobs with slightly varying parameters.

The Belgian business Robovision employs AI-based computer vision techniques and DL in the roots of controlled plants and which is being applied in agriculture-related enterprises around the world. A few decades ago, the business was also participating in a robotic initiative at the Audi production facility in Brussels as part of this research effort that exploited some IoT and AI algorithms.

1.3   Strategies of AI with the IoT

There are plenty of other implementations where AI and the IoT collaborate, such as in practice as we have seen or in more long-term fully independent scenarios (e.g., automated vehicles), in augmented AI or self-governing intellectual ability, and in industrial applications, exploration and production, home automation, avionics, transportation, industrial unmanned aerial system implementations, protection, infrastructure, or many wearable devices.

Nowadays, the foremost use of AI and the IoT can be found in preventing wasted time through advanced analytics, enhancing productivity, increased information sources via mesh IoT application information, investigation (as demonstrated by biotech companies for instance), and so on. Regarding international data corporations, one research company anticipated that, by 2020 to 2022, cognitive/AI skills will underpin 100% of all effective IoT endeavors, though that proportion appears to be high.

The issue of the IIoT and ML merging with each other concerns the most important applications across sectors and use scenarios, such as the latest technological trends, which are where user, consumer, owner, and patient satisfaction can be found. In other instances (in particular, Maersk in IoT and AI logistics), use instances, commercial prospects, and consumer value proposals are focused on "Building the IoT," where AI is referred to as the brain and the IoT is referred to as the body. "IoT is the body that provides AI's brain the power to operate,". The IoT also supplies the data that AI requires to make sound judgments.

1.3.1   AI and the IoT: Numerous Technology Advancements and Stages

Intelligent machines (a phrase integrating AI and automated systems approaches), the IoT, as well as other innovations are represented at differing stages in numerous emerging sectors as follows [37]:

- **More sophisticated architectural frameworks** in microprocessor architecture, non-volatile storage (with incorporated storage devices to improve the IoT performance of the device), and embedded semiconductor optoelectronic devices.

- **New prediction techniques for IoT** sensory information flood that can take advantage of growing parallel processing capacity (which is related to the preceding point) and techniques in system design (e.g., DL).
- **AI inside systems at the transmission side** as connections are getting more complicated, including in the context of 5G and the IoT, where top companies highlight spatial multiplexing in upcoming 5G technology.
- **What companies refer to as "real intelligent systems,"** in which machine intellectual ability is supposed to merge with AI and ML methodologies.

But there is a lot more, including IIoT privacy and semantic interoperability, semantic services, enhanced knowledge, expanded dispersed IoT infrastructure, identification, and statistics.

The expansion of business (implementations and latest scenarios) and the growing number of levels where AI is administered and introduced into the IoT to achieve its complete capacity are not separate. We are seeing an increase in the use of the IoT in conjunction with other technologies. And this is not surprising. Executives have recognized this progression, while not all options have been identified. On the degree of AI and IoT utilization, Vodafone noted in the 2017–2018 edition of its IoT Survey that 79% of respondents believed that, by 2022, more than half of enterprises will utilize ML to make some sense of IoT information.

When we examined the AI and IoT market in September 2017, all the top companies noted that IoT technologies and services are integrated into an ever greater and larger range of services and use instances, as highlighted in the IIoT reference. This also applies to the IoT. There is also: next-generation access control; robotic systems; innovative aspects of AI (which persist) such as DL, emerging structures in AI and ML, and developed sensors with engrained operations designed to allow for enhanced efficiency; and organizational techniques (AI is evolving and improving virtually all applications in industrial ecosystems, from PLC, human–machine interface applications, and industrial production implementation structures for information systems, as well as the latter in conjunction with blockchain technology and the IoT) [38].

1.3.2 Merged AI with the IoT

The use of the IoT is altering the corporate environment today. The IoT is assisting in the significant gathering of a massive amount of information from many sources. On the one hand, there is the wrapping around of the plethora of data flowing from innumerable IoT devices; on the other hand, this complicates data collection, processing, and analysis. To realize the growth and full capability of IoT systems, investing in innovation will be required. The combination of AI and the IoT has the potential to reshape enterprises and ecosystems.

An AI-enabled IoT develops autonomous robots that replicate intelligent human behavior and improve coordination with little or no human intervention. Combining these two streams serves both the general public and professionals. Although the IoT

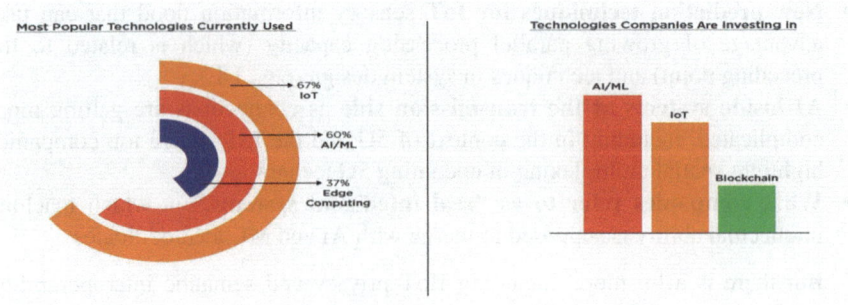

Fig. 1.1 Most popular technologies on the market

is concerned with members directly over the network, AI enables things to benefit from information and observations.

1.3.3 The IoT with AI is Becoming Increasingly Prevalent

Many companies have indeed integrated AI and the IoT into their services and activities. It was also discovered that AI and the IoT are the leading innovations that businesses are employing to boost productivity and gain competitiveness [39]. Figure 1.1 depicts the details of the most popular technologies currently used in the market.

As per the IBM Global C-suite research project, C-suite leaders help to develop their businesses through digitizing interactions between people. The IBM Academy examined a group of C-suite managers and discovered that 19% of participants (classified as top achievers known as reinventors) are very able to enjoy the benefits of enhanced IoT with AI. Figure 1.2 illustrates the level of current IoT adaptation to AI.

Many entrepreneurs and major corporations favor AI technologies for realizing the full potential of the IoT. Google, Facebook, eBay, and Salesforce have begun to integrate AI algorithms into various IoT networks.

1.3.4 Where Can AI Help in Enabling the IoT?

At its foundation, the IoT is about sensors installed in devices that provide streams of data via network connectivity. As shown in Fig. 1.3, all IoT-related operations must go through five fundamental steps: generating, transmitting, collecting, analyzing, and responding. The value of the "act" is dependent on the preliminary study. As a result, the specific purposes (especially of the IoT) are established during the evaluation phase. This is where AI methods come into play [40].

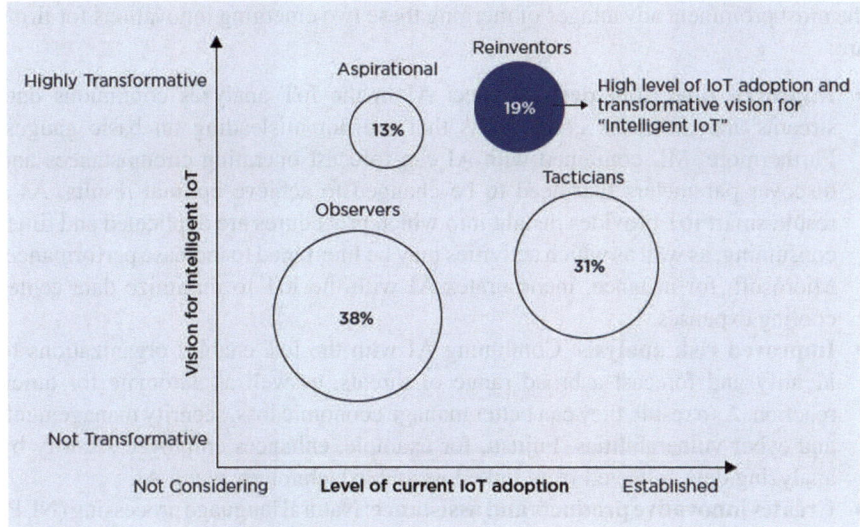

Fig. 1.2 Level of current IoT adaptation to AI

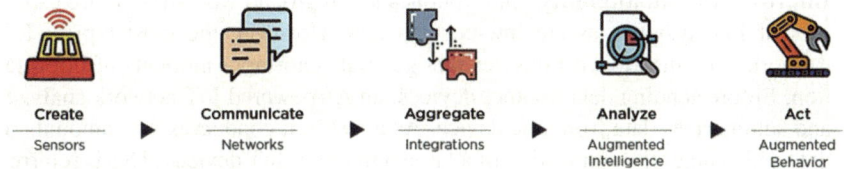

Fig. 1.3 IoT-related services

Although the IoT offers information, AI gains the ability to unlock replies, providing both innovation and knowledge to drive intelligent decisions. Organizations can make educated judgments since the sensor information can be examined using AI. Both AI and the IoT are effective at achieving the aforementioned agile solutions:

- To manage, analyze, and derive useful insight into the data;
- To ensure quick and precise research;
- To better predict for localized and centralized knowledge;
- To balance customization with secrecy and privacy protection.

1.3.5   Advantages of AI Merged with the IoT

Businesses and consumers profit from the IoT and AI in a variety of ways, including pre-emptive intervention, tailored experiences, and cognitive technologies. Some of the most prominent advantages of merging these two emerging innovations for firms are:

- **Improved operating performance**: AI in the IoT analyzes continuous data streams and discovers connections that are not misleading on basic gauges. Furthermore, ML combined with AI can forecast operating circumstances and discover parameters that need to be changed to achieve optimal results. As a result, smart IoT provides insight into which procedures are duplicated and time-consuming, as well as which activities may be fine-tuned to increase performance. Microsoft, for instance, incorporates AI with the IoT to minimize data center cooling expenses.
- **Improved risk analysis**: Combining AI with the IoT enables organizations to identify and forecast a broad range of threats, as well as automate for quick reaction. As a result, they can better manage economic loss, security management, and cyber vulnerabilities. Fujitsu, for example, enhances employee security by analyzing data collected from linked wearable technology using AI.
- **Creates innovative products and assistance**: Natural language processing (NLP) involves improving the ability of humans to interact with machines. Without a doubt, the IoT and AI can immediately develop new goods or improve existing services by allowing businesses to efficiently collect and analyze data.
- **Improves IoT adaptability**: Smartphones and high-end workstations are examples of IoT systems, as are low-cost devices. However, the most typical IoT network contains low-cost devices that generate enormous amounts of information. Before sending data to other devices, an AI-powered IoT network analyzes and summarizes data from one device. As a result, it condenses vast amounts of data and enables the connection of a large number of IoT devices. This is referred to as adaptability.
- **Reduces excessive system failures**: System failures can lead to expensive unscheduled outages in various industries, such as offshore petroleum and heavy industry. Planned maintenance using AI-enabled IoT enables you to anticipate equipment downtime and plan organized maintenance operations. As a result, clients may avoid the negative impacts of an outage.

1.3.6 Scenarios of AI with the IoT in Reality

Let's take a deeper look at companies that have improved user engagement and created innovative business models employing AI-powered IoT:

- **Using automation in industry**: Production is one of the businesses that has adopted new automation, AI, facial detection, DL, robotics, and much more. Factory bots are becoming smarter with the help of implanted sensors that ease information transmission. Furthermore, because the bots are fitted out with AI systems, they may learn from fresh data. This method not only keeps costs down but also improves the production process in real time.

- **Self-driving vehicles**: The best illustration of the IoT and AI functioning with each other is Tesla's self-driving automobiles. Self-driving vehicles use AI to predict the behavior of traffic and pedestrians in a variety of situations. They can, for instance, ascertain road markings and climate, optimize speed, and become intelligent with every journey.
- **Retail analytics**: Industrial analytics uses a plethora of datasets from cameras and sensors to track consumers' movements and forecast when they will arrive at the checkout aisle. As a result, the system may recommend variable staffing to minimize transaction time and maximize cashier efficiency.
- **Smart home automation**: This technology is an excellent illustration of IoT driven by AI. Depending on its customers' work schedules and environmental requirements, mobile connectivity allows the monitoring and regulation of temperature from any location.

Altogether, the IoT combined with AI can pave the way for more innovative products and experiences. One should combine AI with incoming information from IoT devices to get more value from the system and help businesses grow.

1.4 Conclusion

The implementation of AI with the IoT carries the potential for several industrial and business-level applications. Industries in a range of businesses, including production, entertainment, and on-demand medicine, have emerged to recognize the potential of technology in increasing efficiency and competitiveness.

References

1. Melo-Dias, C., & Silva, C. F. (2019). Teoria da aprendizagem social de Bandura na formação de habilidades de conversação. *Psicologia: Saúde e Doenças, Lisboa, 20*(1), 101–113.
2. Krupiy, T. (2020). A vulnerability analysis: Theorising the impact of AI decision-making processes on individuals, society, and human diversity from a social justice perspective. *Computer Law and Security Review, Southampton*, 38.
3. Mackenzie, A. (2015). The production of prediction: What does ML want? *European Journal of Cultural Studies, Boston, 18*(4–5), 429–455.
4. Ayvaz, S., & Alpay, K. (2021). Predictive maintenance system for production lines in manufacturing: A ML approach using IoT data in real-time. *Expert Systems with Applications, Louisiana*, 173.
5. Russell, S., & Novig, P. (2010). *AI a modern approach* (3rd Ed., p. 1132). Pearson Education, Inc. Accessed on March 29, 2021.
6. Anyoha, R. (2017). Can machines think? In: *Harvard University the graduate school of arts and sciences*. Science in the News
7. Siebert, J. U., Kunz, R. E., & Rolf, P. (2020). Effects of proactive decision making on life satisfaction. *European Journal of Operational Research, Poznan, 280*, 1171–1187.
8. Esposito, A., Esposito, A. M., & Vogel, C. (2015). Needs and challenges in human computer interaction for processing social-emotional information. *Pattern Recognition Letters*, 1–11.

9. Wang, J. X. (2021). Meta-learning in natural and AI. *Current Opinion in Behavioral Sciences, Michigan, 38*, 90–95.
10. Chowanda, A., Sutoyo, R., Meiliana, & Tanachutiwat, S. (2021). Exploring text-based emotion recognition ML techniques on social media conversation. *Procedia Computer Science,* 2021179, 821–828.
11. Ivanova, E., & Borzunov, G. (2020). Optimization of ML algorithm of emotion recognition in terms of human facial expressions. *Procedia Computer Science, Manchester, 169*, 244–248.
12. Bar-Anan, Y., Wilson, T. D., & Hassin, R. R. (2010). Inaccurate self-knowledge formation is a result of automatic behavior. *Journal of Experimental Social Psychology, Canterbury, 46*, 884–894.
13. Windasari, N. A., Lin, F. R., & Kato-Lin, Y. C. (2021). Continued use of wearable fitness technology: A value co-creation perspective. *International Journal of Information Management, Swansea.*
14. D'alfonso, S. (2020). AI in mental health. *Current Opinion in Psychology, Amsterdam, 36*, 112–117.
15. Langer, A., Feingold-Polak, R., Mueller, O., Kellmeyer, P., & Levy-Tzedek, S. (2019). Trust in socially assistive robots: Considerations for use in rehabilitation. *Neuroscience and Biobehavioral Reviews, Beer-Sheva, 104*, 231–239.
16. Noriega, M. (2020). The application of AI in police interrogations: Na analysis addressing the proposed effect AI has on racial and gender bias, cooperation, and false confessions. *Futures, Bristol,* 117.
17. Keskinbora, K. H. (2019). Medical ethics considerations on AI. *Journal of Clinical Neuroscience, Istanbul, 64*, 277–282.
18. Nilsson, N. J., & Cook, S. B. (1984). AI: Its impacts on human occupations and distribution of income. *Computer Compacts, 2*(1), 9–12.
19. Um, Q., Chen, Y., & Wang, J. (2019). Deciphering brain complexity using single-cell sequencing. *Genomics Proteomics Bioinformatics, Hong Kong, 17*, 344–366.
20. Kaltenthaler, E., & Cavanagh, K. (2010). Computerised cognitive behavioral therapy and its uses. *Progress in Neurology and Psychiatry, Pennsylvania, 14*(3), 22–29.
21. Bolte, A., Goschke, T., & Kuhl, J. (2003). Emotion and intuition. *Institute of Psychology,* Braunschweig University of Technology, Braunschweig, Germany.
22. Crowder, J. A., & Friess, S. (2010). Artificial neural diagnostics and prognostics: Self-soothing in cognitive systems. In *International Conference on AI, ICAI'10,* July 2010.
23. Crowder, J. A. (2010). Flexible object architectures for hybrid neural processing systems. In *International Conference on AI, ICAI'10,* July 2010.
24. Crowder, J. A., & Carbone, J. (2011). *The great migration: Information to knowledge using cognition-based frameworks.* Springer.
25. Crowder, J. A. (2011). The artificial prefrontal cortex: Artificial consciousness. In *International Conference on AI, ICAI'11,* July 2011.
26. DeYoung, C. G., Hirsh, J. B., Shane, M. S., Papademetris, X., Rajeevan, N., & Gray, J. R. (2010). Testing predictions from personality neuroscience. *Psychological Science, 21*(6), 820–828.
27. Marsella, S., & Gratch, J. (2002). A step towards irrationality: Using emotion to change belief. In *1st International Joint Conference on Autonomous Agents and Multi-Agent Systems, Bologna, Italy,* July 2002.
28. Miller, E. K., Freedman, D. J., & Wallis, J. D. (2002). The prefrontal cortex: Categories, concepts, and cognition. *Philosophical Transactions of the Royal Society B: Biological Sciences, 357*(1424), 1123–1136.
29. Newell, A. (2003). *Unified theories of cognition.* Harvard University Press.
30. Damasio, A. (1994). *Descartes's error: Emotion, reason, and the human brain.* Gosset/Putnam.
31. Davis, M., & Whalen, P. J. (2001). The amygdala: Vigilance and emotion. *Molecular Psychiatry, 6*, 13–34.
32. Eichenbaum, H. (2002). *The cognitive neuroscience of memory.* Oxford University Press.
33. Kosko, G. (1986). Fuzzy cognitive maps. *International Journal of Man-Machine Studies, 24*, 65–75.

34. LaBar, K. S., & Cabeza. (2006). Cognitive neuroscience of emotional memory. *Nature Reviews Neuroscience, 7*, 54–64.
35. LeDoux, J. E. (2000). Emotion circuits in the brain. *Annual Review of Neuroscience, 23,* 155–184.
36. LeDoux, J. E. (2002). *Synaptic self: How our brains become who we are.* Viking.
37. Levine, P. (1997). *Walking the tiger: Healing Trauma.* North Atlantic Books.
38. Yang, Y., & Raine, A. (2009). Prefrontal structural and functional brain imaging findings in antisocial, violent, and psychopathic individuals: A meta-analysis. *Psychiatry Research, 174*(2), 81–88. https://doi.org/10.1016/j.pscychresns.2009.03.012.PMID19833485
39. Ashcroft, M. (1997). *Human memory and cognition.* Prentice Hall Professional.
40. Nass, C., & Moon, Y. (2022). Machines and mindlessness: Social responses to computers. *Journal of Social Issues, 56*(1), 81–103.

Chapter 2
Artificial Intelligence for Understanding Human Behavior and Psychology

2.1 Introduction

In open spaces, for example, the capacity to estimate human activity and related situations might be critical [1]. Recognizing how somebody behaves while sitting on the verge of a station platform or trying to defuse a crisis before it grows might have a significant influence on protecting others [2]. It is no surprise that the emphasis on public health and safety is at an all-time maximum, so gaining access to impartial knowledge may be extremely valuable to security firms wanting to mitigate the risks of public health and safety from a public strategic viewpoint [3]. But, if history has taught us anything, it is that excellent, dependable knowledge is tough to obtain [4]. Emergent AI technology such as robots, advancements in computer vision, and high-tech biometrics are just a few examples of potential developments. This might aid us in the pursuit of comprehending human nature [5]. What is the need to develop emotional intelligence? The next subsection provides more insight on what an individual think and feel about it [6].

2.1.1 Getting Rid of "the Present Human Prejudice"

How could emerging AI applications serve to enhance the degrees of knowledge of human activity [7], and how might this transform into anything relevant from the standpoint of emotional intelligence? Artificial emotional intelligence (AEI) is a field that can provide in-depth research and analytics concerning emotions and personal characteristics without the effect of human prejudice [8], which frequently complicates such investigations and the resulting information [9]. Using technologies that can eliminate human participation might take threat detection to a whole new level, particularly when utilized to precisely interpret subconscious facial movements in real time (when they are occurring) and then transform them into a spectrum of more profound emotions [10].

© The Author(s), under exclusive license to Springer Nature Singapore Pte Ltd. 2023
G. Chhabra et al., *Artificial Intelligence to Analyze Psychophysical and Human Lifestyle*,
https://doi.org/10.1007/978-981-99-3039-5_2

This would produce the correct representation when utilized with the appropriate qualities (in authenticity) [11]. In these circumstances, the principal emotions deciphered by the algorithm are those best known in the language of thoughts and feelings: anger, disgust, contempt, happiness, sorrow, surprise, and fear [12]. As a consequence of these reactions, such technologies may identify several essential traits such as trust, enthusiasm, sincerity, anxiety, excitement, stress, and sadness. Identifying when a person exhibits these characteristics in society might be a sign of possible threat or danger [13].

2.1.2 Standing in a Group

Panic is a significant issue. Understanding whether someone is afraid of a scenario before it happens might be really useful knowledge [14]. Anger or disdain are two more feelings that may be utilized to the benefit of large groups since they can help you anticipate antisocial conduct [15]. Authenticity is another trait that may be utilized to identify situations such as stealing or even someone looking forward to taking things [16], particularly if they exhibit exceptionally low levels of honesty [17]. In the instance of shown features such as sadness or stress, security staff would be able to assess those who may be in danger of suicide ideation and engage them before it becomes too late.

Of course, like any such innovation, the goal is protection instead of recovery, or, at the very least [18], the ability to take appropriate action at a particular point in time. Detecting uneasiness through facial gestures is particularly beneficial since the data may be used to examine any potential behavioral linkages [19], such as an "assaulter" expressing indications of anxiousness. Ensuring the safety of the public has never been more important, but using AEI innovation in conjunction with observing excessive reality and antisocial behavior [20], for example, could provide relevant data to be used to avoid incidents such as attacks on the public, criminal behavior, or even suicide attempts [21].

2.1.3 Risk Management and Vision

Through the interpretation of real features, innovation can now notify security personnel in real time of extreme behavior [21], such as highly concentrated quantities of rage in a group, or excessive degrees of anguish or sadness when sitting at railway stations [22]. This increased knowledge is crucial in terms of recognizing the risk of certain circumstances and having the vision to manage them before they start to go wrong [23].

When spotting a potential suspect, AEI innovation can provide a critical layer of knowledge that was previously inaccessible [24], for example, determining how anxious someone is and whether they are displaying any clear (or possibly less visible) indicators of despair or discomfort [25]. If they provide more control and can integrate this additional layer of information proof with their current or supporting information [26], they may be capable of preventing certain situations from occurring [27].

Progressing beyond the simple decoding of emotions provides more control and requires solutions that go further [28], employing incomplete image recognition, reliable camera shots, and cutting-edge pixelated actual data to unveil traditional personality and behavioral traits [29], ensuring the identification of indications concealed from human eyes. This was originally thought to be very hard to do.

2.1.4 Emotional Needs and Psychological Behavior

One may anticipate AEI technology to be deployed as a substantial advantage to private space, in which day-to-day hazards are increasingly combatted, and to community security over the coming year [30]. This technological advancement contributes to the continual trend identification and analysis that currently exists [31]. The combination of identifying traits and feelings with face identification transforms crowd surveillance and monitoring from a reactive to a proactive operation. Security professionals may now be certain that they are functioning with the extra advantage and backing of mental and physiological information as well as a visual trail, thanks to developments in AEI technology [32]. This helps to discover wanted or accused persons as well as recognizing those who are going to commit an infraction, which is crucial in today's environment [33].

2.1.5 The Importance of AI in Psychology

The term "AI" is commonly used to refer to both the "smart and autonomous systems fueled to execute tasks that would ordinarily involve human intellect" and the diverse areas of study involved in developing such technology [34]. AI is already a regularly used term for everything from robotics to software deployed in systems. And, depending on the situation and the observer, it can signify varying complexities and efficiency [35], but it re-creates either complicated human behavior or specialized intelligent operations.

One of the most modern concerns for AI is psychology, particularly psychological health. As AI expands its scope, it is becoming extremely important that psychologists, psychiatrists [36], and counselors comprehend the technology's current capabilities and upcoming promise to revolutionize mental healthcare.

AI could emulate a professional with abilities that exceed those of its intellectual equivalent. Furthermore, the accompanying instances of modern technology examine people by observing their human perceptions [37]:

- Ultraviolet photography is used to detect temperature differences;
- To validate a patient's identification, biometric authentication is used;
- To analyze facial expressions and eye movements, sensing devices are used;
- Audio evaluation is used to detect small changes in speech features;
- Olfactory receptors (smell) are assessed so as to detect impairment.

Although AI could perform treatment, e-therapy, and evaluations on its own, it could also aid professionals before, throughout, and after appointments [38]. An inspection system, including an increase in heart rate or temperature, reacts differently to complicated questions and can provide the therapist with significant and informative supplementary information [39]. Not only that, but levels of data, maintaining records management, and initiating autonomous follow-up steps will save real professionals considerable time.

2.1.6 AI as a Knowledge-Based Technology

Knowledge-based systems were among the first applications of AI in the healthcare profession. Although not everyone thinks that these systems are AI, technologies aid decision-making by integrating professional knowledge and skills [40]. While such technologies have been available for a few decades, the architecture has evolved from mostly regulated logic to generating judgments based on machine learning and fuzzy control (the term used by experts in the area to deal with incomplete facts).

It is not hard to envisage innovations like voice recognition, Amazon Echo, or Android Auto as being able to offer psychological consultations or professional guidance at a low cost [41], thanks to advancements such as introducing additional voice recognition and computational linguistics to knowledge-based systems. Further facilities are available from AI. Using its collection of knowledge in conjunction with private details, it also assesses healthcare problems and identifies probable incompatibilities with medical interventions.

Furthermore, AI-enabled healthcare support networks provide expanded capacity, managing a larger amount of highly complicated information than their traditional equivalents and providing data access to all users throughout the day. The burden of time-limited psychosocial support may be considerably alleviated, and AI can enable more targeted interaction with individuals who need it and where it is needed [42].

2.2 Artificial Environments

Augmented worlds, or machine virtual social worlds, provide a secure, cost-effective setting for individuals to examine their difficulties. The surroundings may be rendered more realistic for humans by being immersed, by customizing situations, and by increasing or decreasing stresses [43]. Virtual friends, such as virtual animals, likewise improve well-being while alleviating loneliness in easily accessible settings.

Augmented reality projects the potential flexibility of virtual reality onto the real environment. It takes advantage of the processing capability of smartphones and mobile devices to securely create connections with the origin of their fear or fitness trainers. Exposure therapy discusses how individuals might recover when confronted with their concerns [44].

2.2.1 Gaming for Computer Systems

Game consoles have effectively boosted customer involvement and therapy commitment in hesitant individuals. By giving a discrete and game-based learning treatment to patients, AI-enhanced activities can avoid the stigma of mental illness therapy and deliver realistic circumstances customized to patients' requirements [45]. Virtual Life, an interactive online platform, has been extensively trialed as a medium for digital counseling and guided gaming to allow patients to learn new skills.

2.2.2 Instances of AI Applications in Psychology

AI technology that complements or indeed substitutes the psychologist, therapist, and perhaps other mental health professionals is not science fiction and may be attainable in the coming years [46].

2.2.2.1 Psychological Pattern Identification and Algorithmic Research

Research into the recognition and algorithmic analysis of psychological indicators analyzes linguistic, body gesture, and interactive content to discover signs of human suffering using pattern recognition, object tracking, and computational linguistics. This innovative system evaluates combat veterans from conflict zones and identifies those who need more psychiatric care [47]. The approach will incorporate information from face-to-face consultations with data on napping, dining, and internet activities to provide a patient's health description and psychological indications.

2.2.2.2 AI and Information Science Research Lab

Harvard University's computer science and AI research labs have effectively employed AI to scan recorded footage and discover small variations in a person's heartbeat and blood supply that are imperceptible to visual inspection. While it is particularly useful throughout the treatment program for detecting behavioral clues, it may also be used in clinics to track trauma patients' respiration or small newborns under stress [48].

2.2.2.3 Watson Medical Services

Watson Medical, IBM's intelligence analytical tool, has become widely available and comes pre-loaded with scientific journals to function as a consultation as well as a medical professional. This AI's great goal is to use information, innovation, and skills to replace or promote quality mental and physical care, conduct diagnostics, and offer remedies [49].

2.2.2.4 RP-VITA

The United States Food and Drug Administration has certified the RP-VITA robots for wireless connectivity among health practitioners and individuals. This constantly tracks individuals quite well when retrieving personal health information. The approach is interdisciplinary, offering assistance with psychiatric, neurological, cardiological, and intensive care evaluations [50].

2.2.3 Analysis System for Psychological Diagnosis

The Psychiatric Medical Intelligent System encodes expert information about mental health illnesses using modern AI systems, which it then utilizes to evaluate and recommend therapies. The AI understands individuals' demands using a mixture of regulation and fuzzy logic, deciding on possible treatments that fit particular limits and are suited for other medical problems. Integrating the advantages of psychological understanding with AI-enabled innovation enhances health treatments and wellness. It is projected to grow quickly due to the added benefits of being cost-effective and accessible anywhere [51].

2.2.3.1 Use of AI for Psychological Assessment

By integrating approaches such as data mining (the generation of new knowledge through the deep study of huge amounts of information) and insightful analysis, AI technology provides useful therapeutic tools. AI can detect current and foreseeable issues, as well as test and confirm forecasts and solutions. AI found some characteristics related to suicidal ideation and behavior when extracted data from 707 people with suicidal inclinations in Metropolitan Madrid [52] and Peru. The discoveries prompted a set of preventative treatments for at-risk people that lowered suicidal behavior and increased "psychological health, emotions of self-worth, and motivation for life".

In 2017, Kravets et. al., developed a framework that has used fuzzification to replicate psychological conditions, effectively assessing sick people and testing their psychiatric diagnoses based on flawed awareness. A suitable AI model enables you to piece together scattered data, construct thought processes, experiment with their authenticity, and recommend treatments [53].

2.2.3.2   AI Applications in Psychology

Psychology seeks to comprehend the complexities of cognition by conducting investigations, evaluating, and developing hypotheses about how the human psyche manages and interprets complex data through concentration, storage, and perception. The goals of AI and cognitive psychology are similar in that they both attempt to understand the nature of intelligent behavior, with the former seeking to develop such mechanisms using advanced capabilities [54]. While there are important variations between mathematical modeling and AI, both are essential tools for examining the evolution of intelligent thought and the information ecosystem in the emerging discipline of cognitive science.

Quantitative data is defined as "the process of designing machines to simulate or duplicate elements of human intellectual performance." In contrast, the basic processes of AI often exhibit little relation to the methods utilized by the human mind. The AI developer's purpose is to generate an output that seems knowledgeable instead of establishing computational models that assist us to comprehend cognitive abilities [54]. These processes do not have to be essentially equivalent to those of humans. However, there appears to be one paradigm that bridges the difference between the two methods.

The network of synapses within the initial motivated nodes of the mind begins to correspond. "Artificial neural frameworks are often made up of densely interconnected systems of basic units that display training" and describe cognition without particular rules. Although, a very sophisticated human brain effectively reproduced some brain functions (such as image recognition), the jury is still out on whether such models can describe the cognitive process [55].

Deep learning methods, influenced by cognitive psychology theories and methodologies, have shown some effectiveness in describing how toddlers acquire object identification and provide an excellent illustration of the advantages of merging competencies and understanding from different fields.

2.3   The Top Four AI-Powered Psychology Tools

While the application of AI in psychology is still a new phenomenon, the widespread availability of smartphone apps ensures that some of us have the resources necessary to operate the rising number of AI-inspired psychological tools. A few tools are discussed below [56].

- **Woebot**: This was a Google Play Honore in 2019 and encourages participants to think about circumstances by utilizing tools influenced by cognitive behavioral therapy (CBT) [57]. The emotion monitor then displays the positive improvements achieved over weeks and months.
- **Youper**: This offers a tailored psychological health aid to support the reduction of stress, tension, and sadness. Through a succession of quick conversations, the application monitors and reduces stress using approaches from numerous treatments, notably CBT and meditation.
- **Replika**: This is an AI-enabled chatbot that offers emotional support and imaginary companionship to persons struggling with mental health issues, stress, or other difficulties [58].
- **Tess**: This is a web-based psychological health bot that uses AI to provide users with healthy cognitive strategies. Instead of an application, it fosters resistance by using content chats via Whatsapp, Text, and web services [59].

2.4 Related Works

AI is a potential strategy for assisting and, in some cases, replacing certain procedures in psychiatric evaluation and therapy. Technology provides an opportunity to give new sorts of therapy (such as interactive multimedia as well as sports) and the potential to fulfill and interact with people that are difficult to access or interact with. Such novel techniques can also allocate the time and resources of counselors and therapists to engage in more essential or specialized care. However, legitimate values cannot be avoided. There is currently no advice on how to design such technologies or incorporate them with the activities of medical practitioners, pre-existing information and technology, or regulatory regimes [60].

Identifying and deciding on the amount of personal oversight necessary before, throughout, and after meeting clients is another concern when using innovative approaches. At the very least, any evaluation or therapy must protect and defend the privacy and individuality of the patient. However, if the hazards of unintentional or purposeful abuse, as well as ethical considerations, are properly controlled, AI offers a useful way to treat mental health on a widespread basis. It also allows for the collection and analysis of enormous volumes of information to increase the experience and wisdom of psychological symptoms and health effects [61].

2.4.1 How Is a Psychologist Supplemented by AI?

For the time being, total replacement of one by the other is not conceivable, yet collaboration between AI and a psychologist could be viable. This could occur, for instance, via extensive video assessment or by taking variables into account in a psychological assessment (such as fluctuations) and differences in the benchmarks of facial gestures. It has also been observed that, for the time being, the subjective knowledge of relationships between people is a deficiency in AI, owing to its essentially human nature [62].

It is critical to recognize that, despite the psychologist's chosen function, a wide variety of abilities are necessary, including active listening skills, the ability to conduct subjective investigations, and flexibility in individual/group evaluation. All of these serve as the foundation for the framework of psychological evaluation, which is a way to explore the psychology practitioner and which, owing to its complexities, cannot be fully executed by cognitive computing.

Unlike many other specialties, where the components of research can be incorporated nearly completely and objectively, psychology has as its purview of research brain activity and its various forms of expression. It is dynamic and ever-changing. An AI would be so advanced that it would be able to execute, for example, a psychological evaluation with the productivity and efficiency of a good psychologist. Nevertheless, this is only a distant possibility for the time being, because even recent research that attempts to understand the complex developing brain hardly ever prospers or indeed unravels its practically limitless abstract ideas and characterizations.

Regarding the foregoing, however, there is no method for an AI to construe all human subjective nature. A few applications, such as Fear Fighter and Beating the Blue, have already been enhanced and applied as techniques in the therapy of emotional and behavioral abnormalities (moderately severe) and are broadly used in the UK. The above tools are also used in other therapies, including those for relationship dysfunction, mental health conditions, and drug addiction. Both are predicated on CBT's development of the scientific foundation of this psychotherapy's ability to blend significantly with mathematical fundamentals, thereby opening a new field: computerized cognitive behavioral therapy (CCBT). Regardless of the requirements to access such programs, "testing" is required so that those who use them have a well-before assessment and can use the most effective intervention mode of communication for every case. It is important to mention that the National Institute for Health and Care Excellence (NICE), a part of the body of the Board of Health in London, recommends this mode of treatment.

Communication between humans and advanced analytics is advantageous and is found in automobiles, TVs, cellular phones, smartwatches, and other devices daily. This integration happens for the satisfaction of those who use such equipment as well as for numerous different specific purposes such as tracking health and quality of life. For court room defendants, AIs have been used in questioning; for instance, to produce less prejudiced and exclusionary examination [63]. The morally correct and emotional ramifications of the relationship between individuals and AI can indeed be frightening, based on the circumstances.

When it comes to producing screening tests as an effective process or evoking testimonies in interrogation methods, automatons are more credible than individuals in both regions. The difficulty becomes more serious when the ramifications of this overconfidence are investigated, for while AIs may be more completely unbiased than individuals. This is because those who create the automated system are eventually impacted by cultural preconceptions. Similar to the directory, the dataset is used to feed the automated system, which, for instance, has race and ethnic biases.

As a result, it is critical to "humanize" the equipment to acknowledge human traits in the methodologies, such as the prospect of judgment mistakes. Awareness of this element should reduce the majority's typical presumption that AI is error-free, while also emphasizing that a living person's individuality cannot yet be fully replicated by learning algorithms.

2.4.2   AI and Human Awareness

Individuals implement goals and regulations on machines mindlessly. In a nutshell, individuals react to indications that trigger different elements, identifiers, and aspirations from a previous time instead of all those that apply to the current time. To illustrate, three aspects (triggered elements, identifiers, and aspirations) are to be assumed when seeking to understand human conceptions of AI. In a first study, individuals misuse sociological phenomena by implementing traditional gender roles into machines and culturally recognizing them [64]. A second study states that individuals start engaging in social machine behaviors, such as politeness and reciprocity [65]. A third study demonstrates humans' hasty intellectual responsibilities by observing what they are supposed to identify [66]. It concludes that humans use interpersonal commands suitable for interpersonal interactions rather than for personal communication.

Gender made no substantial change, but people's paired features were influenced by sexual identity and perfectibility. The authors in [64] discovered a significant similarity between "neutral" and "personable" for men, "intelligible" and "enjoyable" for both men and women, and "efficient" and "personable" for men, demonstrating that individuals are ready and able to designate human attributes to machines. Nevertheless, situations that confound must be considered. The level of representation of organizations affects how individuals understand each other's character traits, such as the connector and the machine, which had a high association for comprehension and sociability. However, only the connector demonstrated a strong relationship between being capable, gentle, and reliable. Due to the work of these researchers, one could assert that how AI is presented to individuals influences how AI is interpreted. Even an infotainment system in a vehicle that is given a unique model seems to create a different interpretation. Numerous factors influence the subjective experience of machines and AI systems. There is still ongoing research on how AI should be proffered so that it is better interpreted by individuals.

2.5 Conclusion

Even though AI is successfully established nowadays, it has yet to start generating what is identified as "awareness." A wearable capturing a heartbeat and recommending that its user rest if his or her breathing exercise is raised at multiple intervals is considered a facet of AI. Despite being innovative in comparison to 20 years ago, it is not yet an autonomous, adaptable, and self-aware unit like a living being.

It has been observed that AIs can outperform sustainably grown humans in particular tasks such as data collection and interpretation, whether they are ordinary, interpersonal, or psychological citizens. Nevertheless, regarding propagating living-person preconceptions, these techniques are unable to evaluate the results collected in a manner that generates more difficult operations, such as conducting a psychosocial evaluation, although it has already been conceived in science fiction and can be understood as an approximation of the long run. Despite the emergence of digitalized therapeutic interventions such as Defeating the Blues and Fear Fighter, they are incapable of performing more complicated operations such as psychological evaluations or even comprehensive cognitive therapy; they still require complexity to continue operating and are restricted to very different tasks.

Eventually, it is expected that AI will have the capability to develop identities and hence act as psychological AIs in the coming years. Will they be able to be assessed mentally and emotionally? To whom would they present their results and evaluations? Is it feasible to use AI for medicinal purposes? Could psychological disorder handbooks and categorizations contain the character traits of these novel life forms?

References

1. Melo-Dias, C., & Silva, C. F. (2019). Teoria da aprendizagem social de Bandura na formação de habilidades de conversação. *Psicologia: Saúde e Doenças, 20*(1), 101–113.
2. Krupiy, T. (2020). A vulnerability analysis: Theorising the impact of AI decision-making processes on individuals, society, and human diversity from a social justice perspective. *Computer Law and Security Review, 38.*
3. Mackenzie, A. (2015). The production of prediction: What does machine learning want? *European Journal of Cultural Studies, 18*(4–5), 429–455.
4. Ayvaz, S., & Alpay, K. (2021). Predictive maintenance system for production lines in manufacturing: A machine learning approach using IoT data in real-time. *Expert Systems with Applications, 173.*
5. Russell, S., & Novig, P. (2010). *AI a modern approach* (3rd edn., Vol. 1132). Pearson Education, Inc. Accessed on March 29, 2021.
6. Anyoha, R. (2017). Can machines think? In *Harvard university the graduate school of arts and sciences.* Science in The News.
7. Siebert, J. U., Kunz, R. E., & Rolf, P. (2020). Effects of proactive decision making on life satisfaction. *European Journal of Operational Research, 280*, 1171–1187.
8. Esposito, A., Esposito, A. M., & Vogel, C. (2015). Needs and challenges in human computer interaction for processing social-emotional information. *Pattern Recognition Letters*, 1–11.

9. Wang, J. X. (2021). Meta-learning in natural and AI. *Current Opinion in Behavioral Sciences, 38,* 90–95.
10. Chowanda, A., Sutoyo, R., Meiliana, & Tanachutiwat, S. (2021). Exploring text-based emotion recognition machine learning techniques on social media conversation. *Procedia Computer Science, 179,* 821–828.
11. Ivanova, E., & Borzunov, G. (2020). Optimization of machine learning algorithm of emotion recognition in terms of human facial expressions. *Procedia Computer Science, 169,* 244–248.
12. Bar-Anan, Y., Wilson, T. D., & Hassin, R. R. (2010). Inaccurate self-knowledge formation as a result of automatic behavior. *Journal of Experimental Social Psychology, 46,* 884–894.
13. Windasari, N. A., Lin, F. R., & Kato-Lin, Y. C. (2021). Continued use of wearable fitness technology: A value co-creation perspective. *International Journal of Information Management.*
14. D'alfonso, S. (2020). AI in mental health. *Current Opinion in Psychology, 36,* 112–117.
15. Langer, A., Feingold-Polak, R., Mueller, O., Kellmeyer, P., & Levy-Tzedek, S. (2019). Trust in socially assistive robots: Considerations for use in rehabilitation. *Neuroscience and Biobehavioral Reviews, 104,* 231–239.
16. Noriega, M. (2020). The application of AI in police interrogations: Na analysis addressing the proposed effect AI has on racial and gender bias, cooperation, and false confessions. *Futures, 117.*
17. Keskinbora, K. H. (2019). Medical ethics considerations on AI. *Journal of Clinical Neuroscience, 64,* 277–282.
18. Nilsson, N. J., & Cook, S. B. (1984). AI: Its impacts on human occupations and distribution of income. *Computer Compacts, 2*(1), 9–12.
19. Um, Q., Chen, Y., & Wang, J. (2019). Deciphering brain complexity using single-cell sequencing. *Genomics, Proteomics & Bioinformatics, 17,* 344–366.
20. Kaltenthaler, E., & Cavanagh, K. (2010). Computerised cognitive behavioral therapy and its uses. *Progress in Neurology and Psychiatry, 14*(3), 22–29.
21. Bolte, A., Goschke, T., & Kuhl, J. *Emotion and intuition.* Institute of Psychology, Braunschweig University of Technology, Braunschweig, Germany. annette.bolte@tu-bs.de
22. Crowder, J. A., & Friess, S. (2010). Artificial neural diagnostics and prognostics: Self-Soothing in cognitive systems. In *International Conference on AI, ICAI'10,* July 2010.
23. Crowder, J. A., & Friess, S. (2010). Artificial neural emotions and emotional memory. In *International Conference on AI, ICAI'10,* July 2010.
24. Crowder, J. A. (2010). Flexible object architectures for hybrid neural processing systems. In *International Conference on AI, ICAI'10,* July 2010.
25. Crowder, J. A., & Carbone, J. (2011). *The great migration: Information to knowledge using cognition-based frameworks.* Springer Science.
26. Crowder, J. A. (2011). The artificial prefrontal cortex: Artificial consciousness. In *International Conference on AI, ICAI'11,* July 2011.
27. Crowder, J. A. (2011). Metacognition and metamemory concepts for AI systems. In *International Conference on AI, ICAI'11,* July 2011.
28. DeYoung, C. G., Hirsh, J. B., Shane, M. S., Papademetris, X., Rajeevan, N., & Gray, J. R. (2010). Testing predictions from personality neuroscience. *Psychological Science, 21*(6), 820–828.
29. Marsella, S., & Gratch, J. (2002). A step towards irrationality: Using emotion to change belief. In *1st International Joint Conference on Autonomous Agents and Multi-Agent Systems,* Bologna, Italy, July 2002.
30. Miller, E. K., Freedman, D. J., & Wallis, J. D. (2002, August). The prefrontal cortex: Categories, concepts, and cognition. *Philosophical Transactions of the Royal Society of London. Series B, Biological Sciences, 357*(1424), 1123–1136.
31. Newell, A. (2003). *Unified theories of cognition.* Harvard University Press.
32. Damasio, A. (1994). *Descartes's error: Emotion, reason, and the human brain.* Gosset/Putnam.
33. Davis, M., & Whalen, P. J. (2001). The amygdala: Vigilance and emotion. *Molecular Psychiatry, 6,* 13–34.
34. Eichenbaum, H. (2002). *The cognitive neuroscience of memory.* Oxford University Press.

35. Kosko, G. (1986). Fuzzy cognitive maps. *International Journal of Man-Machine Studies, 24*, 65–75.
36. LaBar, K. S., & Cabeza. (2006). Cognitive neuroscience of emotional memory. *Nature Reviews Neuroscience, 7*, 54–64.
37. LeDoux, J. E. (1996). *The emotional brain.* Simon and Schuster.
38. LeDoux, J. E. (2000). Emotion circuits in the brain. *Annual Review of Neuroscience, 23*, 155–184.
39. LeDoux, J. E. (2002). *Synaptic self: How our brains become who we are.* Viking.
40. Levine, P. (1997). *Walking the tiger: Healing trauma.* North Atlantic Books.
41. Yang, Y., & Raine, A. (2009, November). Prefrontal structural and functional brain imaging findings in antisocial, violent, and psychopathic individuals: A meta-analysis. *Psychiatry Research, 174*(2), 81–88. https://doi.org/10.1016/j.pscychresns.2009.03.012.PMID19833485
42. Ashcroft, M. (1997). *Human memory and cognition.* Prentice Hall Professional.
43. Nass, C., & Moon, Y. (2000). Machines and mindlessness: Social responses to computers. *Journal of Social Issues, 56*(1), 81–103.
44. Altun, K., & Barshan, B. (2010). Human activity recognition using inertial/magnetic sensor units. In A.A. Salah, T. Gevers, N. Sebe, & A. Vinciarelli, (Eds.), *Human behavior understanding.* Lecture Notes in Computer Science (Vol. 6219, pp. 38–51). Springer.
45. Yüksek, M. C. (2011). *A comparative study on human activity classification with miniature inertial and magnetic sensors.* M.Sc. Thesis, Bilkent Univ., Dept. of Electrical and Electronics Eng., Ankara, Turkey.
46. Webb, A. (2002). *Statistical pattern recognition.* Wiley.
47. Yüksek, M. C., & Barshan, B. (2011). Human activity classification with miniature inertial and magnetic sensor signals. In *Proceedings of the 19th European Signal Processing Conference,* Barcelona, Spain, August 29–September 1 (pp. 956–960). EURASIP.
48. Kotsiantis, S. B. (2007). Supervised machine learning: A review of classification techniques. *Informatica, 31*, 249–268.
49. Duda, R. O., Hart, P. E., & Stork, D. G. (2001). *Pattern classification* (2nd ed.). Wiley.
50. Wu, W. H., Bui, A. A. T., Batalin, M. A., Liu, D., & Kaiser, W. J. (2007). Incremental diagnosis method for intelligent wearable sensor system. *IEEE Transactions on Information Technology in Biomedicine, 11*, 553–562.
51. Jovanov, E., Milenkovic, A., Otto, C., & de Groen, P. C. (2005). A wireless body area network of intelligent motion sensors for computer-assisted physical rehabilitation. *Journal of NeuroEngineering and Rehabilitation, 2*(6).
52. Riviere, C. N., Ang, W. T., & Khosla, P. K. (2003). Toward active tremor canceling in handheld microsurgical instruments. *IEEE Transactions on Robotics and Automation, 19*, 793–800.
53. Kravets, A., Poplavskaya, O., Lempert, L., Salnikova, N., & Medintseva, I. (2017). The development of medical diagnostics module for psychotherapeutic practice. In Creativity in Intelligent Technologies and Data Science: Second Conference, CIT&DS 2017, Volgograd, Russia, September 12–14, 2017, *Proceedings 2* (pp. 872–883). Springer International Publishing.
54. Yurtman, A. (2012). *Detection and classification of human activities using wearable sensors.* M.Sc. Thesis, Bilkent Univ., Dept. of Electrical and Electronics Eng., Ankara, Turkey, September.
55. Hauer, K., Lamb, S. E., Jorstad, E. C., Todd, C., & Becker, C. (2006). Systematic review of definitions and methods of measuring falls in randomized controlled fall prevention trials. *Age and Ageing, 35*, 5–10.
56. Noury, N., Fleury, A., Rumeau, P., Bourke, A. K., Laighin, G. O., Rialle, V., & Lundy, J. E. (2007). Fall detection—Principles and methods. In *Proceedings of the 29th Annual International Conference on IEEE Engineering in Medicine and Biology Society,* Lyon, France, August 22–26 (pp. 1663–1666). IEEE.
57. Kangas, M., Konttila, A., Lindgren, P., Winblad, I., & Jämsä, T. (2008). Comparison of low-complexity fall detection algorithms for body attached accelerometers. *Gait & Posture, 28*, 285–291.

58. Lee, J., & Ha, I. (2001). Real-time motion capture for a human body using accelerometers. *Robotica, 19*, 601–610; Shiratori, T., & Hodgins, J. K. (2008). Accelerometer-based user interfaces for the control of a physically simulated character. *ACM Transactions on Graphics (SIGGRAPH Asia 2008), 27*, article 123.
59. Savva, N., Scarinzi, A., & Bianchi-Berthouze, N. (2012). Continuous recognition of player's affective body expression as the dynamic quality of aesthetic experience. *IEEE Transactions on Computational Intelligence in AI and Games, 4*, 199–212.
60. Kleinsmith, A., Bianchi-Berthouze, N., & Steed, A. (2011). Automatic recognition of non-acted effective postures. *IEEE Transactions on Systems, Man, and Cybernetics, Part B, 41*, 1027–1038.
61. Siewiorek, D. (2012). Generation smartphone. *IEEE Spectrum, 49*, 54–58.
62. Nguyen, A., Moore, D., & McCowan, I. (2007). Unsupervised clustering of free-living human activities using ambulatory accelerometry. In *Proceedings of the 29th Annual International Conference on IEEE Engineering in Medicine and Biology Society*, Lyon, France, August 23–26 (pp. 4895–4898). IEEE.
63. Wang, Z. L., Jiang, M., Hu, Y. H., & Li, H. Y. (2012). An incremental learning method based on probabilistic neural networks and adjustable fuzzy clustering for human activity recognition by using wearable sensors. *IEEE Transactions on Information Technology in Biomedicine, 16*, 691–699.
64. Keyes, O. (2018). The misgendering machines: Trans/HCI implications of automatic gender recognition. *Proceedings of the ACM on human-computer interaction, 2*(CSCW), 1–22.
65. Nass, C., & Moon, Y. (2000). Machines and mindlessness: Social responses to computers. *Journal of social issues, 56*(1), 81–103.
66. Sanchez, M., Exposito, E., & Aguilar, J. (2020). Autonomic computing in manufacturing process coordination in industry 4.0 context. *Journal of industrial information integration, 19*, 100159.

Chapter 3
Wireless Body Area Networks in Healthcare

3.1 Introduction

Recent developments in wireless information exchange and electronics have made possible the development of tiny and intelligent sensors that can be used on, around, in, or transplanted in the human body, making omnipresent healthcare a promising new technology with the potential to enhance the effectiveness, accuracy, and accessibility of medical treatment. With the potential for substantial improvements in healthcare delivery and monitoring, wireless body area networks (WBANs) are now an important area of study and advancement in this setting. WBANs are made up of many kinds of different biological sensors. These sensors may be implanted beneath the skin or made to be worn on various regions of the body. There are certain specifications for each one, and they all serve distinct purposes. These gadgets monitor the physiological responses of patients and may also pick up on human states like anxiety, tension, and happiness. They connect to a dedicated destination network, which has a higher processing power. Its function is to relay the patient's biosignals to the treating physician so that he or she may make an accurate diagnosis and provide effective treatment.

The three levels of communication inside a body area network (BAN), between BANs, and outside of BANs are laid out in Fig. 3.1 as part of the WBAN common architecture. Communications inside a WBAN's master node are referred to as intra-BAN communications, and they occur between individual wireless body sensors and the network's central hub. In inter-BAN communications, the central hub exchanges data with individual endpoints like laptops, smartphones, and home service robots. The beyond-BAN layer is responsible for establishing the connection between the individual's device and the web. Several methods, such as Bluetooth and IEEE 802.15.4, provide interaction between various components via the exchange of data. Most of the needs of WBAN applications have been met by IEEE 802.15.6, which was developed with them in mind.

Figure 3.1 depicts the general architecture of a WBAN [1]. However, when compared to competing systems that allow WBANs, its performance is lacking in

G. Chhabra et al., *Artificial Intelligence to Analyze Psychophysical and Human Lifestyle*, https://doi.org/10.1007/978-981-99-3039-5_3

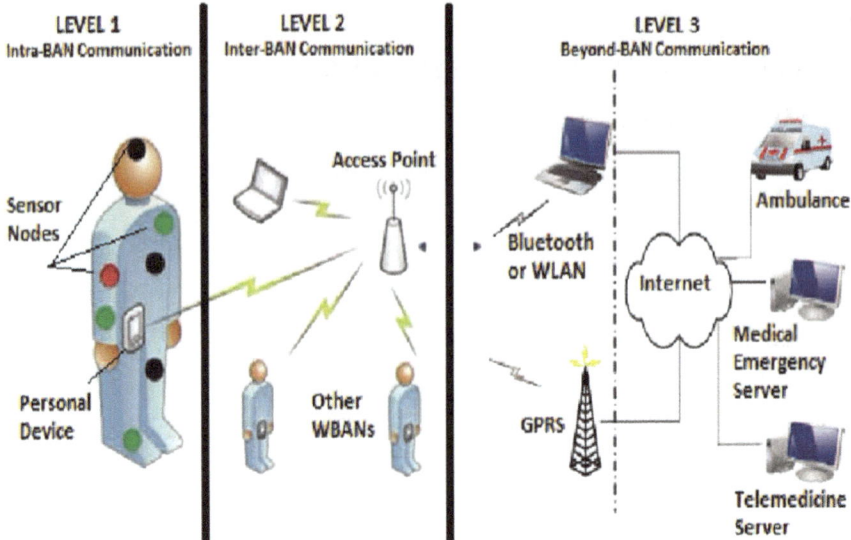

Fig. 3.1 Architecture of a WBAN

certain instances. Wi-Fi, Bluetooth, and mobile networks are all viable options for implementing WBAN applications because of their unique properties that enable them to fulfil the requirements of a variety of different uses. The goal of the many areas that WBAN apps extend to is to better the lives of its users. The primary way to classify these uses is according to whether or not they have a medical or other practical purpose. Medical aid in times of calamity, such as terrorist attacks, earthquakes, and bushfires, is only one of many non-medical uses for motion and gesture detection. The majority of medical apps focus on healthcare for sick and elderly people. Biofeedback applications that regulate states of emotion and supported living programs that enhance the lives of disabled people are just a couple examples. Others comprise: disease detection and monitoring; home care for the elderly; rehabilitation following surgery; and assisted living programs that reduce isolation and improve independence. Biokinetic sensors are able to gather the signals from human body movements such as angular rate of rotation or acceleration and are typically used in conjunction with physiological sensors to detect vital signals, such as electrocardiography, blood pressure, and temperature for health monitoring. When paired with body sensors, ambient sensors provide information about the surrounding environment, such as temperature, pressure, light, and humidity. As these sensors work in monitoring the environment, they can provide useful supplementary data for medical treatment and sometimes for medical diagnosis as well, which is commonly the case in a domestic setting. However, various technical constraints, such as node movements and temperatures, low node capacities, and node placements in terms of processing and energy consumption, must be considered during the conceptualization of WBAN applications. Considerations such as limited coverage area and data rate, which are intrinsic to wireless technology, must also be included in connections between in-body and on-body nodes. For some medical applications, the requisite data rates and latencies are laid forth in ISO/IEEE 11073. In addition, WBAN apps may have more prerequisites that are intrinsic to the medical function of the application and to the state of the patient. Applications that depend on implanted sensors, for instance, need methods that minimize energy consumption to lengthen battery life, whereas highly critical applications, such as operations on elderly cardiac patients, need to attain maximum throughput and the shortest delay. These claims and needs have prompted us to investigate the various WBAN implementations and emphasize the criteria for their operation. We will also investigate the various technologies in use, and will make an effort to match WBAN applications with the most suitable technologies in order to maximize the quality of service. Here is how the chapter is laid out. Section 3.2 discusses the principal types of WBAN applications. In Sect. 3.3, we examine the various WBAN technologies. In Sect. 3.4, we provide the criteria for each class of medical application and examine the most suitable technologies that may meet those needs.

3.2 Applications of WBANs

WBANs have many novel and fascinating uses. Among these uses are those in smart healthcare, supported living for the aged, emergency response, and even interactive gaming. Many studies have divided WBANs' potential uses into two categories: medical and non-medical, as previously mentioned [1, 2]. For medical purposes, the authors of [3] differentiated between intra- and extracorporeal uses. We now provide an overview of the major types of medical applications, and will deal with the specifics of QoS needs of such applications.

3.2.1 Remote Medical Monitoring and Telemedicine

With an aging global population and escalating healthcare expenses, telemedicine networks have advanced to provide a variety of medical services. Telemedicine permits scientists, doctors, and medical professionals from all over the globe to assist a greater number of patients by delivering treatment remotely by utilizing integrated health information systems and communications technology. In reality, the signals provided by body sensors enable efficient data processing, resulting in trustworthy and precise physiological estimates, and allowing a remote medical professional to give real-time suggestions as a medical prescription. The diagnosis process, chronic disease management, and post-operative recovery monitoring are all areas that may benefit from such a smart healthcare system. In general, patient monitoring software regulates critical signals and gives the patient immediate feedback and data that aids in his or her recovery. There is no need to restrict the patient's regular activities or risk seriously harming him if we keep him under a doctor's observation while he is in his natural physiological setting. Patients with certain disorders may benefit from in-hospital monitoring whereas those who need to be in the hospital for intensive treatment and observations, sometimes for an extended length of time, may benefit more from daily-life activity monitoring. At the same time, data on a number of different health indicators are being tracked in real time. The focus of in-home monitoring for post-surgical recovery is on patients after they've been discharged following an operation/surgery. It is possible to better disclose organ failures and diagnose emergencies more quickly with the use of data collected continuously by a WBAN because of its ability to assess physiological parameters. Such a remote monitoring system is preferable in terms of security, convenience, and cost [4–6]. There have been several proposals in the literature in this area. Some of them have attempted to research individual illnesses while others have sought to build a general framework that could accommodate the vast majority of cases [7]. Remote patient-monitoring applications include those for Parkinson's [8], cancer detection [9], diabetes [10], artificial retinas, asthma, Alzheimer's, and cardiovascular diseases [11–13].

3.2.2 Therapy and Rehabilitation

The purpose of rehabilitation is to help patients regain their pre-disability level of functioning via the use of therapeutic interventions after they have been released from hospital [14, 15]. Rehabilitation is an evolving procedure that modifies the available resources to alter any undesirable motion behavior and bring about the desired outcome. Movement of patients in a rehabilitation course has to be regularly checked and corrected so as to maintain a proper motion pattern to allow a person who has undergone a stroke to achieve the maximum possible degree of independence so that he or she may be as productive as feasible. Therefore, in a home-based rehabilitation plan, detecting/tracking human mobility becomes crucial and important. Rehabilitation is a unique field of study because of its diverse set of sensors, virtual reality integration, real-time input for patients, and multi-sensor data fusion [16].

3.2.3 Biofeedback

The advent of WBANs has made it feasible for individuals to self-remotely monitor their own bodies by gaining access to sensor data. Biosensors, such as those used in temperature analysis, blood pressure detection, electrocardiography, and electromyography, are implanted or externally placed in humans to keep tabs on certain behaviours or pathologies and provide patients with feedback that can be used to better manage their health [17]. Biofeedback is a system that monitors a person's vital signs and other potentially valuable factors and relays that information back to him so that he may learn to regulate his own body's responses to stress and other stimuli, so enhancing his health and overall performance [18–20]. Biofeedback has been around since the 1960s, and it has helped people with problems like migraines and high blood pressure to gain control of their emotions and other involuntary bodily processes. Breathing, heart, muscle, and brainwave monitoring equipment are all examples of biofeedback instruments.

3.2.4 Environment-Assisted Living

Safe and independent aging depends on a number of factors, including the effects of an aging population in general, rising costs in conventional healthcare, and the significance placed by people on maintaining their own autonomy. This area's applications boost the quality of life so people may remain independent for longer with the help of home automation [15]. As an alternative to nursing homes and retirement communities, assisted living communities provide a home for the disabled, elderly, and those who are partially dependent but don't require constant medical attention. Thanks to constant mental and physical monitoring, the characteristics of the living environment may be sensed and controlled by an ambient sensor network, which subsequently transmits the body's data to a central station. From their heart rates, blood pressures, and accelerometer readings, we may infer their general health. In the event of significant changes in the measured parameters or departures from the normal range, the system may connect to a healthcare facility for monitoring and emergency intervention [21].

3.3 WBAN Technologies

WBANs may need many layers of technological complexity. The most prominent technologies suggested for WBANs are analyzed in depth in this section.

3.3.1 Bluetooth

In order to provide the highest possible degree of privacy, Bluetooth technology was developed as a standard for wireless communications over short distances [22]. This allows for a single device to operate as a master and up to seven additional devices to act as slaves inside a single piconet, an ad hoc network. Slaves must synchronize with the master's system clock and hop in accordance with the master's predetermined pattern. In addition, each device may belong to numerous piconets concurrently, when they reach the radio vicinity of other master devices. One of Bluetooth's most alluring features is that it makes it possible for a diverse set of Bluetooth-enabled devices to link up and exchange data from almost any location on the planet. Another essential characteristic is the capability of the devices to converse without the necessity for an insight placement of the linked devices. Therefore, it is extensively utilized for linking a broad range of portable devices to provide data and voice services. Devices that use Bluetooth technology may be found operating in the 2.4 GHz Industrial, Scientific, and Medical (ISM) band, where they hop between 79 individual 1 MHz channels at a notional rate of 1600 hops per second to avoid interference. As per the norm, there are three distinct categories of wireless equipment, each with its own range and transmission power specifications (between 1 and 100 m). The highest data rate is 3 Mbps.

3.3.2   Bluetooth Low Energy (BLE)

This is an offshoot of the original Bluetooth standard and was developed to be a more practical solution for WBAN applications due to its lower power requirements and ability to operate with a lower duty cycle. BLE was developed to link wirelessly with the tiny devices of mobile terminals. Such devices are generally too small to tolerate the energy consumption and expenses associated with a normal Bluetooth radio and at the same time these devices are great candidates for healthcare applications. The theoretical maximum throughput for BLE is 1 Mbps. Because there are fewer channels involved in the pairing process, synchronization may be completed in milliseconds rather than the seconds it takes with Bluetooth. This aids latency-critical BAN applications, such as emergency responses and raising the alarm, and boosts power efficiency. The minimized latency, data rate, and power consumption helps BLE to be suited for better communication between the access point and worn sensor nodes. However, the adaptive frequency hop spread spectrum enables the BLE devices to exist with wireless networks. Since the technology runs in the 2.4 GHz ISM band, the interference with other devices can be a concern. Additionally, Bluetooth is more useful at handling applications with power requirements, network coverage, and varying data rates. However, it is more practical for short-term broadband applications where two or more peer-to-peer devices can communicate; for example, the personal servers of two or more WBANs or between a PC and a WBAN [23].

3.3.3   Zigbee and 802.15.4

The Zigbee standard specified the Zigbee12. This is a type of wireless technology which is commonly employed in a low-power battery-based environment [24]. It is intended for radio-frequency applications that demand a long battery life and a low data rate, and which facilitates implementation, due to its security support (128 bit), to ensure integrity, conduct authentication, and privacy of communications. Zigbee-enabled devices may function for years without requiring battery replacement because of their sleep mode [25]. There are two distinct components to Zigbee technology. To begin, the Zigbee alliance defines the network, security, and application software layers as the application layers. Secondly, the physical and medium-access control layers are defined by the IEEE 802.15.4 standard. This standard specifies the use of unslotted/slotted carrier sense multiple access with collision avoidance (CSMA/CA) mechanisms for wireless channel access and the allocation and management of guaranteed time slots (GTSs). Wireless Zigbee products use the 868 MHz, 915 MHz, and 2.4 GHz spectrums. Therefore, Zigbee's interference with wireless local area network (WLAN) transmission is a major drawback for WBAN applications, particularly in the 2.4 GHz frequency range where a great number of wireless devices operate. Zigbee's low data rate (250 Kbps) is another drawback that prevents it from being suitable for large-scale and real-time WBAN applications. Although the low data rate makes it impractical for usage in healthcare settings with numerous patients at once, it is perfect for individual use (single patient).

3.3.4 IEEE 802.11

IEEE 802.118 specifies the requirements for WLANs. Wi-Fi is a wireless networking technology that, whether used with an access point or in ad hoc mode, enables users to access the World Wide Web at broadband speeds in accordance with IEEE 802.11 standards. Its high-speed wireless networking, which enables videoconferencing, phone conversations, and video streaming, makes it perfectly suited for huge data transfers. The fact that Wi-Fi is built into every smartphone, tablet, and laptop is a huge advantage, but their excessive energy consumption is a major disadvantage.

3.3.5 IEEE 802.15.6

The WBAN standard, IEEE 802.15.6, enabled communications inside and around the human body for a wide range of medical and non-medical uses. There are several different frequency bands used for data transmission in the IEEE 802.15.6 standard. These include the narrowband (NB), which uses the 400, 800, and 900 MHz as well as the 2.3 or 2.4 GHz bands, and the ultra-wideband (UWB), which uses the 3.1 GHz to 11.2 GHz, whereas human body communication uses frequencies around 1050 MHz. This standard is a breakthrough in the field of wearable wireless sensor networks (WSNs) since it supports a plethora of data speeds, low energy consumption, a large number of nodes (256 per BAN), a broad range of possible applications, and varying node priority to suit a multiplicity of needs. A slotted Aloha access process or CSMA/CA manages channel access. Since it offers three different security schemes, it allows for the customization of security parameters. The IEEE 802.15.6 standard supports data transfer speeds of up to 10 Mbps while using negligible amounts of energy. Furthermore, it can take into account certain bodily motions, though this is not sufficient for upcoming WBAN applications which need such scenarios as sitting, lying, running, swimming, jogging, and standing. This specification, with its maximum achievable throughput of 680 Kbps, can meet the throughput needs of the vast majority of WBAN applications. However, it cannot accommodate the requirements of new applications that need flawless audio and video transmissions.

3.3.6   Different Radio Technologies: 7.3.6

Other radio technologies are also effective and may be employed in the creation of WBAN applications. High bandwidth is made available via UWB technology, which is used in small range communication systems. UWB offers the sole dependable form of localization, which is especially critical for interior localization in assisted living institutions and hospitals. The intricacy, however, makes it inappropriate for use in wearable devices. One additional growing standard for health and wellness monitoring apps is the ANT protocol10. Several producers of sensors back the ANT protocol, which is slow and uses little energy. Because of its ultra-low power consumption, Zarlink technology is well-suited to medical implant applications that operate at low frequencies and data rates. Using long wave magnetic signals, the Rubee active wireless protocol can transmit and receive small data packets (just 128 bytes in size) via a local area network. Operating a Rubee does not need direct visual contact between two devices. Patient monitoring and other mobile healthcare applications may benefit greatly from Rubee's extended battery life, ultra-low power consumption, consistent operating providence, and high security level.

3.4   Technologies Versus Applications

The medical applications built on WBANs show significant potential in enhancing people's lives and meeting the numerous needs of the elderly, allowing them to age in place with peace of mind and good health. Wireless technologies are used for communicating between sensors and between the base station and sensors since Bluetooth technology is a highly easy method to transmit information. Although IEEE 802.15.6 is meant to serve a broad range of medical professionals who are looking for applications, the most generally adopted and utilized standards are IEEE 802.15.1 (Bluetooth) and IEEE 802.15.4 (often referred to as Zigbee). However, there are other factors to think about as well, such as data rate and interference caused by the presence of many technologies. Based on the needs of a certain WBAN application, the most suitable radio technology may be selected. We will break down the needs of various types of medical applications that make use of wireless technology and highlight those that can meet those needs [6].

Depending on the specifics of the operating environment and the nature of the WBAN application, these demands may vary. In fact, the goal of many rehabilitation-focused apps is to track a patient's motor functions while he or she undergoes treatment. Examples of possible therapeutic uses include development based ones, such as motor rehabilitation, intellectual disability, or brain damage therapies (accident rehabilitation, stroke rehabilitation, illness rehabilitation, or surgical rehabilitation). As several sensors are used, the precise body location for the nodes and electromagnetic interference should be taken into account at network layers to support secure transmission. Furthermore, sensors should sample at high frequencies to accurately acquire the observed phenomena. In order to retrieve reliable medical data, the system must demonstrate great precision in its data gathering and processing. It should also offer real-time communication, with a money-back guarantee for any delays, to provide honest feedback to the service user during treatment and follow-up, enabling patients to adjust their movements instantaneously. As the health of patient populations is involved, the system must promise the delivery of alerts, such as falls by the elderly when exercising, though within strict delay restrictions. Energy misgivings can be considered for elderly or permanently damaged patients to avoid bothersome charging processes.

Biofeedback also provides users with the capacity to continuously and effectively monitor health factors including body/intra-body temperature, cardiac rate, and arterial blood pressure. Human biological factors must be monitored closely to guarantee healthy living and proper conduct. Thus, the parameters must be captured as precisely and reliably as feasible. Even when implementation feeds these bioinformatic tools back to the user, the wireless communication adopted must take into consideration the unique attributes of such a medium, like entanglements. Sensor node energy limits should be carefully considered in such applications. In reality, battery life is shortened due to the small size of the sensors; and if a sensor fails, an important piece of information about the patient's health is lost. In addition, there are more issues in efficiency, cost, and user interface that must be designed for when implementing these physiological applications. In order for this kind of application to be useful, raw sensor data must be converted into information that can be understood by both patients and medical professionals. The use of Bluetooth-enabled mobile devices, such as a smartphone, is fundamental to many of the proposed solutions. Other methods include the patient carrying a portable device (like a personal digital assistant) that is in constant contact with the sink node. Modern personal digital assistants (PDAs) have sufficient computer capability to handle some data and have many gigabytes of flash storage. The foundation of the proposed interconnected system is a practical wireless architecture that makes use of wireless and Bluetooth connections. Wearable sensors may provide data to a PDA using Bluetooth's short-range communication. A PDA's embedded micro-database is responsible for managing the obtained patient data, which will then be sent wirelessly to a distant server over a WLAN and, if necessary, treated by medical professionals [25].

Healthcare surveillance and e-health services are two examples of what an ambient assisted living (AAL) system may provide. When it comes to healthcare expenses, nothing beats AAL's ability to help seniors maintain their dignity and their independence (aging in place). Patients' activities and lifestyle may be tracked with the use of smart homes fitted out with a variety of acoustic, vibration, and visual sensors. Security and privacy are major concerns in AAL systems since the data delivered are often very sensitive and individual. Therefore, it is imperative that all information transmission adheres to strict standards of privacy, security, and accessibility. The IEEE 802.15.6 standard offers three distinct degrees of security that may be implemented to ensure safe and effective transmissions. An assurance of real-time data is essential in case of emergency. Since telemedicine deals with people's health records, it also deals with very private and crucial information. While Wi-Fi lacks the ability to guarantee packet delivery times, Zigbee with its beacon technology enabled may give such assurances and therefore enable real-time communication. One potential drawback of Zigbee is its very modest transmission speed.

3.5 Conclusion

We highlight the quality-of-service requirements of some of the most important WBAN applications below. The goal is to provide enough wireless technology for use in such systems. A selection of suitable means of interaction through electronic media has been provided. Depending on the needs of the application and the layer in the architecture at which the radio will be installed, the most suitable radio technology for WBANs may be chosen:

1. Intra-BAN communication involving sensor systems and a parent node, where throughput, latency, and power considerations may be present in a typical WBAN design. Collisions and external interference are common in two types of inter-BAN communications.
2. Communication systems between the primary server and one or more network connections—3G, cellular, Zigbee, Bluetooth, and WLAN are all examples of wireless technologies that could be used for inter-BAN communication.
3. Beyond-BAN communications are necessary to allow authorized health practitioners (such as a doctor or nurse) to remotely monitor a patient's medical records via a cellular network or the World Wide Web.

References

1. Ullah, S., Higgins, H., Braem, B., Latre, B., Blondia, C., Moerman, I., & Kwak, K. S. (2012). A comprehensive survey of wireless body area networks. *Journal of Medical Systems, 36*(3), 1065–1094.
2. Tobon, D. P., Falk, T. H., & Maier, M. (2013). Context awareness in WBANs: A survey on medical and non-medical applications. *Wireless Communications, IEEE, 20*(4), 30–37.

3. Boulemtafes, A., & Badache, N. (2016). Design of wearable health monitoring systems: An overview of techniques and technologies. In *mHealth ecosystems and social networks in healthcare* (pp. 79–94). Springer International Publishing.

4. Chen, M., Wan, J., Gonzlez, S., Liao, X., & Leung, V. (2014). A survey of recent developments in home M2M networks. *Communications Surveys & Tutorials, IEEE, 16*(1), 98–114.

5. Chakraborty, C., Gupta, B., & Ghosh, S. K. (2013). A review on telemedicine-based WBAN framework for patient monitoring. *Telemedicine and e-Health, 19*(8), 619–626.

6. Zhou, H., & Hu, H. (2008). Human motion tracking for rehabilitation: A survey. *Biomedical Signal Processing and Control, 3*(1), 1–18.

7. Alam, M. M., & Hamida, E. B. (2015). Strategies for optimal mac parameters tuning in IEEE 802.15. 6 wearable wireless sensor networks. *Journal of Medical Systems, 39*(9), 1–16.

8. Vallejos de Schatz, C. H., Medeiros, H. P., Schneider, F. K., & Abatti, P. J. (2012). Wireless medical sensor networks: Design requirements and enabling technologies. *Telemedicine and e-Health, 18*(5), 394–399.

9. Astrin, A. (2012). IEEE standard for local and metropolitan area networks part 15.6: Wireless body area networks: IEEE std 802.15. 6-2012. The document is available at IEEE Xplore.

10. Jovanov, E., & Milenkovic, A. (2011). Body area networks for ubiquitous healthcare applications: Opportunities and challenges. *Journal of Medical Systems, 35*(5), 1245–1254.

11. Li, H. B., Takizawa, K., & Kohno, R. (2008, October). Trends and standardization of body area network (BAN) for medical healthcare. In *European Conference on Wireless Technology, 2008. EuWiT 2008* (pp. 1–4). IEEE. ISO 690.

12. Adibi, S. (Ed.). (2015). *Mobile health: A technology road map* (Vol. 5). Springer.

13. Kernen, N., Srestniemi, M., Partala, J., Hmlinen, M., Reponen, J., Seppnen, T., Jms, T., et al. (2013, July). IEEE802. 15.6-based multiaccelerometer WBAN system for monitoring Parkinson's disease. In *The 35th Annual International IEEE Engineering in Medicine and Biology Society Conference*, Osaka, Japan.

14. Wang, J., Zhang, Z., Yang, X., Zuo, L., & Kim, J. U. (2013). A novel three-tier diabetes patients monitoring architecture in hospital environment.

15. Rashidi, P., & Mihailidis, A. (2013). A survey on ambient-assisted living tools for older adults. *IEEE Journal of Biomedical and Health Informatics, 17*(3), 579–590.

16. Al Masud, S. M. R. (2013). Study and analysis of scientific scopes, issues and challenges towards developing a righteous wireless body area network. *International Journal of Soft Computing and Engineering (IJSCE)*.

17. Alam, M. M., & Hamida, E. B. (2014). Surveying wearable human assistive technology for life and safety critical applications: Standards, challenges and opportunities. *Sensors, 14*(5), 9153–9209. ISO 690.

18. Pereira, O., Caldeira, J. M., & Rodrigues, J. J. (2011). Body sensor network mobile solutions for biofeedback monitoring. *Mobile Networks and Applications, 16*(6), 713–732.

19. Caldeira, J. M., Moutinho, J. A., Vaidya, B., Lorenz, P., & Rodrigues, J. J. (2010, February). Intra-body temperature monitoring using a biofeedback solution. In *Second International Conference on eHealth, Telemedicine, and Social Medicine, 2010. ETELEMED'10* (pp. 119–124). IEEE.

20. Rodrigues, J. J., Pereira, O. R., & Neves, P. A. (2011). Biofeedback data visualization for body sensor networks. *Journal of Network and Computer Applications, 34*(1), 151–158.

21. Pervez Khan, M., Hussain, A., & Kwak, K. S. (2009). Medical applications of wireless body area networks. *International Journal of Digital Content Technology and its Applications*.

22. Chen, M., Gonzalez, S., Vasilakos, A., Cao, H., & Leung, V. C. (2011). Body area networks: A survey. *Mobile Networks and Applications, 16*(2), 171–193. ISO 690.
23. Jin, Z., Oresko, J., Huang, S., & Cheng, A. C. (2009, April). HeartToGo: A personalized medicine technology for cardiovascular disease prevention and detection. In *Life Science Systems and Applications Workshop, 2009. LiSSA 2009. IEEE/NIH* (pp. 80–83). IEEE.
24. Hadjidj, A., Souil, M., Bouabdallah, A., Challal, Y., & Owen, H. (2013). Wireless sensor networks for rehabilitation applications: Challenges and opportunities. *Journal of Network and Computer Applications, 36*(1), 1–15.
25. Acampora, G., Cook, D. J., Rashidi, P., & Vasilakos, A. V. (2013). A survey on ambient intelligence in healthcare. *Proceedings of the IEEE, 101*(12), 2470–2494.

Chapter 4
Techniques for Behaviour Analysis Using Deep Learning

4.1 Introduction

New norms have been developed for the transportation sector—as a result of the increasing need for transporting both people and products—as well as the development of information and communication technologies. In addition, new transportation paradigms may be established thanks to the development and maturation of sensor technology, which could lead to a deeper comprehension of drivers' actions. The increasing number of cars on the road, particularly in densely populated areas, also presents significant dangers to human health and the natural world. For instance, the European Automobile Manufacturers Association estimated that there were 242.7 million passenger automobiles in use throughout EU member states in 2019 [1]. In the year 2020, the World Health Organization (WHO) estimated that more than 1.35 million people died in traffic accidents globally [2]. We need to take a close look at the environmental impact of automobiles in addition to the rising numbers of vehicles and car accidents. In particular, the European Parliament claimed in 2019 that transportation was responsible for roughly 30% of the total CO_2 emissions [3] in the EU. Considering the above, it is obvious that efforts to study safer and environmentally friendly practices and regulations should be stepped up to better address new environmental and safety issues. To this end, it is right to seek valuable insights and make predictions about potentially dangerous driving behavior in terms of both the environment and driver safety by monitoring and analyzing data emanating from sensors installed inside vehicles.

Over the last several decades, governments all over the globe have taken steps to curb CO_2 emissions and so slow down or possibly avert climate change and its potentially catastrophic repercussions. The EU has specifically approved a number of policies to attain carbon neutrality by the year 2050. One of these initiatives encourages Europeans to switch to hybrids and electric cars and imposes stricter regulations on emissions requirements [4]. There are numerous internal-combustion-based vehicles already on the roads and which need to receive more attention, in addition to the regulations and the move to electric automobiles that already affect

© The Author(s), under exclusive license to Springer Nature Singapore Pte Ltd. 2023
G. Chhabra et al., *Artificial Intelligence to Analyze Psychophysical and Human Lifestyle*,
https://doi.org/10.1007/978-981-99-3039-5_4

future vehicle sales. Gathering and analyzing data directly from the vehicle is crucial for assessing and informing the driver about his or her driving behavior as it impacts fuel consumption, which in turn has a direct impact on the emissions emitted by the automobile. Having this knowledge would give the motorist incentive to drive in a more environmentally friendly manner.

Sensors installed inside motor vehicles provide the information required to conduct such analyses of driver behavior. Modern automobiles are equipped with a wide variety of sensors that track data such as velocity, temperature, and engine revolutions per minute (RPM). Up until recently, these readings were solely useful for in-car diagnostics and wouldn't transfer out of the automobile. Cars are now equipped with networking capabilities thanks to the fast growth of ICT; this allows them to connect with external devices like cellphones, databases, other vehicles (vehicle-to-vehicle communication), emergency call centers, and motorways. By using on-board diagnostic (OBD) modules, data may be sent to external applications from even the earliest car models. In particular, the protocol of OBD II is currently widely utilized for reading diagnostic information. As a result, an older vehicle may be fitted out with a small device that can collect various diagnostic messages and measurements, and then transmit these messages to a smartphone or another network-connected device, where they can be stored and analyzed on an external interface. In addition, there has been a tremendous development in the streaming of data, data storage, and advanced analysis technologies, which has occurred simultaneously with the fast growth of sensor and networking technologies. Also, the real-time analysis of rapidly produced data from various automobiles, with the help of big data and artificial intelligence tools, can be made accessible for commercial use.

Thus, in this study we suggest and offer a new method for uninterrupted data collection, data storage, and data analysis by using cutting-edge streaming processes along with big data, machine learning (ML), and deep learning (DL). All of the data utilized in this analysis came from OBD II devices installed in five cars that belong to a Greek highway administrator and which were driven vast distances by various individuals on a daily basis. This data analysis, which was aimed at categorizing drivers' behavior as environmentally friendly or not, was carried out on a cloud-based platform that was built and released to meet the demands of the fast and large data streams arriving from automobiles by way of an appropriate streaming module. The investigation used supervised ML and DL algorithm benchmarking on a pre-labeled dataset, in addition to popular unsupervised ML approaches for data labeling.

In Sect. 4.2, we survey the state of the art in the field of driving behavior analysis; in Sect. 4.3, we detail the tools and infrastructure used for data collection and analysis; in Sect. 4.4, we present the dataset and the algorithms used to conduct the evaluation; and in Sect. 4.5, we reveal the outcomes of the present chapter.

4.2 Related Work

Driving behavior analysis (DBA) using ML has become more popular in recent years. The increased use of ML algorithms is a rising trend. We can search for recent publications which display the number of appropriate papers collected from SCOPUS using the keyword TITLE-ABS-KEY (keywords related to ML). This area of study has shown significant development over the last decade. The fast development of computer technology and the widespread use of ML techniques bode well for this growing trend. There has also been an increase in opportunities for studying and automating driver behavior because of the digitalization and ICT integration of cars.

Analyzing driving behavior is challenging because of all the variables involved, including road conditions, traffic, the vehicle, and the driver. In light of this, the problem may be posed and addressed in a broad range of ways. To further understand the causes and methods involved in DBA, Alluhaibi et al. [5] did a thorough literature review. The researchers focused on studies that tried to place drivers in aggressive (dangerous) or nonaggressive categories (normal). (i) In-vehicle information storage systems play a pivotal role in modern automobiles. These systems, often designed to engage in CAN-bus (Controller Area Network) and OBD (On-Board Diagnostics) interactions, as well as integrate with other devices and necessary kits within the vehicle, have become indispensable; (ii) sensing based on smartphones in vehicles, principally relying on the resource usage of the wide range of numerous sensors on a phone or tablet in order to gauge vehicle speed; and (iii) behavior monitoring systems are all examples of sensors used for driver behavior categorization, as presented in [5]. The DBA may be categorized as static or real-time, and the outputs vary among approaches, based on the currently available devices and the unique requirements of each situation.

As can be seen in Fig. 4.1, the use of ML has been steadily on the rise over the last several years. Accordingly, Elassad et al. [6] conducted a thorough literature assessment of the relevant research with the aim of presenting solutions and methodologies for DBA via the use of ML. The ML methods employed were broken down into the following categories by the authors of [6] (the proportion of research that uses each methodology is included in brackets): (i) NN (22%), (ii) SVM (24%), (iii) clustering (8%), (iv) fuzzy (3%), (v) IR (1%), and (vi) decision trees (6%). Based on a meta-analysis of 82 articles from 46 journals and conferences, the most common methods found are: (vii) evolutionary algorithms (1%), (viii) ensemble learners (11%), (ix) Bayesian learners (15%), and (x) other methods (2%). In addition, [6] offers in-depth evaluations of the research metrics, such as accuracy, recall, and precision, and organizes the studies into three primary groups according to the DBA dimension, that is driving events and psychological states. Through their thorough literature assessment, Elassad et al. [6] support the developing pattern of ML approaches used for DBA and research gaps with future objectives in this study arena. Furthermore, this study found that the effectiveness of each approach greatly varies depending on the dataset and the setting of the research uses.

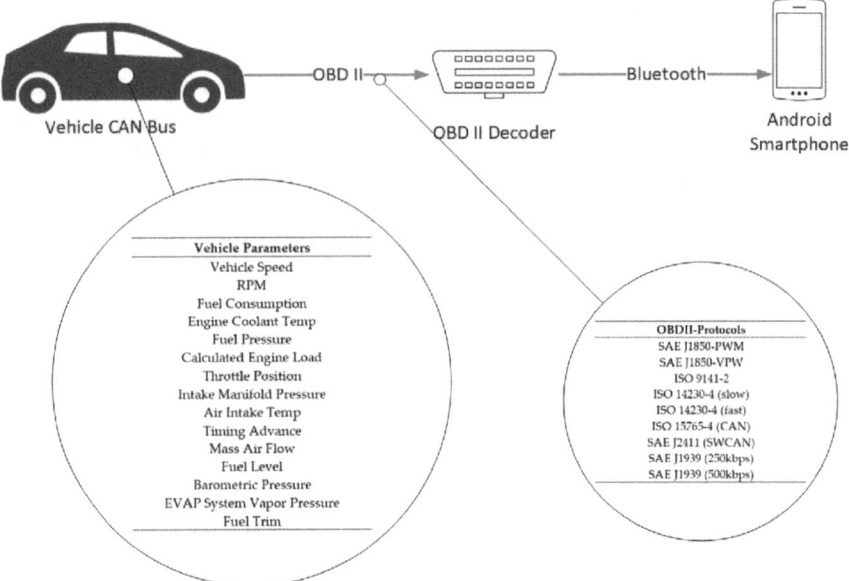

Fig. 4.1 In-car equipment layout

Despite the fast development of ICT technologies that are integrated in cars, fuel utilization is strongly dependent on the behavior of the driver. This makes various DBA addressing scenarios with ecological footprint systems. To this end, Araujo et al. [7] suggest a system that integrates data from the vehicle's OBD II port and the Electronic Control Unit (ECU). Through a fuzzy evaluator, an Android app provides the user with helpful advice about how to alter his or her behavior in light of the recognized car state and the user's input concerning fuel usage [7]. One approach presented by Massoud et al. [8] uses a smartphone and an OBD II adaptor to help the driver reduce fuel use by accessing information from the car's sensors. To be more exact, the authors of [8] consider many factors (such as throttle position, RPM, speed, and automobile jolt) to arrive at a score between 0 and 100. When drivers in the proposed framework engage in environmentally unfriendly behaviors, they are immediately confronted with immediate, actionable, and contextualized feedback. Finally, Massoud et al. [8] advocate for gamifying this process, for example by rating drivers, to provide them with greater motivation to drive in a fuel-efficient manner. Massoud [9] presents a more in-depth analysis of these methods in her PhD dissertation, where she goes into further depth about the underlying algorithms and technology. Chen et al. [10] use machine learning techniques like principal component analysis and multiple linear regression to analyze eco-driving behavior, in order to evaluate driver behavior and offer helpful eco-driving suggestions to enhance their overall skillset. It's important to note that research on eco-friendly driving is still in its infancy, and that more frameworks exist than those already listed. Thus, enviroCar is a crowdsourcing effort that intends to build a public database of vehicle information that can be mined by researchers of all stripes [11]. Delhomme et al. [12] also use a statistical method based on information from 1243 male and female French drivers of varying ages. This research shows that gender, age, and environmental concern all affect how often certain behaviors are recorded and how difficult people find it to anticipate, drive at a constant pace, use the accelerator and brake conservatively, and change gears [12].

Castignani et al. [13, 14] also use smartphone and OBD II in their research, but their suggestion is a more general DBA that doesn't put as much emphasis on ecological parameters. The authors in [13] suggest an Android-based explanation that makes use of information from Android sensors to categorize drivers based on a set of 12 input factors, 18 inference rules, and an evaluator based on fuzzy systems that takes into account normal, moderate, and aggressive driving styles. The Sense-Fleet app, described in [14], was a further effort by the same creators. SenseFleet is a framework that makes use of GPS and OBD II data to identify a variety of events. In addition, as the authors of [14] emphasize, SenseFleet adds a scoring system that, in addition to the number of occurrences, considers information about the surrounding environment, such as the weather, the road, and traffic. Using data collected from an OBD II adaptor, sent through a smartphone to a cloud-based environment, and analyzed there, Abdelrahman et al. performed a series of investigations [15–17]. The SHRP 2 dataset, one of the biggest collections of driving data, was used for these research projects. Techniques based on random forests (RFs) [16, 17] and support vector regression (SVR) [15, 16] performed better than other algorithms in these investigations. Chen et al. [18] conduct another intriguing investigation comparing several machine learning methods using vehicle data. An OBD II connector was put in a research car, and the authors analyzed data from that connection. Comparing the results of the various methods studied, it became clear that the RF strategy was the most effective for this particular dataset [18]. Similarly, Navneeth et al. [19] use a smartphone and OBD II to gather data, which they analyzed by applying ML, specifically the K-Nearest Neighbors (KNN) method, for grouping the driver's behavior and computing a score that shows how unsafe the driver's behavior is. Research conducted by Carvalho et al. [20] on the efficacy of various recurrent neural networks solely made use of information gleaned from the sensors of smartphones, for example, acceleration and location. They took inputs from four distinct driving routes taken by two separate drivers in the same kind of weather, with seven distinct driving events (labels) used in the assessment of the Recurrent Neural Networks (RNNs). They found that the gated recurrent unit performed better than Long Short-Term Memory (LSTM) and simple RNN on this particular dataset [20]. Using dynamic Bayesian networks, Obuhuma et al. [21] analyzed data obtained from an OBD that may be broken down into three categories: cornering, braking, and acceleration. Lindow and Kashevnik [22] undertook a fascinating investigation by performing a comprehensive literature analysis on previous research pertaining to the various data, technologies, sensors, and ML techniques used in the investigation of driver behavior. They also suggest a conceptual architecture that uses cellphones to collect data, a cloud infrastructure to store and analyze that data using ML algorithms, and several kinds of users, like drivers, fleet managers, and operations centers, to get the results [22].

The preceding paragraphs introduce a number of intriguing research projects with similar focuses. The start of this section provided research that looked at the DBA issue from a narrower perspective, without using ML techniques; we then introduced studies that looked at the ecological component of driver behavior. Khandakar et al. [23] introduced a mobile solution that uses a smartphone's OBD II adapter to collect data that can then be analyzed for signs of driving irregularities and distractions. Renininger et al. [24] used a very similar implementation strategy to gather vehicle data and deliver it to a cloud program for data storage and analysis, including additionally a smartphone and OBD II port. Fugiglando et al. [25] developed a somewhat different but still fascinating technique, which involves collecting data from an in-car data logger and then using a system to obtain a score that represents the driver.

The research described in the preceding paragraphs served as inspiration for the current investigation. The goal is to offer a system that can efficiently store, process, and analyze data as it streams in, in order to determine which ML and DL algorithms are best suited for the purpose of behavior classification of a driver. It's important to note that the research relies on data acquired from real cars, which are part of a large highway operator's fleet. The goal is to provide a high-level summary of comprehensive results for the classification of drivers by detailing the in-car hardware, the streaming procedure, and the cloud infrastructure and big data in place and deployed to support the collection of data, data storage, and its analysis requirements for an application. In addition to a technical explanation of the fix, we give an in-depth look into how ML and DL algorithms classify drivers' actions. In this research, well-known ML and DL algorithms were used for the evaluation. The purpose of this research is not to develop a novel algorithm but rather to provide a comprehensive platform for collecting, storing, processing, and analyzing data from automobiles.

4.3 Facilities for Collecting and Analyzing Data

4.3.1 In-Vehicle Equipment

Since its widespread adoption by the automobile industry in 1993, the controller area network (CAN) has been included in every new car to collect information from the car's sensors. ISO11898, the worldwide standard for CAN, was first published in 1993 and amended in 2015. Nearly all modern automobiles include an OBD II interface that may accommodate an OBD II decoder to gather, analyze, and communicate diagnostic information to other devices. The five automobiles used in the experiments all feature a Bluetooth-connected OBD II decoder for use in putting the suggested framework into action [26].

Embedded in the OBD II device is the microprocessor ELM-327 [27]. This is utilized in almost all OBD II decoders on the market today since it translates between the OBD and RS232 protocols. Based on information provided by ELM electronics [28], the ELM-327 is compatible with SAE J1939 (500 kbps), SAE J1939 (250 kbps), SAE J1850-PWM, SAE J2411 (SWCAN), ISO 15765-4 (CAN), ISO 14230-4 (fast), ISO 14230-4 (slow), ISO 9141-2, and SAE J1850-VPW.

Due to its portability and ability to pair with a smartphone through Bluetooth, the Konnwei KW-903 model was chosen as the OBD II decoder for this research. You can see what information may be acquired from the Konnwei KW-903 [29].

Some of these characteristics are retrieved, while others are sent to a hybrid system for data management hosted in the cloud. In Sect. 4.4, we go through the criteria for making this choice. The information from the aforementioned OBD II decoder is sent to an Android 9.0 smartphone over Bluetooth. This information is sent from the Android mobile to the cloud platform through the Internet. An Android app with a standard user interface is employed to gather data from the phone, allowing the consumer to monitor the status of the linking and the measurement in real-time. This app's only purpose is to keep tabs on the status of data transfer from the OBD to the phone and then to the cloud infrastructure. Every five seconds, the system will either automatically transfer data to the cloud-based network, or the driver may choose to do it themselves. Figure 4.1 depicts a schematic of the automobile equipment used in this investigation.

4.3.2 Data Management and Analysis Software Hosted in the Cloud

This research recommends a cloud-based platform with two primary parts: (a) a broadcasting module and (b) a hybrid big data administration and social psychologist. These parts provide an integrated system for receiving, storing, and processing data streams.

4.3.2.1 Streaming Data Module

The data integration component is in charge of maintaining a constant, two-way connection between the motor vehicle, processing subsystem, and hybrid data management. An open-source toolkit, Apache Kafka, is used for analyzing data from this streaming module [30]. Apache Kafka has three core features: (i) publishing (writing) and subscribing (reading) to event streams, (ii) keeping event channels, and (iii) interpreting event streams. Kafka is built to function in a distributed fashion, making it suitable for processing massive data streams. Kafka's distributed architecture allows for high availability and adaptability. Table 4.1 provides a brief overview of some of Kafka's most fundamental ideas and phrases (Fig. 4.2).

Table 4.1 The jargon of Kafka and a description

Kafka term	Description
Topic	Data flow group related to a specific category
producer	Applications which publish messages in one or more Kafka topics
Broker	Applications which receive and transmit a message from a producer to a consumer
Consumer	Applications which subscribe (read) the messages from one or more topics through the brokers

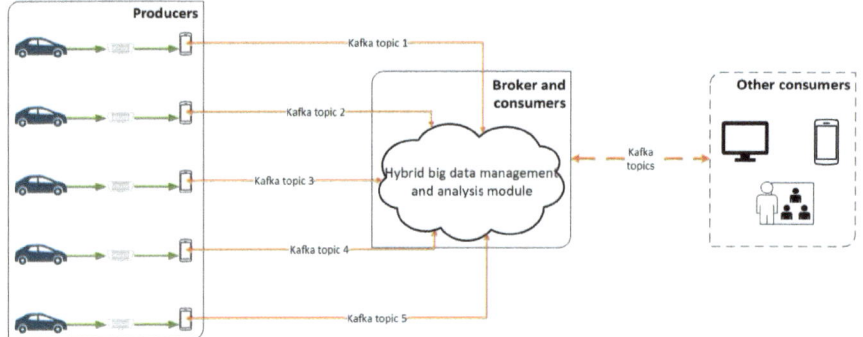

Fig. 4.2 Kafka streaming technique

4.3.2.2 Big Data Analytical Management and Processing Module

As previously indicated, the hybrid big data management and analysis module includes a relational database, a non-relational database, and an analytics engine. To better serve the fundamental needs of a big data platform, this component was developed. Andrew McAfee and Erik Brynjolfsson coined the key ideas of big data [31]—velocity, variety, and volume (the 3Vs)—and informed the creation of this module's major needs and guiding design principles. Specifically, the five cars indicated above (as shown in Fig. 4.2) feed their data into the big data management module that retains the data indefinitely and may accommodate more data streams or vehicles. As a result, this hybrid module adheres to the volume concept. In accordance with the velocity concept, the module was developed to make use of shared hardware resources, hence increasing the overall processing speed of the system. The variety principle, which we leave till last, emphasizes the module's adaptability to different data kinds, the format of which need not be specified in advance to comply with established norms. There are a variety of formats in which we may get data from the cars. In addition, the module may gather, store, and interpret other data formats received from other streams, not only those arriving from automobiles and employed for the objectives of this research.

This module is built and constructed in such a manner that it is very dependable and future-proof, in addition to the 3Vs indicated above. To begin, this component was made to work smoothly and reliably even when not tampered with. This implies that the system can cope with unforeseen circumstances with little or, preferably, no downtime. One way this is accomplished is by giving the platform the ability to detect and respond to software-specific unexpected faults by automatically restarting the affected services and recording the issue in the process. Information technology staff may utilize the data gleaned from this method to better understand what went wrong and how to prevent a recurrence. This module may be deployed to multiple distinct pieces of hardware so as to boost its computing capabilities and availability owing to replication. Its scalability is another noteworthy feature since it allows it to be quickly extended to meet growing storage and analysis demands and to be adapted to uses outside database administration.

The following is a description of the four primary commonly used software components that make up the module under consideration: MySQL, MongoDB, Hadoop, and PySpark [32–35]. These parts make it possible to collect data, keep it safe, and evaluate it without caring where the data came from in the first place. Similarly, this particular technique may host and handle information from diverse areas and not simply vehicle-based data that are employed for the objectives of this research. Finally, this technique is built as a black-box and may be accommodated to a platform/framework, needing nothing other than a single click at the beginning.

MySQL is a popular choice because of its flexibility as a relational database, allowing for analyses and visualization to occur in near real-time. However, the MongoDB is chosen to maintain the obtained data and perform historical and batch analysis on it. Big data management and analysis may all benefit from this hybrid approach to data administration. This method, which incorporates both non-relational and relational databases, allows us to take advantage of big data features like storing and historical analyzing in the training of standard ML metaheuristics and the quick response of networked databases in the visualization of real-time information and the simplification of analysis based on statistical techniques.

The large data operational architecture that supports both the MongoDB and the PySpark analysis module is another fundamental part of the described module. The Hadoop is the most well-acknowledged and highly used framework for large data operations and was chosen for the created solution because of its suitability for its intended purpose. Apache Hadoop integration with the hybrid big data admin-istration and modeling method provides a user-friendly interface for managing the aforementioned database application and any other big data operations, necessitating the use of the cloud-based platform. The analysis of the streaming and stored data is handled by the PySpark data analysis component, which works in tandem with the Hadoop architecture. The PySpark module accepts ML and DL models as input for acquisition of data and returns the results of the analysis and recommendations to the used databases and to the related Kafka topics so that they may be consumed by the appropriate users. The following section will include a more in-depth explanation of the ML and DL algorithms that were developed, deployed, and evaluated during

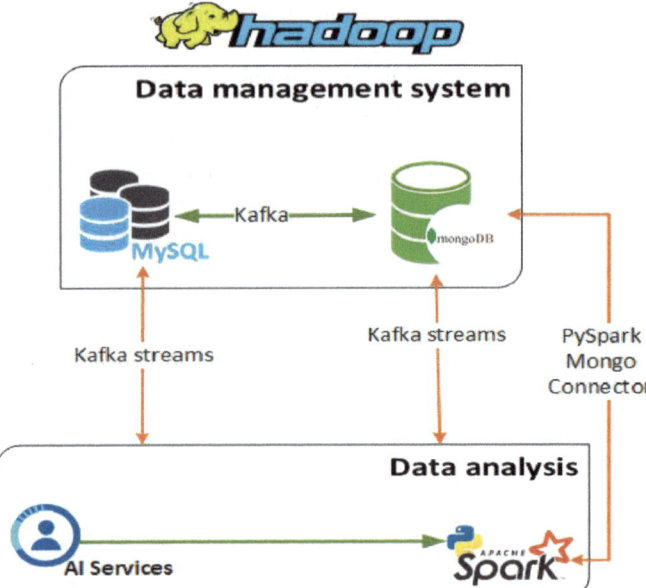

Fig. 4.3 Hybrid model for big data management and analysis

this project, as well as the outcomes that were gleaned from doing so. Figure 4.3 is a conceptual diagram of the hybrid administration and investigation section.

4.4 Dataset and Algorithms/Methods

4.4.1 Summary and Classification of Datasets

After 1996, it became mandatory for all new cars and trucks to be equipped with onboard computers known as OBD sensors, which gather and monitor data on vehicle operations [36]. Five different cars belonging to a major interstate company in Greece provided the data utilized for analysis in this study. There are now 4 million data instances in the current dataset, all of which were acquired at the same time. All the zeros are subtracted out after some preliminary processing on the data, so that we can focus on the intervals during which the vehicles were in use. Therefore, the offered dataset only contains information on moving vehicles. This information is gathered and transferred to the hybrid platform, using a (specified) threshold for recurrent action every five seconds. In addition, as of the time this study was written, the platform had amassed more than 20 million data points in MongoDB, from which the database sample used to train and analyze ML models had been taken using the preparation procedures. The characteristics of the dataset were sent from the cars' OBD devices to the hybrid platform.

The Apache Spark contains one of most significant techniques incorporated into the cloud-based platform, that is, the module accountable for the implementation of the ML algorithms. The primary purpose of combining these elements is to configure a data-frame feature extractor, which can handle the vast amount of information. Any program tasked with managing massive amounts of data would benefit greatly from including a data feature extractor. This improves the model's overall performance from a mathematical standpoint by maximizing its capacity to categorize patterns via the activation of scoring functions. Feature extraction methods are crucial because they simplify the input dataset, which has a major impact on how well the present ML approach performs on loss and accuracy parameters. As indicated, the present technique is critical for the deployment of the suggested algorithm for ML to make similarities more evident, hence increasing the efficacy of the modeling and analysis. Both supervised and unsupervised approaches may use the feature selection procedure to narrow down the number of inputs. What differentiates these two approaches is whether or not the classification algorithm is dependent on the target variable. Filter-based feature selection, which makes use of performance measurement techniques that feature selection approaches, was used in this research as an example of an attribute selection methodology applied to a target variable. In particular, the (feature) extractor portion sorts through the scores of correlations and/or the dependency between the raw response variable to pick out the most important ones. If the platform user has received fresh data in the last 20 s, then the data frame unit that the feature matrix is set up to manage is a heterogeneous time series. PySpark was set up to periodically verify (every 20 s) whether or not the platform consumer had received any new data. This allows for the elimination of superfluous characteristics that might otherwise drive up computational complexity and disorient the training model. As a result, less time and energy are spent computing, and a more manageable subset of data is used for training purposes alone.

After data background subtraction is completed, PySpark receives the data volumes streamed from the vehicles and the final dataset structure is given.

To take a data labeled technique based on the speed OBD and RPM values, we use an ML algorithm like unsupervised clustering on the present database after preprocessing it using the PySpark package. As the cars used in this investigation employ internal combustion engines, these two characteristics were chosen from the pool of accessible information. It is well known that the energy efficiency of engines is very sensitive to both velocity and rotational speed [37]. Increased fuel consumption and carbon dioxide emissions arise from aggressive driving styles, which are often characterized by rapid acceleration followed by a sustained high rate of engine rotation (RPM) [38]. However, it should be noted that all dataset values obtained, are extracted to serve as input values for the unsupervised algorithm for data labeling, even though speed and RPM values are used to display data labels. In technical terms, the clustering process is an unsupervised ML approach that groups instances of data such that related observations are closer together. This makes it possible to find clusters from among the huge quantity of instances of data in the supplied dataset. More-over, this is classified as an "unsupervised" technique, though the training process is not carried out using labeled data. As a substitute, the data are grouped according to their shared characteristics and patterns. Hierarchical clustering, DBSCAN, and K-means are only a few of the many clustering techniques that can be discovered in the research literature. The K-means method was chosen for this investigation since it is both very simple and widely used. The ideal number of clusters, denoted by K, is a crucial aspect of the present algorithm's construction. A centroid is a fictional datapoint created by the execution of the method. These centroid/average data points give insight into the present data's division. To rephrase, we will divide the target dataset into K clusters such that there is minimum separation between cluster axes and instances inside each cluster. Once data from PySpark (Feature Extractor) has been preprocessed, then it can be established how many clusters are necessary for best performance. In order to give this ideal cluster size, K, the so-called Elbow Method is used [39, 40] to minimize the sum of squared errors.

4.4.2 Data Analysis Using Machine Learning and Deep Learning

Predicting a goal value or characteristic, or discovering patterns, are common uses for ML techniques in projects and datasets. To make accurate predictions, using freshly supplied data as input at unique time occurrences [41, 42], these applications employ data to train computers with new patterns. Ensemble techniques, neural networks, discriminant analysis, naive Bayes, support vector machines (SVMs), decision trees, and linear regression (LR) are some of the most widely used ML algorithms. In order to train using the supplied labeled training dataset, this work employs supervised ML. LR, random forests, and SVMs are the techniques investigated with respect to the accuracy and loss of the presented model(s).

Recently, DL's rise to prominence may be attributed to the impressive results it achieves in data-intensive training scenarios. Object, signal, and/or picture recognition are all examples of tasks that benefit from the usage of DL algorithms' ability to handle increasingly complicated datasets and structures. RNNs, multiple layer perceptron (MLP), and supervised learning are all examples of popular DL methods (deep Q networks).

New ML model training using ML methods is more efficient and uses less computing resources, leading to faster execution times. To enhance the model's precision, feature preprocessing should be applied to the investigated dataset to minimize its complexity and give better patterns for the learning method.

However, unlike ML techniques, DL algorithms have a longer execution time and higher hardware and computer resource requirements. To accomplish higher-level computer vision algorithms incrementally, DL approaches are considered as subcategories of the larger ML domain [41, 42]. This reduces the need for additional work when using feature preprocessing techniques. Each node/hidden layer in a DL architecture supplies a weight that represents the relationship between the change of the weights and the model's output as the model is trained.

In circumstances where the input size grows as the time increases, as in the above-discussed example, where the sensors of OBD devices from the automobiles continually communicate data, DL delivers superior outputs in loss and accuracy, in comparison with other classic ML approaches. In addition to this, the improvement of training outcomes in terms of time [41, 43] is directly attributable to the development of parallel computing technologies and its incorporation of robust Graphics Processing Units (GPUs) into very highly configured infrastructures. The existence and significance of preprocessing, particularly the removal of specific insignificant features, with the goal of reducing the dataset size and, consequently, simplifying the procedure, is another significant consideration when shortlisting computer or deep learning methods. DL approaches, on the other hand, do away with the need for the extraction of features by automatically identifying high-level characteristics in the given dataset, therefore providing new and insightful information about the data [42].

Two of the most popular DL methods, MLP and RNN algorithms, were implemented and compared in this study alongside three classic learning algorithms: random forest, SVM, and logistic regression. The cars will remain to transmit data again to the cloud-based platform. Therefore, implementing a wide range of algorithms is necessary to deliver varied benchmarking outputs for the present dataset. Figure 4.4 shows that although standard ML techniques might anticipate their performance to degrade as datasets grow in size, DL techniques are not predicted to be negatively impacted by this trend. Given that the data quantity is still below a certain value, the recommended architecture may assess and pick the best suitable model by considering the dataset size and real data format. The present research gives various comparison findings for several models. Furthermore, as mentioned by [44], to the best of our knowledge there is no direct comparative research between ML and DL models for the analysis of driver behavior.

These algorithms were evaluated on several parameters, such as loss and validation loss, accuracy and validated accuracy, F1 score, Area Under the ROC (receiver operating characteristics) Curve (AUC), precision, recall, and execution time. For both the loss (training set) and the validation loss (validation data), this measure is computed as the total of the predicted value's distances from the true values [45], which is the fraction of predictions that came true divided by the entire number of forecasts made.

Both the training and validation sets were evaluated using the accuracy metric. The F1-score is computed by taking the product of the precision and recall values, together with the loss and accuracy measures. Rates of true positives in the anticipated and actual positives may be calculated using the precision and recall measures. For this reason, the F1-score is the harmonic mean of accuracy and recall [45]. The true positive (TP) rate and false positive (FP) rate are plotted against one another on a ROC graph's y-axis and x-axis, respectively. At the heart of every ROC graph is a cost–benefit tradeoff (TP vs. FP). The AUC, as described by Hanley and McNeil in [46], is often used to evaluate various approaches based on the ROC curve. Since

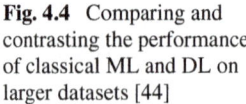

Fig. 4.4 Comparing and contrasting the performance of classical ML and DL on larger datasets [44]

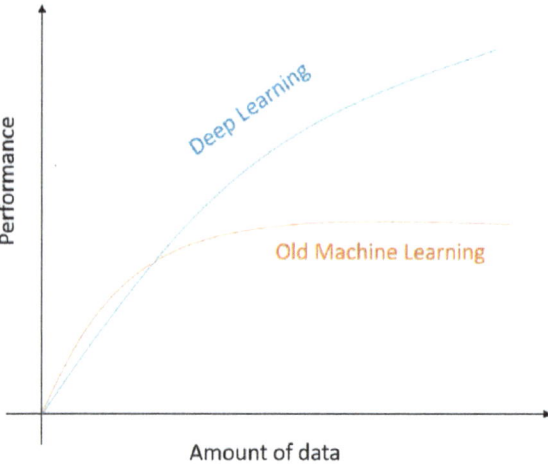

Amount of data

the AUC is the ratio of the area to a unit square, its value can only be between 0 and 1. The AUC is a measure of how well a classifier separates similar instances. It is a statistic that may be used to assess the efficacy of the approaches used to determine whether or not a given data point represents a driver who is friendly toward the environment. Finally, the execution times of each method are shown, together with the evaluation metrics, to shed light on the computational cost and to emphasize the distinction between ML and DL algorithms in this context.

4.5 Conclusions

The goal of this project was to test and evaluate existing ML and DL techniques in order to provide a proof of concept (POC) holistic approach to an analysis of driver behavior based on massive vehicle data streams. To this end, a number of ML and DL techniques were introduced, constructed, deployed, and assessed on large and rapidly changing vehicle datasets. According to the findings, using both ML and DL techniques together is optimal for these datasets. As predicted, the execution time difference between ML and DL algorithms was determined to be the key differentiator between all the known evaluated approaches.

The purpose of this research was to showcase and analyze the architecture and performance of a real-world, deployed platform using actual data streams from vehicles belonging to a large highway maintenance and operation administration in Greece that operates in shifts. Using the results of the current literature analysis performed in Sect. 4.2, the state of the art (SOTA) tools used for the purposes of this chapter were picked with the intention of making the suggested solution as technologically open and future-proof as possible. Accordingly, we have not sought to provide a novel approach for analyzing driver behavior but rather an integration of platforms which incorporates cutting-edge technologies including ML and DL modules, big data infrastructure, and streaming processes for data analysis.

Driver behavior analysis is still a thriving and developing area of study, despite the exponential growth of the autonomous car industry. As a consequence, future work might build on the findings of this chapter by using the training outputs of the ML and DL algorithms under scrutiny to make real-time classifications of drivers based on their behavior behind the wheel. A potential future strategy would build on the clustering analysis discussed above by performing the actual analysis on other values in pairs from the target data (apart from the RPM–Speed OBD pair already supplied) to generate additional labels/profiles using the same reasoning. An algorithmic combination of the existing dataset's labels might lead to a meta-profile engine in the future. The assessment of every driver can be adjusted in real-time by the proposed cloud-based platform based on continuous data streams from automobile sensors. Additional data and methods like complex event processing and semantic technologies might be used to gather even more insightful knowledge, not just about drivers' actions but also about the current state of the roads and traffic. In this context, information gathered either directly from satellites or remotely from highways can be input through multiple data streams. Precise analysis can reveal hidden information and patterns that could provide valuable tips and insights for both drivers and authorities. Increased highway safety, together with improved efficiency in terms of both traffic and the environment, might result from a more comprehensive use of such tools and technology. However, it is also important to study the disadvantages, hazards, and dangers that come with the development of transportation systems at the same time as exploring more innovative ways. The computing efficiency of these approaches, the reliability of the AI making the decisions, and the security measures and precautions all need more study.

References

1. ACEA. (2021). ACEA Report: Vehicles in use Europe. Vehicles in use Europe; European Automobile Manufacturers' Association (ACEA), Brussels, Belgium.
2. World Health Organization (WHO). (2020). World health statistics 2020: Monitoring health for the SDGs, Sustainable Development Goals. World Health Statistics, Geneva, Switzerland.
3. European Parliament CO_2 Emissions from Cars: Facts and Figures (Infographics). https://www.europarl
4. https://www.europa.eu/news/en/headlines/society/20190313STO31218/co2-emissions-from-cars-facts-and-figures-infographics. Accessed on 5 April 2021.
5. Alluhaibi, S. K., Al-Din, M. S. N., & Moyaid, A. (2018). Driver behavior detection techniques: A survey. *International Journal of Applied Engineering Research, 13*, 8856–8861.
6. Elassad, Z. E. A., Mousannif, H., Moatassime, H. A., & Karkouch, A. (2020). The application of machine learning techniques for driving behavior analysis: A conceptual framework and a systematic literature review. *Engineering Applications of Artificial Intelligence, 87*, 103312.
7. Araújo, R., Igreja, Â., de Castro, R., & Araújo, R. E. (2012). Driving coach: A smartphone application to evaluate driving efficient patterns. In *Proceedings of the 2012 IEEE Intelligent Vehicles Symposium, Alcalá de Henares*, Spain, 3–7 June 2012 (pp. 1005–1010).

8. Massoud, R., Bellotti, F., Berta, R., De Gloria, A., & Poslad, S. (2019). Eco-driving profiling and behavioral shifts using IoT vehicular sensors combined with serious games. In *Proceedings of the 2019 IEEE Conference on Games (CoG)*, London, UK, 20–23 August 2019 (pp. 1–8).

9. Massoud, R. (2020). *Eco-friendly naturalistic vehicular sensing and driving behaviour profiling*. Ph.D. Thesis, Queen Mary University of London, London, UK.

10. Chen, C., Zhao, X., Yao, Y., Zhang, Y., Rong, J., & Liu, X. (2018). Driver's eco-driving behavior evaluation modeling based on driving events. *Journal of Advanced Transportation, 2018*, 9530470.

11. Jirka, S., Remke, A., & Bröring, A. (2013). EnviroCar—Crowd sourced traffic and environment data for sustainable mobility. In *Proceedings of the Environmental Information Systems and Services—Infrastructures and Platforms 2013—with Citizens Observatories, Linked Open Data and SEIS/SDI Best Practices*, Neusiedl am See, Austria, 10 October 2013. Retrieved April 26, 2021, from http://ceur-ws.org/Vol-1322/paper_7.pdf

12. Delhomme, P., Cristea, M., & Paran, F. (2013). Self-reported frequency and perceived difficulty of adopting eco-friendly driving behavior according to gender, age, and environmental concern. *Transportation Research Part D: Transport and Environment, 20*, 55–58.

13. Castignani, G., Frank, R., & Engel, T. (2013). Driver behavior profiling using smartphones. In *Proceedings of the 16th International IEEE Conference on Intelligent Transportation Systems (ITSC 2013)*, The Hague, The Netherlands, 6–9 October 2013 (pp. 552–557).

14. Castignani, G., Derrmann, T., Frank, R., & Engel, T. (2015). Driver behavior profiling using smartphones: A low-cost platform for driver monitoring. *IEEE Intelligent Transportation Systems Magazine, 7*, 91–102.

15. Abdelrahman, A., Hassanein, H., & Abu Ali, N. (2018). Data-driven robust scoring approach for driver profiling applications. In *Proceedings of the 2018 IEEE Global Communications Conference (GLOBECOM)*, Abu Dhabi, United Arab Emirates, 9–13 December 2018.

16. Abdelrahman, A., Hassanein, H. S., & Abu-Ali, N. (2019). A cloud-based environment-aware driver profiling framework using ensemble supervised learning. In *Proceedings of the ICC 2019—2019 IEEE International Conference on Communications (ICC)*, Shanghai, China, 20–24 May 2019 (pp. 1–6).

17. Abdelrahman, A. E., Hassanein, H. S., & Abu-Ali, N. (2020). Robust data-driven framework for driver behavior profiling using supervised machine learning. *IEEE Transactions on Intelligent Transportation Systems*, 1–15.

18. Chen, W.-H., Lin, Y.-C., & Chen, W.-H. (2019). Comparisons of machine learning algorithms for driving behavior recognition using in-vehicle CAN bus data. In *Proceedings of the 2019 Joint 8th International Conference on Informatics, Electronics Vision (ICIEV) and 2019 3rd International Conference on Imaging, Vision Pattern Recognition (icIVPR)*, Spokane, WA, USA, 30 May–2 June 2019 (pp. 268–273).

19. Navneeth, S., Prithvil, K. P., Sri Hari, N. R., Thushar, R., & Rajeswari, M. (2020). On-board diagnostics and driver profiling. In *Proceedings of the 2020 5th International Conference on Computing, Communication and Security (ICCCS)*, Patna, India, 14–16 October 2020 (pp. 1–6).

20. Carvalho, E., Ferreira, B. V., Ferreira, J., de Souza, C., Carvalho, H. V., Suhara, Y., Pentland, A. S., & Pessin, G. (2017). Exploiting the use of recurrent neural networks for driver behavior profiling. In *Proceedings of the 2017 International Joint Conference on Neural Networks (IJCNN)*, Anchorage, AK, USA, 14–19 May 2017 (pp. 3016–3021).

21. Obuhuma, J., Okoyo, H., & McOyowo, S. (2018). Driver behaviour profiling using dynamic Bayesian network. *International Journal of Modern Education and Computer Science, 10*, 50–59.

22. Lindow, F., & Kashevnik, A. (2019). Driver behavior monitoring based on smartphone sensor data and machine learning methods. In *Proceedings of the 2019 25th Conference of Open Innovations Association (FRUCT)*, Helsinki, Finland, 5–8 November 2019 (pp. 196–203).

23. Khandakar, A., Chowdhury, M. E. H., Ahmed, R., Dhib, A., Mohammed, M., Al-Emadi, N. A. M. A., & Michelson, D. (2019). Portable system for monitoring and controlling driver behavior and the use of a mobile phone while driving. *Sensors, 19*, 1563.

24. Reininger, M., Miller, S., Zhuang, Y., & Cappos, J. (2015). A first look at vehicle data collection via smartphone sensors. In *Proceedings of the 2015 IEEE Sensors Applications Symposium (SAS)*, Zadar, Croatia, 13–15 April 2015 (pp. 1–6).
25. Fugiglando, U., Santi, P., Milardo, S., Abida, K., & Ratti, C. (2017). Characterizing the "Driver DNA" through CAN bus data analysis. In *Proceedings of the 2nd ACM International Workshop on Smart, Autonomous, and Connected Vehicular Systems and Services; Association for Computing Machinery*, New York, NY, USA, 2017 (pp. 37–41).
26. Cui, H. (2014). Design and research on automotive controller area network bus analyzer. *Sensors and Transducers, 166*, 91–95.
27. ISO ISO 11898-1:2015. (2015). Retrieved April 26, 2021, from https://www.iso.org/standard/63648.html
28. ELM Electronics ELM327 v2.3. Retrieved April 26, 2021, from https://www.elmelectronics.com/ic/elm327/
29. ELM Electronics OBD. Retrieved April 26, 2021, from https://www.elmelectronics.com/products/ics/obd/
30. Professional Bluetooth Elm327 Obd2 Diagnostic Scanner for Android Windows. Retrieved April 26, 2021, from http://www.konnwei.com/product/420.html
31. Apache Kafka Documentation. Retrieved April 27, 2021, from https://kafka.apache.org/documentation/
32. McAfee, A., Brynjolfsson, E., Davenport, T. H., Patil, D., & Barton, D. (2012). Big data: The management revolution. *Harvard Business Review, 90*, 60–68.
33. MySQL. Retrieved April 28, 2021, from https://www.mysql.com
34. MongoDB. Retrieved April 28, 2021, from https://www.mongodb.com
35. Apache Software Foundation Hadoop. Retrieved April 28, 2021, from https://hadoop.apache.org
36. Apache PySpark. Retrieved April 28, 2021, from https://spark.apache.org/docs/latest/api/python/index.html; Rimpas, D., Papadakis, A., & Samarakou, M. (2020). OBD-II sensor diagnostics for monitoring vehicle operation and consumption. *Energy Reports, 6*, 55–63.
37. Abukhalil, T., Al-Mahafzah, H., Alksasbeh, M., & Alqaralleh, B. (2020). Fuel consumption using OBD-II and support vector machine model. *Journal of Robotics, 2020*, 1–9.
38. Zannikos, F., Tzirakis, E., & Stournas, S. (2007). Impact of driving style on fuel consumption and exhaust emissions: Defensive and aggressive driving style. In *Proceedings of the 10th International Conference on Environmental Science and Technology (CEST 2007)*, Kos island, Greece, 5–7 September 2007. Retrieved June 23, 2021, from https://www.researchgate.net/publication/258149928_Impact_of_driving_style_on_fuel_consumption_and_exhaust_emissions_defensive_and_aggressive_driving_style
39. Bholowalia, P., & Kumar, A. (2014). EBK-means: A clustering technique based on elbow method and K-means in WSN. *International Journal of Computers and Applications, 105*, 17–24.
40. Marutho, D., Hendra Handaka, S., Wijaya, E., & Muljono. (2018). The determination of cluster number at K-mean using elbow method and purity evaluation on headline news. In *Proceedings of the 2018 International Seminar on Application for Technology of Information and Communication*, Semarang, Indonesia, 21–22 September 2018 (pp. 533–538).
41. Zhang, L., Tan, J., Han, D., & Zhu, H. (2017). From machine learning to deep learning: Progress in machine intelligence for rational drug discovery. *Drug Discovery Today, 22*, 1680–1685.
42. Korotcov, A., Tkachenko, V., Russo, D. P., & Ekins, S. (2017). Comparison of deep learning with multiple machine learning methods and metrics using diverse drug discovery data sets. *Molecular Pharmaceutics, 14*, 4462–4475.
43. Munir, M., Chattha, M. A., Dengel, A., & Ahmed, S. (2019). A comparative analysis of traditional and deep learning-based anomaly detection methods for streaming data. In *Proceedings of the 2019 18th IEEE International Conference On Machine Learning And Applications (ICMLA)*, Boca Raton, FL, USA, 16–19 December 2019 (pp. 561–566).
44. Alom, M. d. Z., Taha, T., Yakopcic, C., Westberg, S., Sidike, P., Nasrin, M., Hasan, M., Essen, B., Awwal, A., & Asari, V. (2019). A state-of-the-art survey on deep learning theory and architectures. *Electronics, 8*, 292.

45. Mishra, A. (2021). Metrics to evaluate your machine learning algorithm. Retrieved March 22, 2021, from https://towardsdatascience.com/metricsto-evaluate-your-machine-learning-algorithm-f10ba6e38234
46. Hanley, J. A., & McNeil, B. (1982). The meaning and use of the area under a receiver operating characteristic (ROC) curve. *Radiology, 143*, 29–36.

Chapter 5
Artificial Intelligence and Machine Learning Approaches for Understanding Food and Nutrients

5.1 Introduction

Food intake evaluation is critical in scientific study and medical care to understand the link between the nutrition and health issues of an individual or a group. The healthcare industry generates enormous amounts of data on a regular basis. Machine learning (ML) algorithms to extract relevant information, detect patterns, and anticipate diseases are increasingly being used as an example of AI technology. Food calorie monitoring is increasingly popular as more people become concerned about maintaining a healthy weight, eating a balanced diet, and avoiding obesity. The rate of adult obesity is growing alarmingly. Obesity is caused by a discrepancy between a person's food intake and the amount of calories they receive from their diet. Increased calorific consumption has been linked to a number of disorders. Cancers of the breast, colon, and prostate are all linked to obesity. The second largest cause of cancer is an excess of calorific consumption, after smoking and being overweight/obese. Dietitians have concluded that a set amount of calories must be consumed every day to maintain a healthy calorie balance in the body. More than 110% of the world's adult population is overweight or obese, according to the World Health Organization. Excess weight is a medical disorder characterized by an abnormally high level of body fat that has the potential to harm one's health. A person is considered obese if the amount of food he or she consumes each day is greater than the amount of energy he or she expends. To lose weight and maintain a healthy diet and weight, for the average person, daily consumption measures are essential. Obese people cannot lose weight through diet or improve their health without tracking their daily food intake in real time. For example, a user's record of food consumption in the last 24 h can be analyzed, or a clinical display can have some impact; but these approaches often lead the patient's unease to be forgotten or publicize that the user does not want to utilize these programs. Recently we have seen an increase in the use of smart devices in daily life, including the treatment of numerous diseases [1]. It is our hope that by measuring the daily intake of food quality and ingredients, we will be able to help both healthy people and obese people to find a healthy dietary balance. Users will

G. Chhabra et al., *Artificial Intelligence to Analyze Psychophysical and Human Lifestyle*, https://doi.org/10.1007/978-981-99-3039-5_5

be able to determine a food item's contents by submitting a photograph of it to the system. Convolution neural networks will be used to identify the food items in the photograph.

5.2 Literature Review

In (2019), techniques using machine learning (ML) are introduced for the calculation of food nutritional values and food recognition. Using ML, the author in [2] has developed an entirely new technique for accurately classifying food photos and estimating culinary qualities. In the prototype's training phase, the system used a convolutional neural network to classify food into specified categories using picture recognition to calculate a person's calorie intake.

An image processing technique is presented by the author in [3] to recognize photographs of foods consumed by users. The proposed algorithm can tell users how many calories they will eat per meal based on the photographs they have provided. Using a combination of texture and color data, this method generates a feature vector and uses a support vector machine (SVM) to categorize the photos. Image analysis and nutritional evaluation using deep learning (DL) models was used for recognizing food. After identifying a picture as a particular food item, the database is queried for the nutritional information, brightness pattern, and thermal image of each of the constituents in the identified item. After the image has been segmented into candidate ingredient borders, the mathematical reasoning that supports their heat pattern and intensities is used to classify each boundary into an ingredient. Food recognition and dietary evaluation using vision-based methods: results of an investigation.

5.3 Overview of Medical Artificial Intelligence (AI) Research

AI has increasingly created much buzz in the healthcare sector, sparking a discussion on whether AI specialists could ever completely replace human doctors. AI has the ability to assist doctors in making better clinical decisions and perhaps take the role of human judgment in particular healthcare settings (e.g., radiology). AI in healthcare has been made possible by the rapid development of big data analysis tools and the rising availability of healthcare data. It is possible to use AI to uncover clinically significant information in large amounts of data, which can then aid clinical decision-making [4–6].

People are unanimous in their belief that they enjoy eating. Smartphones and other low-cost picture capture equipment (e.g., point-and-shoot cameras) have led to an increase in the list of food photographs on the internet, as well as the popularity of new food-focused social networks. It is not just for the web and social networks that automatic food classification is becoming a hot study area (e.g., for advertising purposes). Indeed, academics (from a variety of disciplines) are interested in food because of its significance from the perspectives of medicine, society, and anthropology. Images of food can help people better understand their relationship with their food. To treat obesity, specialists (e.g., nutritionists) can employ automated food classification to construct diet monitoring systems that provide objective measures for assessing the food intake of patients [4, 5]. In contrast, food classification is a challenging issue for vision systems and an interesting challenge for computer vision researchers. Food has a great degree of deformability and variety by its very nature. In the Pittsburgh Fast-Food Image Dataset (PFID), there are quantifications of the same food [6]. Classic approaches to image classification fail miserably when applied to food images [6]. Food classification has been the subject of several studies [5–10]. As with any new field, the majority of studies offer a new dataset comprised of numerous food categories in addition to the categorization algorithm. As a result, it is difficult to locate studies that compare multiple procedures on the same dataset, although several approaches have been published. This makes it impossible to determine the unique characteristics of the various procedures and the most effective method for classifying foods up to this point. Other cutting-edge algorithms have been evaluated on PFID, an established and open food dataset with a well-defined testing procedure [5, 6].

5.3.1 AI/ML Techniques for Food Recognition and Nutrition Estimation Comparison

Using the time-honored method of the Gabor filter, researchers [11] identified distinct food items and then categorized them using an SVM to treat persons who are obese. The Gabor filter is a linear texture analysis filter that scans the image in certain directions in a restricted region across the points for any particular frequency content. To arrive at the nutrient content of each food item, a portion of that food was mapped to the nutrition charts. For the assessment of food amounts, a thumb was placed next to each food item while the photo was taken, making it easy for the algorithm to calculate life-size quantities of the food items, resulting in an accuracy increase of approximately 86%.

5.3.2 An Artificial Intelligence Technique for Food Recognition

Here the user is afforded the luxury of having the Meal Planning system furnish them with one or more days' worth of meals at their convenience. The components of the meal are constructed using nutritional information; however, this information is primarily limited to a calorie count. When utilizing Meal Planner, it is also anticipated that the user will enjoy food in some capacity. This can be challenging for many cancer patients to consume food because they experience nausea, sores in the mouth and throat, and changes in their taste buds. However, to keep their energy levels constant, they must eat. The MARY method broadens the scope of meal planning by taking into account the possibility that the user might not want to eat but still need to ingest some food. The components that make up MARY are a user interface, two databases, and two AI modules. Users' overall preferences as well as the specifics of their meals can be gleaned through the usage of web-based portals. In addition to a permanent collection of dishes and recipes, there is also a user database that stores information on the preferences of the people who use the service. This database may be accessed by logging into the website. A food scorer and an AI component work together to choose individual elements of a meal in sequential order.

Additionally, the database specifies food groupings so that food items/recipes can be grouped together for further analysis and comparison. Vegetables, fruit, steak, poultry, pasta, spicy food, and tomato-based dishes are just a few examples of food groupings. Users' data are stored in a second database, which has one item per user. A person's tastes fall into one of three categories i.e. hypogeusia is a diminished sense of taste, ageusia is the complete loss of taste, and dysgeusia is an alteration or distortion in the perception of taste. Nutrients are important, as in nausea, and the need for high-calorific yet easy-to-consume food is also important. The score algorithm uses these metrics to determine how important each factor is. The metrics are filled in on the user's first session with MARY, but they can be changed at any time if the user so chooses. A terrible day's sickness may have a greater impact than a desire to minimize recently consumed foods (Fig. 5.1).

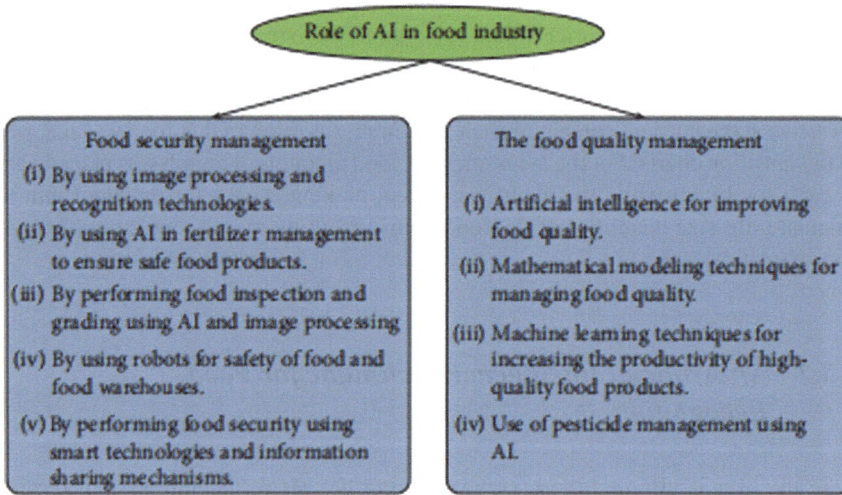

Fig. 5.1 Role of AI in the food industry

5.3.3 Machine Learning Techniques for Food Recognition

An emerging research area in ML is DL. To solve a wide range of complicated problems, it mimics the organization of the human brain to achieve immediate analysis of complex input data. Neural networks rely heavily on autoencoders to complete the translation of learning tasks [12]. An autoencoder was proposed by Rumelhart in 1986 and applied to the analysis of high-dimensional data. On the basis of a better autoencoder prototype, a denoising autoencoder (DAE) was proposed in 2006 [13]. Because of this, the Backpropagation (BP) algorithm is no longer subject to the risk of falling into a local minimum, which is an undesirable outcome. DAE was developed in 2008 by Vincent et al. [14], which adds distorted vectors to enter information to avoid overfitting. Bengio [15] first summarized DL architectures and developed an all-purpose approach for creating neural networks out of stacked autoencoders in 2009. The contractive autoencoder (CAE) was proposed by Salah et al. [16] in 2010 to limit the rise and fall of dimensions. An autoencoder for convolutional neural networks (CNNs) was first presented by Jonathan et al. [17] in 2011. Using a DAE, Liu [19] was able to solve the local extremum problem and the diffusion gradient problem in 2015 by encoding and decoding layers one at a time. To improve autoencoder learning, Deng [20] presented the combined method of a sparse minimized denoising autoencoder (Sm DAE) (Fig. 5.2).

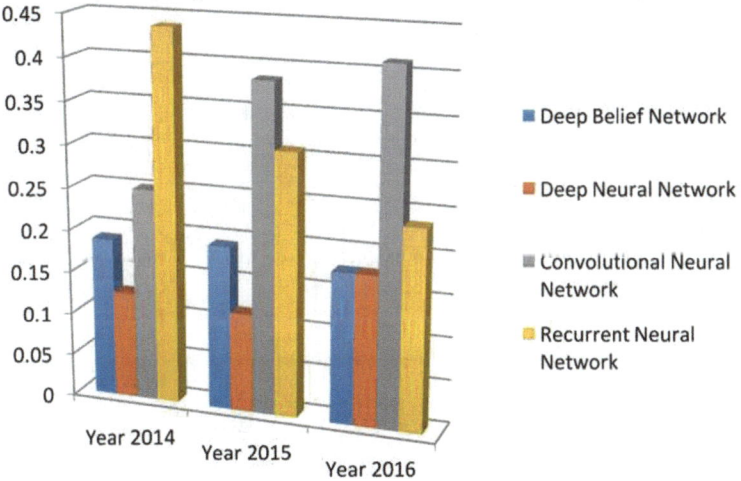

Fig. 5.2 The four most common deep learning algorithms used for food food recognition [19]

5.3.4   Convolutional Neural Network (CNN) Model

Neural networks are mathematical models that are inspired by the functioning of the human brain and are aimed at emulating the behavior of neurons and synaptic connectivity. Using a labeled dataset, a CNN is primarily a supervised learning-based technique. These models are utilized in the training process to produce weight matrices that can mimic human brain behavior. A multilayer perceptron is the ancestor of the typical artificial neural network, which in turn evolved into a CNN. The preconization of patterns, particularly in the area of image processing, is the main emphasis of this field's development. To do this, CNNs create feature maps, which exponentially lower the number of trainable parameters [5]. There are currently many CNN-based architectures for classifying images, such as VGC-16, Inception, and YOLO.

To categorize the food of interest, CNNs are employed as the methodology of choice. Due to its multilayer structure, it can identify objects with the least amount of preprocessing, analyze visual data, and extract features. The four main layers are the convolution layer, pooling layer, activation layer, and fully linked layer (Fig. 5.3).

In ML, a pretrained network model is used to get around the problem of the system becoming stuck on a local solution while it is still learning. These models are capable of performing ML so that they can react instantly to various facts. We employed a CNN model to extract the distinctive characteristics from an object by using a variety of food items from our created dataset [5]. This is a method for transferable learning-based food recognition and for extracting features.

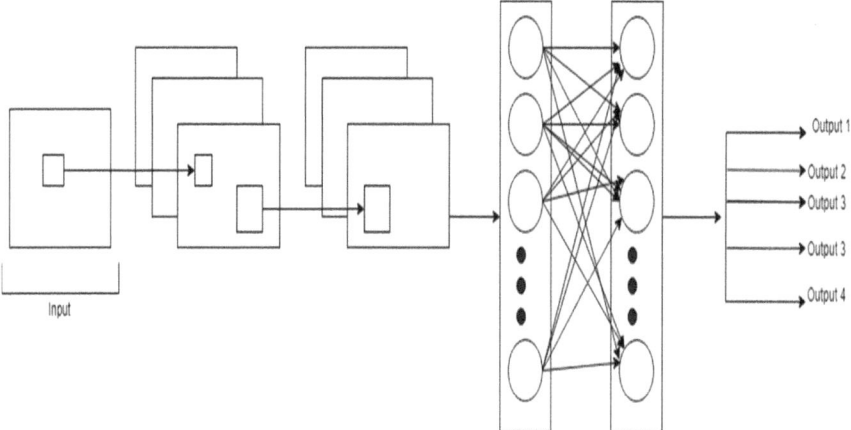

Fig. 5.3 Generalized CNN architecture

5.4 Conclusion

An in-depth look at AI and ML in the food industry has been offered in this chapter. Currently, the food business relies on AI at the most basic level. As their potential to advance sanitation, waste management, and food safety grows, AI and ML are playing a more significant role in society. AI and ML will have a significant impact on the food processing sector in the future because of the enormous potential to increase productivity while also improving the health of consumers. Human errors in the manufacturing process, as well as excessive amounts of food waste, are being reduced by the use of AI and ML in food production and restaurants. Reduced packaging and delivery costs, improved customer satisfaction, faster service, voice search, and more customized orders are all made possible by this technology. Large food processing plants can also profit from these advantages, which will have a long-term impact.

5.5 Future Recommendations

It is necessary to understand calorie intake and its importance, especially after the COVID pandemic. Different researchers have identified different methods for obtaining information on foods and calorie values, and a huge gap has been identified among individuals. By adding new calories to measure nutritional attributes and combining them with DL techniques, it is possible to broaden the basic understanding of calorie calculations among users.

This is revolutionary technology that will be applied to dietary and calorific monitoring once it demonstrates good performance in such health-related applications for which it is being developed. Additionally, "eating journal automated food detection" could assist with the traditional problem of the self (i.e., a written diary). In addition to its potential to predict sales and increase yield, AI can improve company strategy in addition to its other capabilities. In the food business, AI is largely accepted because of its simplicity, precision, and cost-effectiveness.

References

1. Jia, W., Zhao, R., Yao, N., Fernstrom, J. D., Fernstrom, M. H., Sclabassi, R. J., & Sun, M. (2009). A food portion size measurement system for image-based dietary assessment. In *IEEE 35th Annual Northeast conference on Bioengineering.*
2. Pouladzadeh, P., Kuhad, P., Peddi, S. V. B., Yassine, A., & Shirmohammadi, S. (2016). Food calorie measurement using deep learning neural network. In *Conference Record - IEEE Instrumentation and Measurement Technology Conference.*
3. Spector, R. (2009). Science and pseudoscience in adult nutrition research and practice. In: *Skeptical Inquirer.*

4. Yang, S., Chen, M., Pomerleau, D., & Sukthankar, R. (2010). Food recognition using statistics of pairwise local features. In *IEEE Conference on Computer Vision and Pattern Recognition* (pp. 2249–2256).
5. Chen, M., Dhingra, K., Wu, W., Yang, L., Sukthankar, R., & Yang, J. (2009). Pfifid: Pittsburgh fast-food image dataset. In *IEEE International Conference on Image Processing* (pp. 289–292).
6. Jimenez, A. R., Jain, A. K., Ceres, R., & Pons, J. L. (1999). Automatic fruit recognition: A survey and new results using range/attenuation images. *Pattern Recognition, 32*(10), 1719–1736.
7. Joutou, T., & Yanai, K. (2009). A food image recognition system with multiple kernel learning. In *IEEE International Conference on Image Processing* (pp. 285–288).
8. Matsuda, Y., Hoashi, H., & Yanai, K. (2012). Recognition of multiple-food images by detecting candidate regions. In *IEEE International Conference on Multimedia and Expo* (pp. 25–30).
9. Matsuda, Y., & Yanai, K. (2012). Multiple-food recognition considering co-occurrence employing manifold ranking. In *International Conference on Pattern Recognition*.
10. Pouladzadeh, P., Shirmohammadi, S., & Al Maghrabi, R. (2014). Measuring calorie and nutrition from food image. *EE Transactions on Instrumentation and Measurement, 63*(8), 1947–1956.
11. Sun, W., Zhao, H., & Jin, Z. (2017). An efficient unconstrained facial expression recognition algorithm based on stack binarized autoencoders and binarized neural networks. *Neurocomputing, 267*, 385–395. https://doi.org/10.1016/j.neucom.2017.06.050
12. Rumelhart, D., Hinton, G., & Williams, R. (1986). Learning representations by back-propagating errors. *Nature, 323*(6088), 533–536. https://doi.org/10.1038/323533a0
13. Hinton, G., Osindero, S., & Teh, Y. (2006). A fast learning algorithm for deep belief nets. *Neural Computation, 18*(7), 1527–1554. https://doi.org/10.1162/neco.2006.18.7.1527
14. Yu, J., & Liu, G. (2021). Extracting and inserting knowledge into stacked denoising autoencoders. *Neural Networks, 137*, 31–42. https://doi.org/10.1016/j.neunet.2021.01.010
15. Bengio, Y. (2009). Learning deep architectures for AI. *Foundations and Trends® in Machine Learning, 2*(1), 1–127. https://doi.org/10.1561/2200000006
16. Al Machot, F., Ullah, M., & Ullah, H. (2022). HFM: A hybrid feature model based on conditional auto encoders for zero-shot learning. *Journal of Imaging, 8*(6), 171. https://doi.org/10.3390/jimaging8060171
17. Cireşan, D., Meier, U., Masci, J., & Schmidhuber, J. (2012). Multicolumn deep neural network for traffic sign classification. *Neural Networks, 32*, 333–338. https://doi.org/10.1016/j.neunet.2012.02.023
18. Ren, X., & Li, L. (2017). Research on passenger volume demand prediction for external passenger transport hub based on genetic neural network. *DEStech Transactions on Engineering and Technology Research*. https://doi.org/10.12783/dtetr/ictim2016/5536
19. Jiang, F., et al. (2017). Artificial intelligence in healthcare: Past, present and future. *Stroke and Vascular Neurology, 2*(4), 230–243. Retrieved July 11, 2022, from https://doi.org/10.1136/svn-2017-000101
20. Lu, Y., Stathopoulou, T., Vasiloglou, M., Christodoulidis, S., Stanga, Z., & Mougiakakou, S. (2021). An artificial intelligence-based system to assess nutrient intake for hospitalized patients. *IEEE Transactions on Multimedia, 23*, 1136–1147. https://doi.org/10.1109/tmm.2020.2993948

Chapter 6
Artificial Intelligence and the Internet of Things for Improving Health and Nutrition

6.1 Introduction

Devices that are connected to the Internet of Things (IoT) and artificial intelligence (AI) can now make remote monitoring in the healthcare industry a reality. This not only provides physicians with the tools necessary to perform their work more effectively but also offers new prospects for enhancing the safety and health of patients. As a consequence, interactions involving physicians have become much easier and more effective, leading to an increase in patient participation and satisfaction. The health of patients can be monitored remotely, which shortens their time spent in hospital and avoids the need for them to be readmitted. The IoT and AI are having a significant impact on the healthcare business as a whole, in addition to reducing the costs of healthcare and improving treatment outcomes [1].

The IoT and AI have both clearly had a significant effect on the environment inside which people as well as devices interact with a range of health care solutions. As a result, that environment has been redefined as a result of their combined effects. Applications that are created for them have the ability to help us provide superior medical care, which may include improved nutrition, not only for patients but also for medical professionals and healthcare centers [1].

Wearables equipped with the IoT and AI, in addition to other home monitoring equipment, allow doctors to keep a closer eye on the health of their patients. This monitoring system is able to keep track of whether a patient is adhering to their prescribed course of treatment or whether they require immediate medical attention. The IoT allows medical professionals to maintain a more watchful eye over their patients and to connect with them in real time, which benefits both parties. The data collected by IoT and AI devices provide doctors with the information they need to select the most effective course of treatment for their patients as well as achieve the outcomes they want [1].

G. Chhabra et al., *Artificial Intelligence to Analyze Psychophysical and Human Lifestyle*, https://doi.org/10.1007/978-981-99-3039-5_6

6.2   AI and the IoT in Healthcare Nutrition

6.2.1   The IoT in Healthcare Nutrition

With the IoT there is a convergence of pervasive communication, networking, and computational capabilities with ambient intelligence. The IoT when referring to applications within healthcare nutrition technology is called the Internet of Medical Things (IoMT). It is anticipated that the number of health devices equipped with internet connectivity will increase by approximately 10 billion over the course of the next decade. According to Cisco's projections, a single IoT device will be capable of producing 847 zettabytes (ZB) of data annually by 2021. The IoT is poised to overtake most other data sources, in terms of raw volume, at some point in the not too distant future. In regard to supplying caregivers with essential patient health information, the IoT not only delivers essential data about the patient but also provides essential data that can assist in improving healthcare nutrient supplies so that problems can be treated at an earlier stage [2].

6.2.2   AI in Healthcare Nutrition

Patients and medical professionals alike have the opportunity to learn which types of medical image analysis and diagnosis are made simpler with the assistance of AI. The area of healthcare nutrition has grown to become one of the most important fields of AI, in large part as a direct result of Watson, the intelligent cloud developed by IBM. It is now possible to provide patients with individualized care due to the implementation of machine learning, which is one component that would be included in intelligent healthcare solutions. Patients might see substantial improvement as a result of this [3].

The IoT and AI are having a huge impact on the nutrition and healthcare businesses, both of which are under continuous cost-cutting pressure, yet simultaneously seeking to handle an increasingly sick population. Using these technologies, we can take advantage of our ever-changing and interconnected world. Patients, doctors, payers, and medication manufacturers will all profit from more interconnection inside a single ecosystem [4]. Devices such as smart medication, wearable sensors, and monitors can collect real-time medical data, which can then can be analyzed by AI systems to identify health problems, make treatment suggestions, and spot trends. Due to the increased likelihood of treatment adherence on the part of patients and the speed with which new technologies are developed, improved outcomes are achieved [4–6].

6.3   Major Applications of AI and the IoT in Smart Nutritional Healthcare

Being part of an IoT, which envisions a society where everything is hooked up to the internet, every physical object will be able to be identified and made available online. The subsequent step is then to embed AI into systems that are part of the IoT. These systems may collect, process, or exchange data through the use of a data communication system. This is called an IoT framework as it relies on several pieces of technology to solve real-world issues, such as sensors, network connections, AI, and cloud computing, including big data. These products as well as systems have been designed and developed to offer the highest level of functionality and control that is humanly conceivable [2, 5, 7]. AI as well as the IoT are increasingly being used in the creation of new medical tools and systems that focus on the needs of the patient from initial diagnosis, via treatment, to follow-up care. This is done to best serve patients, hospitals, and the healthcare system as a whole. On the other hand, AI-enabled medical IoT devices will make healthcare, including nutritional therapies, more proactive than preventive. Figure 6.1 shows an IOT framework that includes AI.

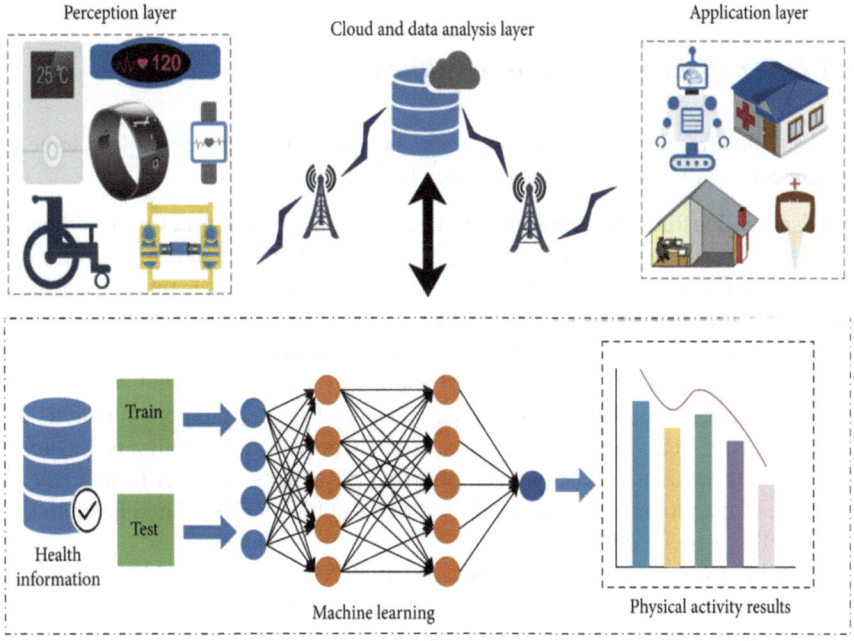

Fig. 6.11   IOT framework that includes AI in healthcare [8]

6.3.1 IOT Applications in Healthcare

- **Location-based real-time services**. In the age of the IoT, healthcare providers can keep tabs on the whereabouts of their patients. This is especially helpful when a patient needs emergency medical attention. IoT devices can also be used to monitor environmental conditions, such as room temperature, in real time [9].
- **Improve patient experience**. The use of IoT devices improves patient satisfaction, who may use them to adjust the temperature and lighting in their rooms, talk to loved ones through videocalls, and use an intercom to summon nurses, thanks to the seamless connectivity between their gadgets. It is also possible for medical staff to easily access patient data saved on IoT devices from the cloud [10].
- **Hygiene compliance**. One of the best ways to prevent illness is to wash your hands frequently. Systematic assessment of the cleanliness of healthcare workers is made possible by the use of hand hygiene monitoring devices. In its simplest form, IoT devices for hand hygiene simply sound an alarm if a member of the medical team approaches a patient's bed without first washing their hands.
- **Remote monitoring**. The IoT can be used to monitor health remotely. Many people worldwide lose their lives since they do not receive medical care in a timely manner. Complex algorithms can be applied and analyzed by IoT devices.

6.3.2 Applications of AI in Healthcare

Medical picture analysis and diagnosis can be aided by AI and could lead to better patient care and higher staff productivity [11].

- **Disease identification/diagnosis**. One of the numerous healthcare difficulties to which machine learning is being applied is identifying and detecting diseases as well as other medical issues. Cognitive computing and genomic tumor sequencing will be combined in a collaborative venture between IBM's Watson Health and Quest Diagnostics, known as IBM Watson Genomics.
- **Personalized treatment/behavioral modification**. Personalized medicine, or better therapy based on an individual's health data and predictive analytics, is indeed a hot study subject and closely tied to better diagnosis of illness. Sustained learning now dominates this field, allowing physicians to select from a smaller range of diagnoses, such as to assess patients at higher risk related health issues as well as genetic information.
- **Drug discovery and development**. A variety of uses for machine learning in clinical development exist now, from next-generation sequencing to precision medicine. Machine learning systems could be utilized for early drug screening and preliminary testing, as well as ways to predict a drug's success rate based on a variety of biological characteristics. Both Microsoft and MIT are working on initiatives that use machine learning techniques to help us better understand

the world around us. They also engage in activities aimed at cancer therapy and leukemia research.

- **Creating electronic smart records**. With the massive amounts of healthcare and medical data now available, this same integration of digital electronic healthcare records is becoming essential for the machine learning apps within the creation of automated guided records that are required for the built-in AI as well as the machine learning which assist in keeping medical records, analyzing health conditions, and suggesting treatment plans.
- **Automation**. Robotic surgeons equipped with machine learning systems could be used in the healthcare sector in the future. Robotic surgeons may one day be totally automated, removing the need for human intervention in surgical procedures, thanks entirely to advances in machine learning techniques.
- **Radiation treatments**. Early results from an AI system that could aid in the planning of radiotherapy treatments for patients with head and neck cancer are encouraging.
- **Benefits of using the IoT in the healthcare industry**. Due to its complexity, the amount of responsibility, and rigorous rules, advances in nutritional healthcare must go a long way before they are completely adopted [12]. As a result of the flaws as well as inefficiencies in this industry, things have changed. The IoT could help us solve these and other healthcare issues. This business has long struggled with low drug adherence, lack of treatment control including off-patient monitoring tools, as well as underserving patients and professional shortages [12]. An IoT for healthcare may be the answer to many of these issues.
- **Benefits of using AI in the healthcare industry**. There are numerous opportunities for nutritional health systems to utilize AI and deliver more effective, efficient, and precise therapies to their patients [13]. AI has the potential to revolutionize the healthcare industry as the amount of data collected grows [12, 14]. This is predicated on the ability of AI tools to provide proactive, sophisticated, and often concealed insights that improve diagnostic and therapeutic decision-making [13]. Improvements in treatment, management of chronic disease, early risk identification, workflow automation, and optimization can all benefit providers and patients when AI is used in these areas.

6.3.3   Architecture of AI and the IOT in Healthcare Systems

As a way to link the patient, provider, and hospital, an AI and IoT-based architecture has been proposed. With the use of AI and the IoT, healthcare providers may better diagnose and treat patients and prevent disease before it even occurs. The use of AI and IoT-based infrastructures enhances the management of smart nutritional health. Figure 6.2 depicts the healthcare system's AI and IoT architecture.

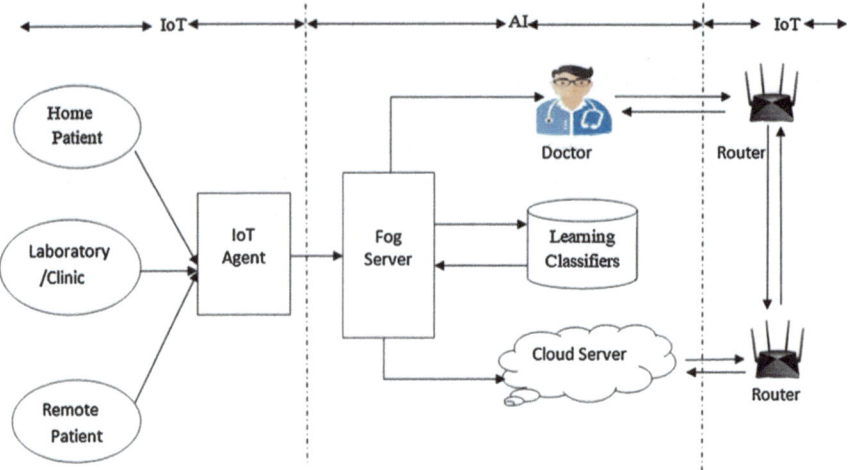

Fig. 6.2 Architecture of AI and the IOT in the healthcare system [14]

6.3.4 AI and IoT Techniques for Food Recognition and Nutrition Estimation

An accurate calculation of a person's daily nutritional intake is a useful strategy for maintaining health and preventing sickness [15]. To obtain a comprehensive estimation of calorie intake, our study serves as a foundation for modern, computer-assisted, remote, nutritional management systems [15]. Using an artificial neural network trained to classify food based on the extracted image parameters, we segment the food in the image and extract image characteristics, such as the region, which proves to be a major, minor axis convex area; we then use these parameters to classify the food. AI and the IOT are utilized to develop simple and easy-to-use software that allows users to shoot real-time images of food and obtain accurate nutritional and calorie information. More pressure and flow estimations and a wider range of food categories will be added to these systems in the future, further increasing their accuracy.

6.3.5 Comparison of AI and the IOT in Nutritional Healthcare

AI in healthcare refers to a variety of different types of cognitive technology that can be used in clinical contexts [16]. AI can be defined as the ability of computers as well as other machines to learn, understand, and act in ways that humans can. In other words, AI in nutritional healthcare uses machines to study and act on medical data to forecast a given outcome.

IoT-connected gadgets have enabled remote monitoring inside the nutritional healthcare sector, unlocking the capacity to keep people healthy while also empowering doctors to provide exceptional care [16].

The healthcare of the future, from robotics and drones to machine learning–based data analytics, will include predictive modeling [16], numerous IoT applications, and involve a wide spectrum of technology.

Unmanned aerial vehicles (UAVs), telemedicine mobile tools, and remote medical tracking technologies—as well as the expanding significance of IoT in healthcare—are just some of the boosters of medical technology development from the initial days of quarantine [16].

This means that AI-based applications in nutritional healthcare, as stated by domain experts, can be divided into three types: descriptive, predictive, and prescriptive. InnoBRIDGE 2019, our annual conference, journals, training programs, group meetings, and webinars, as well as our latest delegation in Sweden under the auspices of InnoBRIDGE 2019, are all part of our ongoing endeavor to acquire and disseminate new information. InnoBRIDGE USA 2020 is our next project, which has been requested by our stakeholders [16].

6.3.6 The AI Diet Algorithm

The AI Diet is an algorithm that informs you how to eat well to survive longer and have a better life. As is well known, an algorithm is a procedure or set of rules performed by a computer for use in calculations for problem solving. The the AI Diet is therefore entirely based on scientific evidence. This has allowed the algorithm to be developed free from the opinions of the scientists who created it. This is easily achievable thanks to cutting-edge algorithms that include not only body composition but also compliance, bodyweight change rate trends, hunger, and weariness in their diet recommendations. The most important thing to remember is that this is not merely a data collection exercise. An algorithm continuously monitors these data points' trends with one another and makes adjustments based on that analysis.

6.4 Future Recommendations

The human touch of doctors, nurses, and allied health workers is being replaced by gadgets and information technology in the field of healthcare nutrition. mHealth, eHealth, cybersecurity, big data, blockchain, and the IoT are all buzzwords in today's healthcare industry. These emerging fields, such as AI, are also known as aided intelligence, deep learning, big data, and other terms. Many people use these terms without understanding their meaning, use, or limitations. In the process, it is developing a new network of service providers. As long as we do not become slaves to technology and instead govern it for the benefit of both physicians and patients, all of this is fine and excellent. There is little regard for evidence-based medicine, human touch, or compassion in regard to diagnosing today's patients. AI and the IoT in nutritional healthcare are the main focus of this issue. In future, researchers may discuss healthcare's unmet needs and how they lead to innovation, as well as the fundamentals of healthcare and how technology can be used to improve healthcare again for the average person at a reasonable cost.

6.5   Conclusion

Medical practice has evolved and continues to evolve. With the advent of medical IoT devices, patients are beginning to accept the shift. Medical device manufacturers are working to provide solutions that are more precise, intelligent, and personalized, while healthcare providers are beginning to use linked healthcare to improve quality, remain competitive, and improve treatment outcomes. Wearable technology, on the other hand, has the potential to revolutionize the entire digital healthcare industry. Developers of wearable technology must embrace its potential for delivering improved outcomes for patients, regulators, and healthcare service providers. An effective hospital will result from utilizing technology to improve clinical outcomes as well as the management of drugs and diseases.

References

1. Wipro. (2022). IoT in healthcare industry. IoT applications in healthcare – Wipro. Wipro.com. Retrieved July 08, 2022, from https://www.wipro.com/business-process/what-can-iot-do-for-healthcare
2. Rodrigues, J., et al. (2018). Enabling technologies for the internet of health things. *IEEE Access, 6*, 13129–13141. Retrieved July 08, 2022. https://doi.org/10.1109/access.2017.2789329
3. Kamble, R., & Shah, D. (2018). Applications of artificial intelligence in human life. *International Journal of Research -GRANTHAALAYAH, 6*(6), 178–188. https://doi.org/10.29121/granthaalayah.v6.i6.2018.1363.
4. Zeadally, S., & Bello, O. (2021). Harnessing the power of internet of things based connectivity to improve healthcare. *Internet of Things, 14*, 100074. https://doi.org/10.1016/j.iot.2019.100074
5. Liao, Y., de Freitas Rocha Loures, E., & Deschamps, F. (2018). Industrial internet of things: A systematic literature review and insights. *IEEE Internet of Things Journal, 5*(6), 4515–4525. https://doi.org/10.1109/jiot.2018.2834151
6. Mande, S., & Rao, J. (2017). Nobel Prize in physiology or medicine 2016. *Resonance, 22*(9), 829–833. https://doi.org/10.1007/s12045-017-0537-3
7. Fadadu, M., & Lotiya, J. (2016). Comparison and performance analysis of various FACTS devices in power system. *International Journal of Engineering and Computer Science.* https://doi.org/10.18535/ijecs/v5i6.06
8. Pradhan, B., Bhattacharyya, S., & Pal, K. (2021). IoT-based applications in healthcare devices. *Journal of Healthcare Engineering, 2021*, 1–18. Retrieved July 08, 2022. https://doi.org/10.1155/2021/6632599

9. Al-Fuqaha, M. G., Mohammadi, M., Aledhari, M., & Ayyash, M. (2015). Internet of things: A survey on enabling technologies, protocols, and applications. *IEEE Communications Surveys & Tutorials, 17*(4), 2347–2376. https://doi.org/10.1109/comst.2015.2444095

10. Riazul Islam, S., Kwak, D., Humaun Kabir, M., Hossain, M., & Kwak, K.-S. (2015). The internet of things for health care: A comprehensive survey. *IEEE Access, 3*, 678–708. https://doi.org/10.1109/access.2015.2437951

11. Eledlebi, K., Alzubaidi, A., Yeun, C., Damiani, E., Mateu, V., & Al-Hammadi, Y. (2022). Enhanced Inf-TESLA protocol: A continuous connectivity and low overhead authentication protocol via IoT devices. *IEEE Access, 10*, 54912–54921. https://doi.org/10.1109/access.2022.3177268

12. DIGITEUM (2020). Benefits of using IoT in healthcare industry: 7 use cases | Digiteum. Digiteum, 2020. Retrieved July 08, 2022, from https://www.digiteum.com/iot-benefits-health care-industry/

13. Sanaz Cordes. (2021). 5 benefits of using AI in healthcare. Wwt.com. Retrieved July 08, 2022, from https://www.wwt.com/article/5-benefits-of-using-ai-in-healthcare

14. Kishor, A., & Chakraborty, C. (2021). Retrieved July 08, 2022, from https://www.researchg ate.net/figure/The-architecture-of-the-proposed-AI-and-IoT-based-healthcare-model_fig2_3 52975738

15. Aditya Gulhane1 and Dr S V Rode, Ijarsct.co.in (2022). Retrieved July 08, 2022, from https://ijarsct.co.in/Paper4459.pdf

16. InnoHEALTH. (2021). AI and IoT in healthcare: Need of future - InnoHEALTH magazine. InnoHEALTH magazine. Retrieved July 08, 2022, from https://innohealthmagazine.com/2019/ expert-opinion/ai-iot-healthcare-need-future/

Chapter 7
Food Recognition and Nutrition Estimation Using Deep Learning

7.1 Introduction

Eating well is essential to human survival [1]. Products made from natural ingredients can be manufactured to satisfy cravings. Food type, structure, nutrients, and process types are all relevant to what constitutes a healthy diet (natural goods vs. processed food). It's true that people's eating habits differ depending on where they live. Knowing the features of foods (type, makeup, micronutrients, process sorts, etc.) is critical for the inspection, as it ensures consistency and data protection across the world [2]. There is a real-world need for quick, precise, and automated detection of food quality. Numerous cutting-edge techniques, including electronic noses, computer vision, spectroscopy, and spectral imaging, have been widely used to recognize food characteristics [3, 4]. Using this method, it may be possible to collect massive amounts of digital data about the qualities of food. Data analysis using these methods is essential since the vast amount of information includes so much repetition and meaningless detail [5]. The issues of dealing with this large volume of data, of extracting meaningful features from the obtained data, and of using these methods in reality are urgent and vital [6, 7].

There is a wide variety of methods for analyzing data, including partial least squares (PLS), artificial neural networks (ANNs), support vector machines (SVMs), random forests (RFs), and k-nearest neighbors (KNN). The amount of data that has to be modeled has exploded in recent years [8–10]. Methods for feature extraction include principal component analysis (PCA), independent component correlation (ICA), wavelet transform (WT), scale based feature translation (SIFT), resilient speedup features (RSUs), and the histogram of a directed gradient [11]. These methods have been shown to be effective when dealing with such information. Recent years have seen a surge in interest in the machine learning approach known as deep learning (DL) [12], due to its impressive capabilities. More individuals than ever are considering it for their own projects, and its potential applications span fields as diverse as remote sensing, agricultural development, medical research, robotics, healthcare, behavior identification, and speech recognition. There are many areas

© The Author(s), under exclusive license to Springer Nature Singapore Pte Ltd. 2023
G. Chhabra et al., *Artificial Intelligence to Analyze Psychophysical and Human Lifestyle*,
https://doi.org/10.1007/978-981-99-3039-5_7

where DL has proven to be superior [13], including the development of DL interpretations of knowledge (even for the separation of multidomain features and capabilities), change learning, working with massive amounts of data, increased academic output, and allowing for greater accuracy. When it comes to automatically learning in-depth features of digital input data for use in subsequent classification and regression tasks, the vast majority of the examined papers agree that coevolutionary neural networks (CNNs), and their derivative algorithms, are the most employed methodologies. A CNN is a powerful technique for analyzing the massive volumes of data produced by quality and safety food assessment technologies (electronic nose, video cameras, spectrophotometer, etc.) [14]. A CNN was first designed to process pictures (two-dimensional data), but it has since been modified to process one- and three-dimensional data [15, 16].

In this chapter, the authors will look at the structure, training method possibilities, and final evaluation results of DL for the processing of the food picture, spectrum, text, and other information that has recently been published on the mobile App.

7.2   Background Theory

7.2.1   Differentiating, Clustering, and Choosing Features

Efficiency, stability, and practicality are all enhanced in classification algorithms when just a few key features are considered. So, there is a lot of effort put into finding the right features to employ when developing classifiers. Most recently [17], a simplified categorization of algorithms was proposed. Approaches that are close to achieving the same aim include wrapper approaches, vector supports, the hidden Markov model, a and feature extraction prototype [18, 19]. Most of the time, they choose clustering functions in an effort to increase variety. These approaches have a three-step foundation: first, a tracking algorithm is chosen to establish a feature space; second, features are clustered; and third, the representative feature of each class is chosen to provide the selection result [20, 21]. The representative characteristic of a classification model is often the most important aspect of the label itself. They used a packing technique to hierarchically cluster the features into groups with similar characteristics, and then chose the top features from each group to comprise the final feature subset [22]. This takes more time and introduces a bias in the teaching process, but considerable advantage is initially introduced, and no adjustments to parameters are necessary. This combines hierarchical clustering with sparse K-means in a feature cluster framework. To start, the collection of functions is organized into logical groups. The characteristics that best reflect each cluster are then chosen using a Lasso-style penalty factor [23, 24]. When working in a supervised learning setting, the agglomerative hierarchical clustering approach may be used to partition the eliminated characteristics that are geographically far from one another to narrow down the feature set and arrive at the final number of attributes [7].

In addition to measuring the correlation effect, clustering the relative subsets, and selecting the maximal data coefficients may be used to accomplish the above goals by serving as the representational attribute of each cluster's centroid [25].

Recent years have seen a meteoric rise in the availability of high-dimensional data on the internet. As a result, the sheer volume of input qualities that interest academics present a significant challenge for machine learning platforms [26]. Data pre-processing is essential for the effective use of machine learning methods. When it comes to cleaning and organizing data, functional selection is a go-to [27, 28]. In machine learning, it plays a key role. This method goes under many other names in the disciplines of machine learning and statistics, such as regression models and PCA; the variables depend on the concentration. Data cleansing is the process of identifying and removing outliers, duplicates, and inaccurate information [29, 30]. Data mining algorithms benefit from this procedure since it makes them more efficient. Feature selection methods are those that do not add value to the product, whereas redundant features provide no value beyond what is already provided by the selected features [31, 32].

7.2.2 Recognizing Food

The variety of food items available makes it difficult to determine which one is which, even within the same category. Pairwise local properties of food are identified by exploiting the spatial interactions between eight distinct components [33]. This presents a challenge for fine-grained image categorization. Color, texture, gradients, and SIFT are separated from the first recognized meal by numerous detectors utilizing multiple kernel learning regions (MKL) [34]. The online software serves as a nutritional device and food-recording diary, giving you a general estimate of your diet's overall healthfulness. The Discrete Cosine Transform (DCT) coefficients and abstracted colors are utilized to classify each component of the meal into one of five categories: staple, primary dish, dipping sauce, fruit, and non-food. You may name items and estimate how much of them you'll consume with the help of the tools in Technology Assisted Dietary Assessment (TADA)'s diet evaluation framework [35]. However, there are restrictions on using a checkerboard to determine how much food was consumed while photographing it on white plates. All of the aforementioned technologies perform image identification on servers, which precludes interactive activities due to delays in contact. On the other hand, gadget may recognize food goods in real time on the consumer side, without contacting any other computer resources, allowing for interactive usage [36].

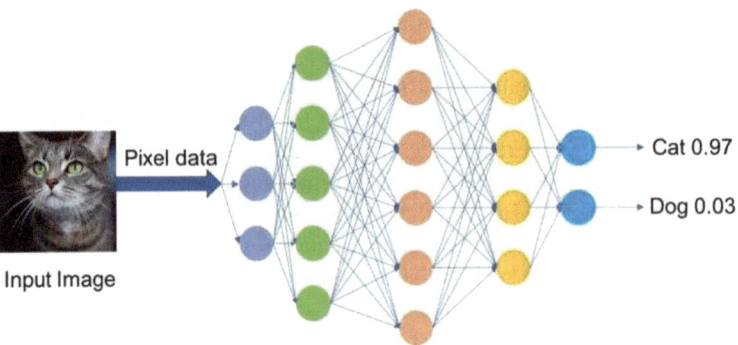

Fig. 7.1 DNN image classification example

7.2.3 Learning at a Deep Level

Several of the approaches described above depend on DL's unique intrinsic properties; thus the authors will give a brief overview of the topic. You may learn more by consulting the cited sources [37]. A DL prediction method, often called a model, is composed of numerous layers, as shown in Fig. 7.1. As the data is transmitted from layer to layer during inference in DL, a series of mathematical operations are performed on the data at each layer. In many cases, the product of one layer is used as the input to the next layer [38]. Data is sent from layer to layer until the final layer processes everything and outputs a function or categories. When a neural network contains several consecutive layers, they call it "deep" [39]. Use of coevolutionary filter operations in arithmetical operations [40] is a popular use of deep neural networks (DNNs) in the images and video processing sectors. One such method is implemented in the form of (CNNs). Predictions of time series are a common use of DNNs and Recurrent Neural Networks (RNNs). The state is maintained by consistently and sequentially projecting inputs utilizing the layer links shown as circles [41]. When training a DNN, calculations are performed in reverse. Many passes are made through the layers, starting at the bottom and working up, in order to boost the arithmetic operations' parameters at each layer given the surface learning labels [42]. The standard method is stochastic gradient descent. Selecting a randomized "mini-batch" of samples at each step and modifying the grades appropriately [43] reduces the likelihood of learning failures (here defined as the difference between predictions and actuals on the ground).

7.2.4 Evaluations of Deep Learning's Performance

The degree to which the desired placement of the item coincides with the position of ground-truth dispersed among several groups of objects is a good indicator for measuring the performance of DL execution and testing [44]. The accuracy of language processing may be evaluated using the understudy score metric [45], which involves a multilingual comparison of a candidate translation with many try to matches of the ground-truth. Throughput, latency, and power consumption are three more generic performance indicators for devices that are not application-specific. DL may be used to carry out learning processes in both a supervised and unsupervised setting. The mean average accuracy of object detection is one metric that may be used to assess accuracy. Then calculate, on average over several item classes, the degree to which projected locations match with ground-truth locations. Machine translation accuracy may be calculated by using a bilingual assessment of the understudy score metric [46].

7.2.5   Food-Related Deep Learning Applications

For applications with many moving parts, such as image analysis or computer vision, DL proved to be the better technique. Recent decades have seen an incredible ascent in the quality of DL-based research. Applications in the food industry, including the cultivation of vegetables, fruits, palm oil, and fish, have benefited greatly from DL's efforts. Several applicable examples will be discussed below.

7.2.6   The Role of Deep Learning in Fruit Processing

The fruit may be eaten uncooked as a human food source. The marketing and cultivation of fruit are both subject to a wide range of challenges, including the control of pests and the elimination of defects such as bruises and rat infestations. But the fruit itself is a result of efficient farming practices. Fruits are chosen based on their ripeness, cleanliness, and nutrient richness. Identifying the quality of vegetables and fruits is a new area of research with its own set of difficulties. Image segmentation sensing techniques paired with DL have recently emerged as a non-critical and robust method of identifying fruit quality, with applications ranging from assortment characterizations to nutritious composition forecasting, infection, and identity damages. Cherries, lemons, dates, walnuts, bananas, avocados, apples, pears, capsicums, mangoes, and many more depend largely on DL for processing [47].

7.2.7   Using Deep Learning for Vegetable Preparation

Vegetables supply a wide variety of necessary elements, making them a cornerstone of a healthy diet. Diseases, infections, pests, damage, and many more may all have negative effects on the value of a business and its consumers' health and happiness.

Most studies have shown that DL is able to effectively evaluate and count a large variety of vegetables, which has been a persistent measurement and assessment challenge [48].

7.2.8　Application of AI to Palm Oil Manufacturing

To boost financial gain, it is necessary to gather data from palm oil plants in agricultural estates. The spotting and incorporation of palm oil into the plantation structure is crucial. The vast bulk of previous research has been on identifying palm oil plants without crowns. Due to a dearth of studies, developments in DL have been used to develop unique systems for identifying both immature and mature oil palms. In an effort to close this knowledge gap [24], researchers have used two independent CNNs [49] to differentiate between juvenile and gowned oil palms.

7.2.9　Fish-Specific Deep Learning

When it comes to getting enough of the proper nutrients throughout the year, fishing has emerged as a vital resource. Even now, DL remains indispensable in the fish-preparation industry. Rauf and co-authors [50] offered their thoughts on the matter. Fish is a classification method for supervised 32-layer VGGNet that uses a subnet hierarchy split into five strictly forbidden subnets. The purpose of this paper was to improve upon the CNN method for identifying fish species by using a DL model relay to improve classification effectiveness by means of highlighting.

They trained the VGGNet system with four CNN layers at a deep degree of supervision using a personal level of training. They made some adjustments to the Pak dataset that allows us to evaluate the effectiveness of the 32-layer CNN prototype. A total of 915 photographs were taken into consideration, organized into six categories and examined from three vantage points. Based on the results of the analysis, the proposed method was shown to have superior performance to the ones already in use [51].

7.3　Literature Review

The Ciocca group [52], included 20 meals—ranging from solid, sliced fruit and vegetables to silky pastes—in a new dataset, which includes products from 11 nations. The authors conducted an experiment using the most popular CNN designs, testing their performance on three different identification tasks: categorizing foods, recognizing food states, and recognizing all foods and states. In this paper, the authors use deep features produced from the CNNs in conjunction with the SVMs as an alternative to the end-to-final classification, since the lack of classified data is usual in practice. Instead, support for such labeling is uncommon. The authors make a variety of analogies between in-depth traits and elements that were clearly created by hand. The results of these experiments show that, across all three classification tasks, the performance of the deep properties of the product category, or the food status at issue, was superior to that of manually crafted features. Finally, the authors evaluated the pervasiveness of the deepest functionality by using a second publicly accessible dataset consisting of food statements. This experiment showed how the features derived from a CNN trained on the suggested dataset achieve state-of-the-art results. This demonstrates how powerful the unique traits are in comparison to the previously unseen information of the CNN [52].

In Srigurulekha et al., new methods for representing food using CNNs are developed. CNNs, in contrast to traditional ANNs, can accurately compute the score work from picture pixels. There are a lot of these layers, and the final yield tensor is built by stringing together the results in chunks. The model is extracted from key photos using a max pooling technique, which is then used for preprocessing. With this suggested strategy, the authors were able to attain an accuracy of 86.85% on the FOOD-101 dataset [53].

Mangosteen identification was performed using DL architectures (CNNs) developed by Azizah et al. [54]. The CNN has established its credibility in the area of image classification. This CNN method employs the four-fold Validation Cross to ensure the integrity of the inputted data. The step of network training in the development of the CNN architecture model is hastened by the initialization of the configuration of the parameters. In tests, the CNN algorithm was very effective in detecting flaws in mangosteen fruit, with an accuracy of 97%.

Using DL, Liu et al. [55] developed new algorithms for visual food recognition with best-in-class accuracy, and they designed a food recognition system to address some of the shortcomings of the traditional mobile cloud computing paradigm, such as long wait times for data and short battery lives for mobile devices. This was accomplished by adopting a service computing model based on edge computing. The authors conducted in-depth analyses supported by empirical data. The investigations have uncovered three points of interest. First, the state-of-the-art minimal energy consumption is maintained; second, existing food accuracy tests are surpassed; and third, the response time is reduced in accordance with the minimum number of current ways.

In this research, Pouladzadeh et al. [56] proposed an auxiliary calorie counting technique to aid patients and doctors in the fight against diet-related health disorders. The research proposes a smartphone software that, when fed a picture of a meal, can calculate how many calories it contains. The authors examined these difficulties and proposed a cloud-assisted mobile food identification system. The findings demonstrate that the recognition step of the cloud-assisted application improves identification accuracy compared to an SVM in non-mixed plates, single meal portions, and mixed food plates. Applying a DNN also increases the accuracy of identifying individual foods to 100%. As stated by Pandy et al. [57], a CNN with several layers was designed specifically for food recognition. Cuisine 101 refers to the fundamental principles and basics of cooking and culinary arts. Cuisine-101 and an Indian food picture library with 50 categories and 100 photographs were each shown. The proposed method relied on the deep architecture of CNN AlexNet. To combine these three networks, the authors built a multistage CNN pipeline (AlexNet, GoogLeNet, and ResNet). Accuracy for the top 1% was 72.13%, for the top 5% it was 91.61%, and for the top 10% it was 99.95%. Excellent prediction findings were attained in this investigation for the Cuisine-101 database at a rate of 73.5%, and for the Indian food database at a rate of 94.4 and 97.6%. The proposed ensemble net achieves better results than the CNN model with a single subnetwork across all levels in both datasets.

To guarantee efficiency gains, Aguilar et al. [58] suggested combining several classifiers that mutually complement each other on the basis of convolutional models. Both the Food-101 dataset, which has information on a wide variety of grain-based meals, and the Food-11 dataset, which contains information about a curated collection of premium foods, were used to evaluate the approach.

Pan et al. [59] introduced a novel system called Deep Food, which uses cutting-edge machine learning algorithms to improve the average accuracy of multi-classification and extract rich and useful features from a DL dataset of photos of food items. Since CNNs are so effective at extracting deep features, they have been the focus of several transfer learning techniques. The classification results for each deep feature set are then utilized to inform a multi-class classification method. The Deep Food scheme is tested using a multi-level dataset that includes 41 food categories and 100 photos for each. Experiments show that Deep Food is effective for multi-class food component categorization. When compared to other research in the field, this model's ability to identify food components is enhanced by the use of ResNet deep feature sets, Information Gain (IG) choices, and the supremacy of Sequential Minimal Optimization (SMO).

Because of the importance of cost, processing speed, and hardware requirements in building practical APPs, Heravi et al. [60] focused on building a basic network. Standard practice in network planning entails decreasing the discrepancy between the two points of reference. However, they proposed a new strategy that integrated data from multiple models into a single large-scale CNN (compressed GoogLeNet architecture with much fewer parameters than the CNN trainer). Teaching assistants in CNN-by-CNN programs have to make an accurate estimate as part of a data transfer activity.

Martinel et al. [61] presented a state-of-the-art subterranean infrastructure developed to suit the food stockpiling scheme. The authors emphasize the vertical characteristics shared by a wide variety of food categories (i.e., 15% of all data in current datasets). To get the end result, they first insert a slice block to store this particular information. Next, they build on the previous progress made with deep waste blocks by combining them into a sliced convolution to determine final grades. Extensive testing against three benchmarks has shown that the proposed method outperforms the current state of the art (e.g., a top-1 accuracy of 90.27% on the Food-101 dataset).

Ciocca et al. [62] investigated CNN-based characteristics for potential use in food identification and recruitment. For this reason, the Food-475 database was initially established. This is the biggest freely available food database, including information on 475 food categories and 247,636 images. They next explain the representation of the food domain in different food databases by looking at the total number of photos, the number of domain classes, and the number of classes. The characteristics are extracted using a CNN with a 50-layer architecture that was trained on food datasets, including representative samples from different food domains. The authors perform tests of functionality related to categorizing food and recovering lost data. Data from the Food-475 database seems to perform better than those from other databases, indicating the necessity for more comprehensive food databases to tackle the obstacles to food identification.

With 13 layers of convolutional neurons, Zhang et al. [63] created a CNN. Images were rotated, gamma correction was applied, and injection noise was employed to boost data. Maximum pooling was compared to average pooling, and found to be equivalent. Specifically, a 128-minibatch size CNN was employed for the falling stochastic gradient with momentum. The average accuracy of the proposed technique is 94.94%, which is an improvement of at least 5% over the best existing methods. Furthermore, the authors verified the optimal setup for this 13-layer model. The Graphics Processing Unit (GPU) will speed up data for training 177 times and for testing by 175 times. The authors discovered that more detailed data would lead to more precise results. Images of fruits may be accurately categorized using this technology.

Williams et al. [64] evaluated the design and performance of a novel pergola-style kiwi harvest robot with autonomous operation. Each of the four robotic guns in the harvester has a unique end-effector built to insure a successful harvest of kiwi fruit. The vision system makes use of current breakthroughs in DNNs and stereos for accurate identification and placement of kiwis under real-world illumination conditions. For the duration of the harvest, four robotic guns are coordinated by a brand-new complicated fruit programming technique. The efficiency of the harvester was evaluated in a commercial orchard via extensive and real-world testing. The provided harvester is able to collect at an average rate of 5.5 s per fruit, allowing it to collect 51% of the all the kiwi fruit in the orchard.

The suggested experiments by Mezgec et al. [65] investigated the integration of a pre-existing food-choice research strategy ("fake food buffet") with a validated one to enable the automated processing and interpretation of data by means of contemporary food-association technology. To do this, they combine Natural Language Processing (NLP), nutritional compatibility, and DL to spot forgeries in the food supply. The first is one of a kind since it employs just a single deep network to perform pixel-level picture segmentation and classification. Its efficacy has been evaluated using pixel-based precision and a cross-sectional area. It starts by figuring out what's in the image, then it compares the composition specifics to known foods, taking into consideration the names and descriptions of the foods. The ultimate accuracy of the DL model trained on fake food photos acquired by 124 research students over 55 food categories was 92.18%, while the food match was performed with an accuracy of 93%.

Reddy et al. [66] developed a calorie-measuring gadget to anticipate the number of calories in a food photo before it is uploaded to a user. This serves several purposes and may be used to keep track of the number of calories consumed each week, as well as the number of calories needed to avoid obesity-related diseases including heart attacks and cancer. The authors have assembled a food image collection from previously available datasets with 20 classes and 500 photos per class to use for complicated image recognition. The authors have built a customized six-layer CNN architecture for feature extraction and picture recognition. The results demonstrate a training accuracy of 93.29% and an experimental accuracy of 78.7% when measuring meal accuracy.

Teng et al. [67] proposed a Chinese food identification architecture as a solution for a small, efficient, neural network with few available resources. The network architecture was developed to simulate and carry out a process pipeline that looks like a bag of features. The proposed architecture, like previous CNNs, optimizes the whole network at once through back propagation, which is critical for recognition accuracy. The authors continue to compare and contrast design with the conventional Bag-of-Features model in an attempt to probe correlations and uncover variables that impact identification precision. This proposed architecture with a five-layer deep CNN achieves the top-1 accuracy of 97.12% and the top-5 accuracy of 99.86% using a freshly constructed Chinese image dataset comprising of 8734 photos from 25 food classes. The results of the experiments show that the suggested CNN compact architecture may effectively address a problem and function in real time.

In [68], the authors compared the newest generation of mobile device food object identification tools. The devices were evaluated using the "food identification" approach. The whole identification process was broken down into six steps: picture retrieval, analysis, segmentation, feature extraction, image classification, and volume estimate. They conduct analyses and classify structures into three groups for the detection of mobile foods: recorders, suggesters, and clinical responses. Separate circumstances apply to each group, and each might provide light on the nature of a given system.

Citing Alajrami et al. [69], deep learning models (CNNs) that are trained and verified have been examined as a potential answer to the problem of individuals being unable to make informed decisions about the shape of tomatoes. In addition, they utilized this trained model to predict the types of (new-to-us) tomato photos that are consistent with the consumption of tomatoes across seven species, using a network of four CNNs and four max polling layers. The overall test reliability was 93%.

7.4 Discussion

More individuals are able to contribute knowledge on food, such as images and textual explanations, thanks to the proliferation of the internet and other social media, mobile applications, and other technologies, leading to the potential for even larger datasets in the future. Experts and institutions from all over the globe conduct their own independent inspections of food quality and safety using their own datasets. One person, a small group of researchers, or a single organization can only gather so much information. Data related to food are expected to be embedded in worldwide databases thanks to new sensors and equipment from foreign clients, investigators, and institutions. These datasets are useful for academics and food research institutions since they can be readily analyzed for further learning.

You can see that researchers in the food recognition domains have used a wide variety of methods and algorithms from what has been discussed so far. After conducting their research, scientists release a set of suggestions. The new research proposal needs to evaluate the similarities and differences between existing food recognition approaches. The study was evaluated with respect to the dataset, algorithms, system, implementation, precision, and the strategy of Significant Satisfied Aims.

Datasets like Mangosteen detection, Food 101, Indian foods, Food-11, and the food dataset are clearly used more often by researchers than the others. CNN, DNN, SVM, PCA, MLP, and KNN are among the most popular algorithms employed in the study of food expressions; however, their use varies greatly from field to field. Instead of relying on a single system, they use a hybrid one that makes use of both mobile and computer technology to carry out their tasks. Moreover, researchers often achieve precision levels of between 70 and 100%. The present day's researchers benefit from the robust structure, framing, and function afforded by this approach and tools. However, the focus of recent study has shifted toward the emerging discipline of food recognition.

7.5 Conclusion

In this chapter, the authos have surveyed numerous recently published articles on the APP pertaining to the DL of food items, describing in depth their overall structure, training methods, and final assessment results for the processing of the food picture, spectrum, text, and other details. The authors have compared the efficiency of DL to that of other conventional methodologies and found that, in the examined experiments, the DL strategy provided superior results.

Food recognition has been a major topic in this chapter. The literature research revealed that many dynamic systems work together to facilitate food recognition. Researchers have successfully used a wide variety of methods and algorithms to reach their goal. The present chapter discussed the current approaches of food choiring (a fake food buffet) and a proven approach for automating data collection and analysis, making use of cutting-edge technology for food association. In addition, the best methods for food recognition include CNNs, DNNs, SVMs, PCA, multi-layer perceptrons, and KNN, and should be used for identifying mangosteens and other foods native to India.

References

1. de Ridder, D., Kroese, F., Evers, C., Adriaanse, M., & Gillebaart, M. (2017). Healthy diet: Health impact, prevalence, correlates, and interventions. *Psychology & Health, 32*, 907–941.
2. Umar Lule, S., & Xia, W. (2005) Food phenolics, pros and cons: A review. *Food Reviews International, 21*, 367–388.
3. Brosnan, T., & Sun, D.-W. (2004). Improving quality inspection of food products by computer vision—A review. *Journal of Food Engineering, 61*, 3–16.
4. Barbin, D. F., Felicio, A. L. d. S. M., Sun, D.-w., Nixdorf, S. L., & Hirooka, E. Y. (2014). Application of infrared spectral techniques on quality and compositional attributes of coffee: An overview. *Food Research International, 61*, 23–32.
5. Zebari, D. A., Haron, H., Zeebaree, S. R., & Zeebaree, D. Q. (2019). Enhance the mammogram images for both segmentation and feature extraction using wavelet transform. In *2019 International Conference on Advanced Science and Engineering (ICOASE)* (p. 100105).
6. Rehman, A., Naz, S., & Razzak, I. (2021). Leveraging big data analytics in healthcare enhancement: Trends, challenges and opportunities. *Multimedia Systems*, 1–33.
7. Abdulrazaq, M., & Salih, A. (2015). Combination of multi classification algorithms for intrusion detection system. *International Journal of Scientific and Engineering Research, 6*, 1364–1371.
8. Cheng, J.-H., & Sun, D.-W. (2017). Partial least squares regression (PLSR) applied to NIR and HSI spectral data modeling to predict chemical properties of fish muscle. *Food Engineering Reviews, 9*, 36–49.
9. Zeebaree, D. Q., Haron, H., Abdulazeez, A. M., & Zeebaree, S. R. (2017). Combination of K-means clustering with genetic algorithm: A review. *International Journal of Applied Engineering Research, 12*, 14238–14245.
10. Dino, H. I., & Abdulrazzaq, M. B. (2019). Facial expression classification based on SVM, KNN and MLP classifiers. In *International Conference on Advanced Science and Engineering (ICOASE)* (pp. 70–75).
11. Mohammad, O. F., Rahim, M. S. M., Zeebaree, S. R. M., & Ahmed, F. Y. (2017). A survey and analysis of the image encryption methods. *International Journal of Applied Engineering Research, 12*, 13265–13280.
12. Obaid, K. B., Zeebaree, S., & Ahmed, O. M. (2020). Deep learning models based on image classification: A review. *International Journal of Science and Business, 4*, 75–81.
13. Kamilaris, A., & Prenafeta-Boldú, F. X. (2018). Deep learning in agriculture: A survey. *Computers and Electronics in Agriculture, 147*, 70–90.
14. Abduallah, W. M., & Zeebaree, S. R. M. (2017). New data hiding method based on DNA and Vigenere Autokey. *Academic Journal of Nawroz University, 6*, 83–88.
15. Jun, Y., Eo, T., Kim, T., Shin, H., Hwang, D., Bae, S. H., et al. (2018). Deep-learned 3D black-blood imaging using automatic labelling technique and 3D convolutional neural networks for detecting metastatic brain tumors. *Scientific Reports, 8*, 1–11.
16. Hinton, G. E., & Salakhutdinov, R. R. (2006). Reducing the dimensionality of data with neural networks. *Science, 313*, 504–507.
17. Zeebaree, S. R., Ahmed, O., & Obid, K. (2020). CSAERNet: An efficient deep learning architecture for image classification. In *2020 3rd International Conference on Engineering Technology and its Applications (IICETA)* (pp. 122–127).

18. Abdulrazzaq, M. B., & Saeed, J. N. (2019). A comparison of three classification algorithms for handwritten digit recognition. In *International Conference on Advanced Science and Engineering (ICOASE)* (pp. 58–63).
19. Osanaiye, B. S., Ahmad, A. R., Mostafa, S. A., Mohammed, M. A., Mahdin, H., Subhi, R., et al. Network data analyser and support vector machine for network intrusion detection of attack type.
20. Darabkh, K. A., Wafa'a, K. K., & Ala'F, K. (2020). LiM-AHP-GC: Life time maximizing based on analytical hierarchal process and genetic clustering protocol for the internet of things environment. *Computer Networks, 176*, 107257.
21. Dino, H., Abdulrazzaq, M. B., Zeebaree, S. R., Sallow, A. B., Zebari, R. R., Shukur, H. M., et al. (2020). Facial Expression Recognition based on hybrid feature extraction techniques with different classifiers. *TEST Engineering & Management, 83*, 22319–22329.
22. Perr-Sauer, J., Duran, A. W., & Phillips, C. T. (2020). Clustering analysis of commercial vehicles using automatically extracted features from time series data. National Renewable Energy Lab (NREL), Golden, CO (United States).
23. Khalifa, I. A., Zeebaree, S. R., Ataş, M., & Khalifa, F. M. (2019). Image steganalysis in frequency domain using co-occurrence matrix and Bpnn. *Science Journal of University of Zakho, 7*, 27–32.
24. Li, K., Feng, Y., Gao, Y., & Qiu, J. (2020). Hierarchical graph attention networks for semisupervised node classification. *Applied Intelligence, 50*, 3441–3451.
25. Guo, Z., Lu, Y., Zhou, H., Li, Z., Fan, Y., & Yu, G. (2021). Anthropometric-based clustering of pinnae and its application in personalizing HRTFs. *International Journal of Industrial Ergonomics, 81*, 103076.
26. Salih, A. A., & Abdulrazaq, M. B. (2019). Combining best features selection using three classifiers in intrusion detection system. In *International Conference on Advanced Science and Engineering (ICOASE)* (pp. 94–99).
27. Chen, R.-C., Dewi, C., Huang, S.-W., & Caraka, R. E. (2020). Selecting critical features for data classification based on machine learning methods. *Journal of Big Data, 7*, 1–26.
28. Zebari, D. A., Haron, H., Zeebaree, S. R., & Zeebaree, D. Q. (2018). Multi-level of DNA encryption technique based on DNA arithmetic and biological operations. In *International Conference on Advanced Science and Engineering (ICOASE)* (pp. 312–317).
29. Zebari, D., Haron, H., & Zeebaree, S. (2017). Security issues in DNA based on data hiding: A review. *International Journal of Applied Engineering Research, 12*, 0973–4562.
30. Gupta, R. (2021). An efficient feature subset selection approach for machine learning. *Multimedia Tools and Applications*, 1–94.
31. Savva, F. (2021). Query-driven learning for automating exploratory analytics in large scale data management systems. University of Glasgow.
32. Mahmood, M. R., Abdulrazzaq, M. B., Zeebaree, S., Ibrahim, A. K., Zebari, R. R., & Dino, H. I. (2021). Classification techniques' performance evaluation for facial expression recognition. *Indonesian Journal of Electrical Engineering and Computer Science, 21*, 176–1184.
33. Chen, J., Zhu, B., Ngo, C.-W., Chua, T.-S., & Jiang, Y.-G. (2020). A study of multi-task and region-wise deep learning for food ingredient recognition. *IEEE Transactions on Image Processing, 30*, 1514–1526.
34. Reddy, V. H., Kumari, S., Muralidharan, V., Gigoo, K., & Thakare, B. S. (2020). Literature survey—Food recognition and calorie measurement using image processing and machine learning techniques. *ICCCE, 2019*, 23–37.
35. Mboya, R. M. (2020). *White maize & food security in sub-Saharan Africa.* Exceller Books.
36. Pike Moore, S. (2020). The ecology of choice: Translation of landscape metrics into the assessment of the food environment using Cleveland, Ohio as a case study. Case Western Reserve University.
37. Ibrahim, R., Zeebaree, S., & Jacksi, K. (2019). Survey on semantic similarity based on document clustering. *Advances in Science, Technology and Engineering Systems Journal, 4*, 115–122.
38. Pedrycz, W., & Chen, S.-M. (2020). *Deep learning: Concepts and architectures.* Springer.

39. Hasan, D. A., Hussan, B. K., Zeebaree, S. R., Ahmed, D. M., Kareem, O. S., & Sadeeq, M. A. (2021). The impact of test case generation methods on the software performance: A review. *International Journal of Science and Business, 5*, 33–44.
40. Abdulrazaq, M. B., Mahmood, M. R., Zeebaree, S. R., Abdulwahab, M. H., Zebari, R. R., Sallow, A. B. (2021). An analytical appraisal for supervised classifiers' performance on facial expression recognition based on relief-F feature selection. *Journal of Physics: Conference Series*, 012055.
41. Yao, Z., Wang, Z., Liu, W., Liu, Y., & Pan, J. (2020). Speech emotion recognition using fusion of three multi-task learning-based classifiers: HSF-DNN, MS-CNN and LLD-RNN. *Speech Communication, 120*, 11–19.
42. Khalid, Z. M., & Zebaree, S. R. (2021). Big data analysis for data visualization: A review. *International Journal of Science and Business, 5*, 64–75.
43. Baccarelli, E., Scardapane, S., Scarpiniti, M., Momenzadeh, A., & Uncini, A. (2020). Optimized training and scalable implementation of conditional deep neural networks with early exits for Fog-supported IoT applications. *Information Sciences, 521*, 107–143.
44. Haider Fawzia, D. A., Mostafac, S. A., Md Fudzeec, M. F., Mahmoodd, M. A., Zeebaree, S. R. M., Ibrahimf, D. A. (2019). A review of automated decision support techniques for improving tillage operations. *Revista AUS, 6*, 219–240.
45. Elhoseny, M., Selim, M. M., & Shankar, K. (2020). Optimal deep learning based convolution neural network for digital forensics face sketch synthesis in internet of things (IoT). *International Journal of Machine Learning and Cybernetics*, 1–12.
46. Eun, D.-I., Jang, R., Ha, W. S., Lee, H., Jung, S. C., & Kim, N. (2020). Deep-learning-based image quality enhancement of compressed sensing magnetic resonance imaging of vessel wall: Comparison of self-supervised and unsupervised approaches. *Scientific Reports, 10*, 1–17.
47. Apolo-Apolo, O., Martínez-Guanter, J., Egea, G., Raja, P., & Pérez-Ruiz, M. (2020). Deep learning techniques for estimation of the yield and size of citrus fruits using a UAV. *European Journal of Agronomy, 115*, 126030.
48. Jin, X., Che, J., & Chen, Y. (2021). Weed identification using deep learning and image processing in vegetable plantation. *IEEE Access, 9*, 10940–10950.
49. Liu, X., Ghazali, K. H., Han, F., & Mohamed, I. I. (2021). Automatic detection of oil palm tree from UAV images based on the deep learning method. *Applied Artificial Intelligence, 35*, 13–24.
50. Rauf, H. T., Lali, M. I. U., Zahoor, S., Shah, S. Z. H., Rehman, A. U., & Bukhari, S. A. C. (2019). Visual features based automated identification of fish species using deep convolutional neural networks. *Computers and Electronics in Agriculture, 167*, 105075.
51. Jalal, A., Salman, A., Mian, A., Shortis, M., & Shafait, F. (2020). Fish detection and species classification in underwater environments using deep learning with temporal information. *Ecological Informatics, 57*, 101088.
52. Ciocca, G., Micali, G., & Napoletano, P. (2020). State recognition of food images using deep features. *IEEE Access, 8*, 32003–32017.
53. Srigurulekha, K., & Ramachandran, V. (2020). Food image recognition using CNN. In *International Conference on Computer Communication and Informatics (ICCCI)* (pp. 1–7).
54. Azizah, L. M. R., Umayah, S. F., Riyadi, S., Damarjati, C., & Utama, N. A. (2017). Deep learning implementation using convolutional neural network in mangosteen surface defect detection. In *2017 7th IEEE International Conference on Control System, Computing and Engineering (ICCSCE)* (pp. 242–246).
55. Liu, C., Cao, Y., Luo, Y., Chen, G., Vokkarane, V., Yunsheng, M., et al. (2017). A new deep learning-based food recognition system for dietary assessment on an edge computing service infrastructure. *IEEE Transactions on Services Computing, 11*, 249–261.
56. Pouladzadeh, P. (2017). A cloud-assisted mobile food recognition system. Université d'Ottawa/University of Ottawa.
57. Pandey, P., Deepthi, A., Mandal, B., & Puhan, N. B. (2017). FoodNet: Recognizing foods using ensemble of deep networks. *IEEE Signal Processing Letters, 24*, 1758–1762.

58. Aguilar, E., Bolaños, M., & Radeva, P. (2017). Food recognition using fusion of classifiers based on CNNs. In *International Conference on Image Analysis and Processing* (pp. 213–224).
59. Pan, L., Pouyanfar, S., Chen, H., Qin, J., & Chen, S.-C. (2017). Deepfood: Automatic multi-class classification of food ingredients using deep learning. In *2017 IEEE 3rd International Conference on Collaboration and Internet Computing (CIC)* (pp. 181–189).
60. Heravi, E. J., Aghdam, H. H., & Puig, D. (2017). Classification of foods by transferring knowledge from ImageNet dataset. In *Ninth International Conference on Machine Vision (ICMV 2016)* (p. 1034128).
61. Martinel, N., Foresti, G. L., & Micheloni, C. (2018). Wide-slice residual networks for food recognition. In *IEEE Winter Conference on Applications of Computer Vision (WACV)* (pp. 567–576).
62. Ciocca, G., Napoletano, P., & Schettini, R. (2018). CNN-based features for retrieval and classification of food images. *Computer Vision and Image Understanding, 176*, 7077.
63. Zhang, Y.-D., Dong, Z., Chen, X., Jia, W., Du, S., Muhammad, K., et al. (2019). Image based fruit category classification by 13-layer deep convolutional neural network and data augmentation. *Multimedia Tools and Applications, 78*, 3613–3632.
64. Williams, H. A., Jones, M. H., Nejati, M., Seabright, M. J., Bell, J., Penhall, N. D., et al. (2019). Robotic kiwifruit harvesting using machine vision, convolutional neural networks, and robotic arms. *Biosystems Engineering, 181*, 140–156.
65. Mezgec, S., Eftimov, T., Bucher, T., & Seljak, B. K. (2019). Mixed deep learning and natural language processing method for fake-food image recognition and standardization to help automated dietary assessment. *Public Health Nutrition, 22*, 1193–1202.
66. Reddy, V. H., Kumari, S., Muralidharan, V., Gigoo, K., & Thakare, B. S. (2019). Food recognition and calorie measurement using image processing and convolutional neural network. In *2019 4th International Conference on Recent Trends on Electronics, Information, Communication & Technology (RTEICT)* (pp. 109–115).
67. Teng, J., Zhang, D., Lee, D.-J., & Chou, Y. (2019). Recognition of Chinese food using convolutional neural network. *Multimedia Tools and Applications, 78*, 11155–11172.
68. Knez, S., & Šajn, L. (2020). Food object recognition using a mobile device: Evaluation of currently implemented systems. *Trends in Food Science & Technology, 99*, 460–471.
69. Alajrami, M. A., & Abu-Naser, S. S. (2020). Type of tomato classification using deep learning.

Chapter 8
A Data-Driven Approach for a Personalized Nutrition and Health Infrastructure

8.1 Introduction

Personalized nutrition (PN) is nutritional advice based on individual data such as that relating to metabolism, biochemistry, and microbiomes. Improving nutrition is central to addressing global development challenges, as nutrition is directly and indirectly linked to the Sustainable Development Goals. Investing in the development of an environment with pertinent laws, rules, and policies is necessary for successful programs to reduce the burden of malnutrition. These interventions need to be quick, dietary-specific, and dietary-sensitive. It is necessary to address the underlying determinants [1]. Nutrition programs are more successful when they are grounded in solid evidence, implemented through multisectoral collaboration, and supported by increased political commitment and investment [2].

Today, we employ data-driven technologies to enhance individual and global nutrition and health outcomes. There are now hundreds of thousands of mobile health apps (mHealth) available for download by individuals in international app stores on topics like fitness, diet, or medical health. These diet and nutrition applications assist people in changing their health-related behaviors, even if additional research is required to determine their overall usefulness. We are in the process of leveraging new technology to restructure the entire global food supply chain so that nutrient-dense foods are cultivated more sustainably and distributed more fairly in order to address nutrition and health on a large scale. The food supply chain uses innovations like Farmwave's pest and disease diagnostics app to promote the production, delivery, and accessibility of wholesome, affordable food. Independent, locally based mobile markets and online shopping platforms are emerging to provide access to food by supplying it directly to communities suffering from food insecurity [3]. New food and nutrition trends appear every year, and in 2022, personalized nutrition is expected to be a big deal. But it is just this that makes it stand out from the competition. The problem is that it isn't even a trend. Rather it gathers information from supermarket loyalty cards, creates coupons for healthy foods, and offers individualized nutrition advice based on customers' purchasing patterns. Data-driven technologies are being

G. Chhabra et al., *Artificial Intelligence to Analyze Psychophysical and Human Lifestyle*, https://doi.org/10.1007/978-981-99-3039-5_8

integrated throughout the whole food system in order to alter customer behavior and address inefficiencies along the food supply chain [4].

8.2   Predictive Models in Nutrition and Health

Efforts should be made to create predictive tools for timely monitoring of individual health responses to food in order to comprehend the underlying dynamics of health, account for inter-individual heterogeneity, and apply personalized diet-based therapies. A systems science viewpoint aids medical professionals in developing individualized dietary strategies, understanding treatment response variability, and tailoring focused treatments [4]. Personalized nutritional approaches may promote the development of information processing representations of digestion, absorption, and metabolism.

These following show connections between molecular activities and medical results:

- Combining data from all relevant scales;
- Creating counter-intuitive hypotheses;
- Experimental confirmation by means of clinical and preclinical research utilizing standardized dietary treatments;
- Advanced machine learning (ML) models are used to connect multiscale models with health outcomes.

We can now extract particular data on consumption for standardized meals, functional foods, and beverage sales reports thanks to big data. Data mining and extraction from databases of insurance claims and electronic health records (EHRs) can be done using initiatives supported by health informatics. Data from EHRs can be combined with expertise from data science, nutrition, and nutrition science to create computer models and synthetic patient cohorts. These synthetic patients can be used as avatars that reflect inter-individual heterogeneity to perform predictive analytics and assess system-level responses to customized nutritional recommendations. These prognostic data can be utilized to clarify the intricate regulatory processes of dietary interventions at the interfaces of the immunological, metabolic, and gut microbiota. The development of health platforms, customization of upcoming dietary advice to promote health, and expedited adoption of recommendations in clinics will all be facilitated by advanced computational methodologies and data analytic platforms [6].

8.3 Data Driven Approaches

When judgments are made based on the analysis and interpretation of hard facts rather than on observation, this is known as a data-driven approach. A data-driven strategy makes sure that plans and solutions are founded on facts rather than speculation, feeling, and anecdotal evidence. "Data-driven" refers to the process of gathering and analyzing data in order to generate conclusions and solutions. Using knowledge from the past and present, a data-driven strategy aids in future prediction. Without data, you run the danger of assuming the wrong things or being duped by prejudiced views. To dominate their industry, businesses today use big data analytics, diagnostic modeling, and data processing.

8.3.1 Healthcare and Data Analytics

As part of the data analytics and management for the healthcare industry, information from every organizational department must be gathered for a central structured data repository. Healthcare professionals can now provide patients with better care by using a holistic therapeutic approach and offering personalized healthcare services. As a result, the answer to the question "What is the role of data analytics in the healthcare industry?" is fundamentally based on the technology's potential to support healthcare organizations in remaining competitive in the increasingly complex market by improving service efficiency and providing higher-quality patient care. Modern software and medical device techniques are needed by healthcare companies today to transform complex data into meaningful insights. Enterprises may now do so owing to data analytics technology by maintaining a highly structured data repository that assists in making wise judgments for boosted productivity and improved service quality. When healthcare organizations integrate data analytics into their systems and feel comfortable using technology, they will begin to receive comprehensive and organized patient data that will start to paint a complete picture of healthcare services. This will enable them to offer totally personalized, thorough, and precise therapy [7].

8.3.2 Role of Data Analytics in Healthcare for Professionals

- **Disease prediction and prevention**. One of the biggest and most gratifying challenges of healthcare data analytics for practitioners is the ability of practice management technology to diagnose diseases early. With the use of ML and the technology's strong analytical capabilities, it is possible to examine enormous volumes of past patient records and pinpoint patterns in patients who have significant illnesses. This increases the likelihood that medical personnel will take preventative measures to help patients lessen difficulties before they become fatal, too complex, or unmanageable.

- **Care coordination**. In emergency care, data analysis is also incredibly helpful, especially when doctors must act rapidly. The doctor has a second chance to save a patient's life thanks to the crucial real-time insight that this technology offers. Technology can assist caregivers in providing better care for their patients and sending alerts about their health, in addition to its function in coordinating treatment in crises.

- **Customer service**. As the healthcare sector embraces value-added business models more frequently, patients will receive better customer service, more individualized care, quicker turnaround times, and overall better and more accurate healthcare services. It is more crucial than ever to take action. Customer care is significantly impacted by data analysis. This technology enables clinicians to add a personalized touch to care and create a seamless healthcare experience by improving billing and payment processes by giving organizations access to structured and filtered data.

- **Financial risk management**. Healthcare businesses are subject to a number of financial hazards, such as unpaid invoices, records that are not used, and decreasing reimbursements. Organizations are now able to use predictive analytics to assess outstanding payments, identify patient insurance coverage, and more. The whole financial flow is improved by the use of data analytics, which is supported by strong artificial techniques.

- **Abuse and fraud**. With the help of data analytics, healthcare organizations can identify and halt fraud and abuse, which improves effectiveness and service level. Fraud of all forms, including human billing errors, unauthorized lab tests, incorrect payments, and insurance claims is especially prevalent in the healthcare industry. Through the use of data analytic technology, hospitals and other healthcare organizations may identify and avoid potential fraud practices (honesty or abuse).

8.3.3 Role of Data Analysis in Patient Care

- **Resident health management**. Population health management (PHM) services are developing as a result of the rise of data analytics technologies in the healthcare sector, including ML, deep learning, and artificial intelligence. With the emergence of PHM, healthcare services are now more concerned with prediction and prevention than with treatment and response. Strong predictive analytics methods can identify patients' risk factors for chronic diseases at an early stage, enabling medical professionals to intervene quickly and prevent issues further down the road. Not only may predictive analytics save lives, but it can also lower the cost of patient care and treatment.

- **Health tracking**. The ability to foresee a patient's health risk before they experience a chronic disease is essential to modern health services. This can only be accomplished by putting effective data analysis technology into use and providing the model with enough training data. This has the ability to precisely evaluate patient medical records, spot crucial trends that hint at potential illness risk, and serve as a tracking mechanism. Healthcare tracking technology has made it possible for healthcare organizations to track important patient health statistics and establish preventative care strategies for early treatment and cure. Healthcare is about giving patients faster, better service. By delivering the proper care at the appropriate moment, technology can also contribute to preventing patients developing chronic conditions.

- **Industry progress.** Data analytics technology has huge potential to create healthcare Business Intelligence (BI) solutions for the future, in addition to the enormous advantages of technology and its capacity to solve present issues facing the healthcare business. The optimal treatment options for a patient's medical history can be determined by using this technology to examine vast volumes of complex medical data.

8.4 Importance of a Data-Driven Approach

Examples of data-driven approaches are becoming more and more common as a result of advancements in technology, computer power, and increased access to vast amounts of data. With the use of our data-driven methodology, pricing, logistics for warehouses, and customer behavior modeling can all be understood and improved.

A data-driven strategy makes optimization considerably simpler than relying solely on intuition. Using data modeling approaches, one can have a fair notion as to the outcomes. Once you know what "data-driven" means, you usually know exactly what is being requested.

The benefits of data-driven decision making are as follows:

- **Promotes transparency and accountability.** Making judgments based on data analysis has a number of benefits, one of which is the elimination of the purely subjective element. Everyone is aware of the decision's rationale. Teamwork and staff morale can be enhanced by greater transparency and accountability. Employees are made more conscious of the value of ongoing data collection and backup by data-driven management. It is acknowledged that a data-driven strategy promotes performance responsibility and has quantifiable objectives and measurable outcomes.
- **Promotes continuous improvement.** The ongoing performance improvement is another benefit of data-driven decision management. Organizations may more readily monitor critical Key Performance Indicators (KPIs), implement gradual changes, and make quick adjustments in response to outcomes. The capacity for scaling inside an organization is also enhanced by a culture of data-driven decision making. This enables the quick implementation of concepts and backup plans without the need for pointless meetings and logistical hassles.

- **Provides strong forecasting insights**. Business executives can use data-driven decision management to glean insightful, practical knowledge. You can compare and test several company strategies with the use of a data-driven strategy. You may determine whether your strategy is working by comparing current data with past trends, or you can start over and reconsider your choices.
- **Aids market investigation**. Data-driven businesses are more inclined to trust and invest in the proper research to guide decisions on innovative product designs, more dependable services, and even radical workplace reforms. Research with a strong data base can assist one to see trends before the market does. Organizations may get ready for the short and long-term future with the help of this streamlined research and historical data.
- **Improves organizational coherence**. Over time, data-driven enterprises promote a culture of uniformity and standardization. People are certain about their choices and completely cognizant of the ramifications of the information gathered. The more people in your organization use data-driven decision-making, the better off everyone is at their jobs individually. Organizations that exhibit consistency across all of their elements are better equipped to consistently profit from dedication, loyalty, and accountability.
- **Other benefits**. The data are made available by Data-Driven Decision Making (DDDM). Data analytics can be used by businesses to find pertinent information about their operations, products, and clients. Data indicate that strategy design is made more precise by DDDM. Executives in the C-Suite like chief officers (e.g., CEO, CIO, CFO, etc.) who have access to reliable data can learn more about how the business is run and have a say in how decisions are made. Quantitative or qualitative data are both acceptable. Customer reviews or, in the context of healthcare, notes from staff members are examples of qualitative data. Statistics and numbers are included in quantitative data. This is either your zip code or billing information. Both types are useful. Decisions are openly disclosed. Organizations may see the data that supports the strategy, allowing them to add more employees.

8.5   Data-Driven Healthcare

The proliferation of data has also changed the healthcare industry. Researchers estimate that patients produced 80 MB of data annually before the epidemic. This amount has unquestionably been surpassed. Data is now being gathered from a variety of sources, including wearable technology, wellness apps, disease registries, demographic health statistics, and personal health information, which includes geographic, financial, and insurance information.

Having access to all of this knowledge gives healthcare administrators a valuable weapon. Applying data can enhance care, streamline administrative procedures, cut costs, and lessen clinical staff burnout. Hospitals are utilizing data analytics and prediction models more frequently to support objective, fact-based plans and choices.

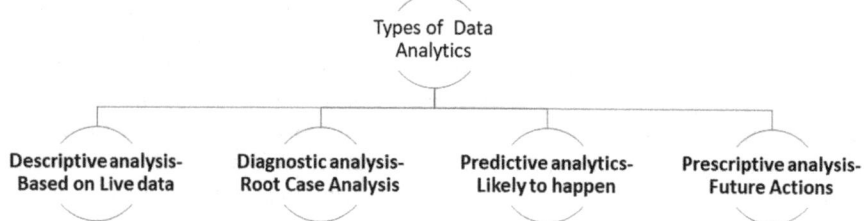

Fig. 8.1 Types of data analytics

As depicted in Fig. 8.1, there are four types of data analysis used for data-driven decision making. A detailed description of these data analysis approaches are discussed Fig. 8.1.

8.5.1   Descriptive Analysis

Descriptive analytics, in its most basic form, describes and depicts a client's or customer's activity. The length of time visitors spent on a website, the pages they stayed on the longest, the links they visited, and the items they bought are a few examples of this information used in marketing. Shopping includes whether a client left her shopping cart unattended, whether she browsed on a desktop or a mobile device, and the date she completed the purchase. Historical patient data are part of descriptive analytics in the healthcare industry. Patient consultations, prescriptions, operations, other treatments, and patient outcomes are all included in these data. They also contain bills and payments, geographical information (which is useful for population health indicators), and more. Business executives can modify their decisions when they comprehend patient and customer behavior. Historical patient data, for instance, can help with screening programs or forecast risk factors for specific diseases.

8.5.2   Analytical Diagnostics

Diagnostic analysis reveals why something happened, whereas descriptive analysis shows a corporation what happened. Business leaders who utilize diagnostic analysis—also referred to as root cause analysis—can better understand why their company or organization produced the outcomes that it did. For instance, by examining what your consumers bought and didn't buy over a specific time period, diagnostic analytics can assist you to determine why your sales are trending upwards or downwards. Diagnostic analytics can help increase understanding from the patient level to the corporate level in the field of healthcare. It can help clinicians, managers, and healthcare executives better comprehend a variety of challenging healthcare issues. Due to the complexity of these issues, diagnostic analysis utilizes artificial intelligence (AI) running on strong computers to evaluate large amounts of data considerably more quickly than humans can. In addition to using algorithms to collect data, AI and ML also employ them to discover relationships and hasten decision making. For instance, AI may gather data from clinical trials, test results, research articles, and other sources and compile them to speed up the creation of new drugs. In identifying false-positive mammograms, AI outperforms radiologists and matches the accuracy of cancer detection. Healthcare is being transformed by this AI and diagnostic analytics combination. AI can analyze massive EHRs and provide data to doctors and patients.

8.5.3 Predictive Analytics

Using both recent and old data, predictive analytics creates models of potential future behavior. To ascertain the likelihood of an event, data scientists employ a variety of approaches including statistical analysis, ML, and data querying. The likelihood is given a score or number. The method of predictive analytics is highly complicated. It is used in financial services, insurance, science, and obviously the healthcare sector. Risk reduction is the main objective of most predictive analytics in a company. One illustration of this is the way insurance firms are lowering the cost of underwriting by using data science, mathematical science, and predictive analytics.

Predictive analytics in healthcare also includes:

- **Patient treatment**. Predictive analytics has been used in healthcare to estimate patient illness risk, find effective patient treatments, and assist clinical personnel in preventing patient deterioration. It can be used to pinpoint dangers related to socioeconomic position and postal code, two social factors that affect health. Through better treatment and prevention, the goal is to enhance patient outcomes.
- **Taking care of patient data**. EHR systems are powerful tools for gathering information about patient care. It can be challenging to use, though, because it incorporates clinical, billing, and other patient information. Security problems may result from improper use of the EHR system. Staff may be relieved of the stress of information overload brought on by EHRs with predictive analytics.
- **Billing and revenue cycle**. During the sales cycle, predictive analytics can be a beneficial tool. Hospitals employ modeling to enhance patient payments and insurance reimbursement. Administrative, financial, and accounting employees can allocate resources more effectively if they have a better understanding of a hospital's or provider's financial status.
- **Personnel optimization**. Clinical staff fatigue and treatment errors might result from a hospital staff shortage. These issues have been brought to light by the pandemic. Hospitals may prepare for an increase in patient flow by identifying

when to ramp up staff with the help of predictive analytics. Bed counts, wage information, and nurse-to-patient ratios are among the statistics.

8.5.4 Prescriptive Analysis

Once leaders have a clear understanding of what occurred, why it occurred, and what might occur, they use prescriptive analysis to develop a strategy. Based on data, it chooses the optimum option. Prescriptive analytics are used by businesses to assist in decision making on ongoing operations and short and long-term objectives.

Prescriptive analytics employs AI and ML, like other data analysis methods, to examine the enormous volumes of information accessible and suggest algorithm-based actions. This can be automatically generated, just like delivery routes. Prescription analytics aids in care improvement and cost reduction. Consider these cases:

- **Information on damage**. Claims templates can be used by insurance firms to support premium increases or new premiums for retirement benefits.
- **Logistics**. Data analytics may be used to model anything from patient transportation to the ordering of supplies, and hospitals can employ prescriptive analytics to identify the best logistics practices and rules.
- **Radiotherapy**. Oncologists can use modeling data to choose the best radiation dosage for a patient.
- **Personnel management**. Data models can be used by hospitals to decide on workforce levels.

8.6   Importance of a Nutrition-Based Approach

The main source of nutrients needed to support life, foster health, proper growth, and development, and guarantee human productivity is food. This supply frequently falls short of meeting all of the nutritional requirements of the world's poorest people, who frequently reside close to farms. The paradox that the poorest people simultaneously have the highest capacity for food production has sparked the growth of eco-nutrition. With a focus on the interactions between agriculture, ecology, and human nutrition, eco-nutrition blends environmental health and human health. Environmental deterioration and decreased food production are caused by a vicious cycle of nutrient depletion, soil erosion, and biodiversity loss. Malnutrition, poor agricultural management, and environmental deterioration are all related. This shows the necessity of implementing eco-nutrition-based solutions. A successful intervention requires a comprehensive approach. Thus, data-driven decision making has transformed the healthcare industry. Without relying on intuition or bias, data analytics provides physicians, clinicians, and administrators with the knowledge they need to enhance healthcare from every viewpoint. They are capable of making decisions based on information that is supportive of their company strategy. Well-managed data manipulation has positive effects on patient outcomes and satisfaction, care quality, and efficiency.

Hospital managers and clinicians across the field are implementing data-driven processes according to the guidelines of experts (by keeping high-quality data, including that of all stakeholders, and investing resources). One can anticipate a wide range of advantages.

8.6.1   Health Data to Improve Treatment Outcomes

Healthcare professionals' ability to give high-quality care to their patients in an effective and efficient manner are already greatly impacted by data analytics. However, their potential to enhance patient outcomes and healthcare procedures will grow as more data kinds become accessible and new tools are created to make analytical results clear and simple for professionals to obtain. The function of data analytics is always expanding.

How technology may be used to solve healthcare provider concerns like staffing, operational efficiency, and improving the patient experience is to understand the potential of data analytics to alter the healthcare business. Understanding what patient-centered care is and how it is influenced by the patient's preferences is the first step.

8.7   Personalized Nutrition Challenges

Personalized nutrition refers to nutritional advice that has been specifically designed to promote health, maintain health, and avoid disease [5]. The four various challenges are listed below and depicted in Fig. 8.2.

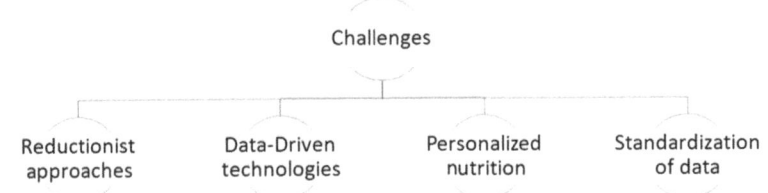

Fig. 8.2 Four challenges to personalized nutrition

Challenge 1: Limitations in Reductionist Approaches and Opportunities for the Adoption of Advanced Computational Data-Driven Technologies

The study of biological pathways at the level of a single gene or protein is largely out of date in nutritional research. There are questions about the dynamic interactions between diet, metabolism, the microbiome, and the host at the cellular and molecular level, as well as about the consequences for personal and individual health. A holistic knowledge of health requires analyzing the connections between nutrition, genes, gene products, health, and environmental exposures, rather than focusing on the impact of specific nutrients or macromolecules on specific genes or gene products [5].

Challenge 2: The Need for a Personalized Infrastructure for Nutrition Computation

Such an infrastructure must be implemented immediately, despite the fact that nutrition research is garnering a lot of support as a result of revolutionary genomic and data science. The difficulties posed by food intake databases must be taken into account in this debate. These databases incorporate functionality that converts chemical components in food into energy and nutritional intakes in order to comprehensively capture complex dietary patterns. Food diaries are one of the techniques now used to monitor food intake; however, it might be difficult to translate food descriptions into energy. To build specialized nutritional databases that can support a setting of common formats, annotations, and network-based systems to improve food monitoring and consumption processes, it may be desirable to make the transfer to an informatics infrastructure. However, there might be differences in how food is described and how data is collected. Techniques for generating compositional values when food is acquired from various locations, such as labs, patients, and hospitals, are included in this.

Challenge 3: The Requirement for Individualized Training and the Standardization of Data

Access to patient records that contain data used to determine patient care is made easier by EHRs and Financial Health Indicators (FHIs). Improvements in patient outcomes and healthcare decision making will result from switching from paper patient records to an electronic format kept in an EHR, which will also result in cost savings. But digitization in electronic form might lead to (i) an incorrect standard format, (ii) inaccurate reporting and insurance company rejection because of insufficient diagnostic code documentation, (iii) a lack of user training a lack of dedication to the situation could lead to further problems), and (iv) inadequately developed technology could result in bugs and issues that result in EHR shortcomings [5].

Challenge 4: Insufficient Data and the Need for Better Techniques

Their high dimensionality and sparsity are two of the main difficulties in processing clinical data from EHRs. The patient's visit or hospital stay is recorded in the EHR along with all clinical events. We examined how changes in nutrition, exercise, and sleep affect blood sugar levels. Through continuous glucose monitoring, a high-density data matrix on glucose levels is used. However, data from EHRs are frequently missing, and the data that are present are heterogeneous, complex, and combined with both organized and unstructured formats. Data inputs to template information such as patient demographics, clinical measures, medication prescriptions, and diagnoses are included in structured data. Unstructured data consist of doctors' handwritten notes. Three major categories can be used to classify the causes of missing data: entirely randomly missing, randomly missing, and non-randomly missing.

8.8 Conclusion

Diet has a significant influence on human health and happiness. A well-balanced diet with sufficient levels of macro- and micronutrients is necessary for the human body to function properly. Health issues like cardiovascular disease, diabetes, obesity, and malnutrition can result from an unbalanced diet. In this chapter, we have looked at cutting-edge computer systems with data processing, sharing, and storage capabilities. We have explored the use of data-driven methodologies that demand the development of a specialized food and health infrastructure system. Based on the longitudinal data collection for physiological measurements, gut flora, and other pertinent biomarker measurements, this chapter will enrich and improve patient treatment.

References

1. Bhutta, Z. A., Das, J. K., Rizvi, A., Gaffey, M. F., Walker, N., Horton, S., et al. (2013). Evidence-based interventions for improvement of maternal and child nutrition: What can be done and at what cost? *The Lancet, 382*(9890), 452–477.
2. Lamstein, S., Pomeroy-Stevens, A., Webb, P., & Kennedy, E. (2016). Optimizing the multisectoral nutrition policy cycle: A systems perspective. *Food and Nutrition Bulletin, 37*(4_suppl), S107–S14.
3. Aitken, M., Clancy, B., & Nass, D. (2017). *The growing value of digital health.* IQVIA Institute for Human Data Science.
4. Schumer, H., Amadi, C., & Joshi, A. (2018). Evaluating the dietary and nutritional apps in the google play store. *Healthcare Informatics Research, 24*(1), 38–45.
5. Ahmed, S., de la Parra, J., Elouafi, I., German, B., Jarvis, A., Lal, V., Lartey, A., Longvah, T., Malpica, C., Vázquez-Manjarrez, N., Prenni, J., Aguilar-Salinas, C. A., Srichamnong, W., Rajasekharan, M., Shafizadeh, T., Siegel, J. B., Steiner, R., Tohme, J., & Watkins, S. (2022). Foodomics: A data-driven approach to revolutionize nutrition and sustainable diets. *Frontiers in Nutrition, 3*(9), 874312. https://doi.org/10.3389/fnut.2022.874312.PMID:35592635;PMCID: PMC9113044
6. Mønsted, T. (2022). A matter of distance? A qualitative study of data-driven early lifestyle assessment in preventive healthcare. In K. Wac & S. Wulfovich (Eds.), *Quantifying quality of life.* Health informatics. Springer. https://doi.org/10.1007/978-3-030-94212-0_19
7. Razzak, M. I., Imran, M., & Xu, G. (2020). Big data analytics for preventive medicine. *Neural Computing and Applications, 32*, 4417–4451. https://doi.org/10.1007/s00521-019-04095-y.)

Chapter 9
Technology for Nutrition, Fitness, and Sports

9.1 Introduction

In the context of athletics, physical fitness, and healthy eating, the study of human anatomy and the science of physical activity are inextricably intertwined [1]. It is the implementation of nutrition information to an effective daily eating plan that provides this same engagement in regular physical activity, aids the repair as well as building showcased hard physical effort, and enhances athletic performance via competitive events, all while simultaneously promoting health and wellness. To be successful, athletes need to have a solid understanding of both of these principles to reach their objectives in the areas of sports, fitness, and nutrition, and to learn the connections between the fields of nutrition and exercise science, emphasizing that regular exercise and healthy eating habits need to work together to produce the best results [2]. At this stage, it is up to each individual athlete to put the knowledge about diet, fitness, and sports that they have recently received to use [3].

Taking part in an endurance sport involves not only physical fitness but also good nutrition, with a particular emphasis on making necessary nutritional adjustments. Targeted fitness development at an early age, especially through adolescence, is considered to be the foundation of leading an active lifestyle, avoiding possible overweight, minimizing motor inadequacies, and ultimately increasing the quality of life [4].

At the conclusion of a competition, athletes are required to have adequate nutrition, to be injury-free, to maintain their attention, and to be ready to participate. In regard to athletic nutrition, it is not just about the number of calories you consume, the amount of protein you consume for muscle growth, or the amount of carbohydrates you consume for energy. The influence that one's diet and eating routines have on athletic performance has attracted much attention in the world of sport. It is the responsibility of sports nutrition specialists to provide broad recommendations that cater to the unique requirements of each athlete in terms of their health, sports, level of physical fitness, nutritional choices, body weight, and composition [5].

Fig. 9.1 Importance of
nutrition and fitness in sports

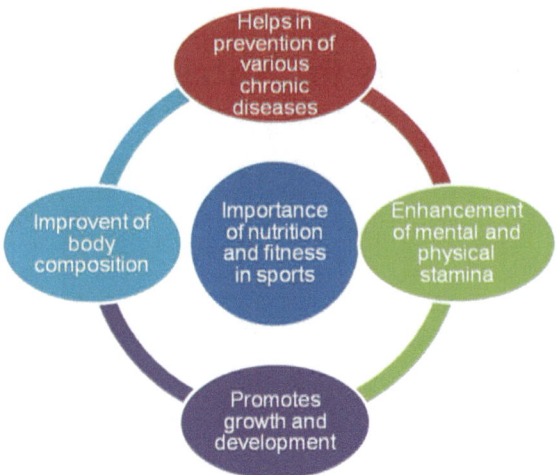

An eating plan can be characterized as a means to feed an athlete's activity and aid the process of rebuilding bodily stores during physical exertion [6]. An athlete's food plan may also be defined as a strategy to fuel their athletic activities. The term "sports nutrition" can also refer to a strategy for enhancing one's general health, level of physical fitness, and sense of well-being. Athletes must contend with a variety of mental and physical hurdles, and if they are not properly nourished, it is possible that these obstacles will not be conquered [6]. Figure 9.1 presents information regarding nutrition, physical activity, and athletic engagement.

9.2 Literature Review

Empirical research on the determinants of dietary interventions, including restriction and supplementation, have given way to direct investigations of the physiological basis of the specific nutrient needs for strenuous physical exercise [7]. This line of research began as an evolution of previous research on the effects of nutritional changes. A person's attempts to train are augmented in various ways by activities such as sports, fitness, and proper nutrition. Even if you alter your workout routine, the amount of fuel your body needs to accomplish it will remain the same. The capacity of an athlete to make it big may be hindered by factors such as injury, weariness, and a lack of recovery as a result of inadequate nutrition [8].

As per the American Dietetic Association, the Dieticians of Canada, and the American College of Sports Medicine, optimal nutrition improves both physical activity and athletic performance, as well as recovery after exercise. In regard to matters of nutrition, timing, and supplements, it is essential to be aware of the substances that are being consumed by the body [9]. According to Slater and Phillips [9, 10], strength and power athletes are primarily concerned with increasing power, which is related to body weight, and is therefore nearly all about resistance training. It is possible for sportsmen and women to increase the hypertrophy of their skeletal muscles; however, the fundamental nutritional issues that they face go far beyond those that are specifically related to hypertrophy. These fundamental nutritional issues include an understanding of sports exercise as well as the diet industry, the strategic timescale of nutritional intake to optimize fueling as well as recovery objectives, and the accomplishment of precompetition overall health needs. Intakes of total calories as well as macronutrients are typically high for strength-power athletes; however, when stated in relation to body mass, these intakes have a tendency to be average. Another consideration is that total calorie and macronutrient intakes are typically high.

If one had the ability to judge the distribution of nutrients throughout the day, particularly before, during, and then after exercise, one would have a better understanding of how to maximize nutrient intake to achieve nutrition-related goals [10]. According to Holway and Spriet's research from [11, 12], meal planning for people with even a moderate amount of energy expenditure should account for an acceptable amount of carbohydrates as well as a protein requirement. Activities that place a premium on power and strength demand the adoption of muscle-building routines that are accompanied by a nutritious diet. The relationship between physical activity and dietary intake is illustrated in Fig. 9.2.

Fig. 9.2 Nutrition-related sports fitness

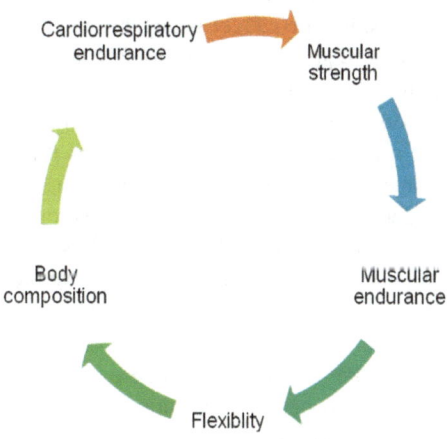

9.2.1 Artificial Intelligence and Machine Learning Techniques for Food Recognition and Nutrition Estimation, their comparison

Because food products are frequently presented in a wide variety of formats, correctly identifying them can be a challenging undertaking. It is difficult to categorize fine-grained photos as well as identify the pairwise distinctive features of food that take advantage of the positional correlations of eight distinct food elements. In the suggested multifood photo identification system, which recognizes the initial food [13], many detectors are able to identify various aspects of the food, including its color, texture, gradient, and even scale-invariant feature transform (SIFT). The internet program acts as both a food-recognition tool and a device that determines nutritional balance. The meal is broken down into five distinct categories based on its discrete cosine transform (DCT) coefficients as well as the extract color of each individual block. These categories are basic, side dish, main dish, fruits, and nonfood. The method that triage amalgamated dermoscopic algorithm (TADA) uses to evaluate diets takes into account both the identification of foods and the calculation of quantities [14]. However, there are several restrictions associated with utilizing white dishes as well as a checkerboard to determine the amounts of food to be consumed. Because of the delays in contact, it is not possible to carry out any operations in an interactive manner in any of the systems that have been described to date. On the client side, our gadget is capable of recognizing foods in real time, and it does so without requiring any additional computer resources. Furthermore, it can be used in an interactive manner [15].

Maintaining a diet that is healthy on a consistent basis is one way to prevent obesity. We present a new method that uses machine learning to automatically categorize images of food and provide predictions about the characteristics of it [16]. We offer a deep learning strategy that is based on such a deep neural network that it can train the convolution neural network (CNN) that is part of the prototype system. The major purpose of the procedure is to improve the overall accuracy of a model that has been pretrained. An example of a prototype system is developed by employing client–server architecture. The client makes a request that image recognition be carried out by the server, which then proceeds to carry out the required processing. The prototype system's three core software components include pretrained CNN models enabling classification, textual data as well as attribute estimation models, and even a server-side module [16]. Training based on machine learning was utilized to increase the categorization accuracy of a variety of foods for which there were hundreds of images.

Since the 1990s, Artificial Intelligence (AI) technology has been applied to the process of determining the degree of uniqueness in food composition and analyzing food composition. When Dettmar et al. [17] employed the Artificial Neural Network (ANN) technique to detect the region of origin of orange juice samples, they did so by employing a set of 16 criteria. The technique of calculation that was utilized had an overall success of 92.5%. In this study, Yang et al. utilized this same isobaric tag for both relative and absolute quantification analytical techniques to evaluate the same differential expression of whey proteins that were found in human and bovine colostrums and mature milk. This was done so that they could compare and contrast the levels of these proteins. This research might be beneficial for foods that are nutritious for infants as well as for dairy products [18]. Moreira et al. [19] used topological maps of such a Kohonen Deep Neural Network (DNN) in their analysis of the method for processing cashew nut samples. This was done to evaluate the methodology. Table 9.1 presents a comparison and contrast between AI or machine learning (ML) techniques as it relates to the reorganization and evaluation of food.

Table 9.1 Comparison of AI and ML techniques in food reorganization and comparison

A multifaceted CNN developed to identify food (reference)	Dataset	Algorithm	System	Accuracy (%)	Significant result
[20]	Create different food	CNN, SVM	Mobile system	–	Newly introduced menu includes 20 various dishes from 11 countries that range from solid, cut through smooth pastes in vegetables and fruit
[21]	Food 101	CNN, SVMs	Computer software	86.85	CNNs are used to create food representations in a new way
[22]	Real-world data	Deep learning	Mobile cloud computing	–	There are already 20 new products on the market, ranging from solid, sliced fruits and vegetables to silky paste
[23]	7000 images	SVM, DNN	Smartphone	100	Suggests a patient and physician-friendly calorie counter to aid the fight against diet-related illnesses
[24]	Food 101, Indian foods	Multilayered CNN	Computer software	97.60	Food can now be identified using a multifaceted CNN

9.2.2 Future Recommendations

The adoption of a healthy lifestyle, the maintenance of a nutritious diet, and the discovery of good methods for stress management all seem to be highly recommended. Additionally, there are some customers who are interested in purchasing nutritional supplements, which can assist them in concentrating better and providing them with more overall energy. Furthermore, adopting specific health and nutrition practices well in advance can truly enhance your ability to extract the utmost value from your workout sessions and help you achieve your highest potential in various areas, including nutrition, fitness, and even sports. This can help you get the most bangs for your buck out of your exercise routines. More specifically, these beneficial effects are due to the fitness and nutrition supplements that are taken before an exercise session. Brands that focus on sports nutrition and physical activity and that sell their wares directly to consumers are discovering that selling their own products directly is an effective way to promote those goods.

9.3 Conclusion

Athletes place great emphasis on their diets; nonetheless, it is vital to build a sports diet that is both effective and favorable so as to realize one's maximum potential and maintain a healthy balance in eating habits. Athletes have the responsibility of ensuring that the meals put into their bodies give them the appropriate nutrients to meet the high levels of energy demand they experience during competition, training, and recovery. If these nutritional requirements are not met, there is an increased risk of both poor performance and health issues. Not only is it advantageous, but it is also risk-free and ethical, to use nutrition in a way that is consistent with the guidelines that have been established. Although there have been thousands of studies that have shown the same effectiveness of creative monohydrate supplemented diets through helping to improve anaerobic capacity, strength, and lean body mass through combination with training, there is indeed much variation within food fads as well as practices that truly are specific to sports, which also indicates that coaches as well as peers have a strong influence on the decisions that athletes make. It is of the utmost importance to educate athletes on the appropriate pattern of dietary intake. It is feasible that poor performance might be caused by failing to eat this same appropriate diet all through the competition as a result of an erroneous belief in the value of markets as well as an ongoing worry of consuming items that are forbidden.

References

1. Congeni, J., & Miller, S. (2002). Supplements and drugs used to enhance athletic performance. *Pediatric Clinics of North America, 49*(2), 435–461. https://doi.org/10.1016/s0031-3955(01)00013-x
2. Yusufov, M., et al. (2016). Baseline predictors of singular action among participants with multiple health behavior risks. *American Journal of Health Promotion, 30*(5), 365–373. https://doi.org/10.1177/0890117116646341
3. Modzelewski, K., Fantasia, K., & Steenkamp, D. (2019). Reconsidering meaningful outcomes in diabetes mHealth research. *US Endocrinology, 15*(2), 74. https://doi.org/10.17925/use.2019.15.2.74
4. Yerrakalva, D., Mullis, R., & Mant, J. (2015). The associations of "fatness," "fitness," and physical activity with all-cause mortality in older adults: A systematic review. *Obesity, 23*(10), 1944–1956. https://doi.org/10.1002/oby.21181
5. Bonci, L. (2010). Sports nutrition for young athletes. *Pediatric Annals, 39*(5), 300–306. https://doi.org/10.3928/00904481-20100422-11
6. Prakash, J. K., Mahendru, D., Mahalmani, V., Sarma, P., & Medhi, B. (2020). Athlete biological passport: Practical application in sports. *Journal of Postgraduate Medicine, Education and Research, 54*(4), 227–230. https://doi.org/10.5005/jp-journals-10028-1380
7. MacDonald, M., Fawkner, S., & Niven, A. (2017). How much walking should be advocated for good health in adolescent girls? *Journal of Physical Activity and Health, 14*(1), 59–66. https://doi.org/10.1123/jpah.2015-0391
8. Williams, C., & Rollo, I. (2015). Carbohydrate nutrition and team sport performance. *Sports Medicine, 45*(1), 13–22. https://doi.org/10.1007/s40279-015-0399-3
9. Burke, L., Hawley, J., Jeukendrup, A., Morton, J., Stellingwerff, T., & Maughan, R. (2018). Toward a common understanding of diet–exercise strategies to manipulate fuel availability for training and competition preparation in endurance sport. *International Journal of Sport Nutrition and Exercise Metabolism, 28*(5), 451–463. https://doi.org/10.1123/ijsnem.2018-0289
10. García-Valverde, A., Manresa-Rocamora, A., Hernández-Davó, J., & Sabido, R. (2021). Effect of weightlifting training on jumping ability, sprinting performance and squat strength: A systematic review and meta-analysis. *International Journal of Sports Science & Coaching, 17*(4), 917–939. https://doi.org/10.1177/17479541211061695
11. Spriet, L. (2019). Performance nutrition for athletes. *Sports Medicine, 49*(1), 1–2. https://doi.org/10.1007/s40279-018-1027-9
12. Chen, J., Zhu, B., Ngo, C., Chua, T., & Jiang, Y. (2021). A study of multi-task and region-wise deep learning for food ingredient recognition. *IEEE Transactions on Image Processing, 30*, 1514–1526. https://doi.org/10.1109/tip.2020.3045639
13. Reddy, V. H., Kumari, S., Muralidharan, V., Gigoo, K., & Thakare, B. S. (2020). A survey of agriculture crop monitoring using IOT based image processing and machine learning techniques. *International Journal of Pharmaceutical Research, 12*(3). https://doi.org/10.31838/ijpr/2020.sp3.057
14. Giller, K. (2020). The food security conundrum of sub-Saharan Africa. *Global Food Security, 26*, 100431. https://doi.org/10.1016/j.gfs.2020.100431
15. Bejko, E., Gupta, A., & Mattar, M. (2020). Not every hot, tender, inflamed joint is infected (or gout)! *Journal of Clinical Case Studies Reviews & Reports, 2*(2), 1–5. https://doi.org/10.47363/jccsr/2020(2)115
16. Salim, N., Zeebaree, S., Sadeeq, M., Radie, A., Shukur, H., & Rashid, Z. (2021). Study for food recognition system using deep learning. *Journal of Physics: Conference Series, 1963*(1), 012014. Retrieved July 7, 2022, from https://doi.org/10.1088/1742-6596/1963/1/012014
17. Meng, L., & Xiang, J. (2018). Brain network analysis and classification based on convolutional neural network. *Frontiers in Computational Neuroscience, 12*. https://doi.org/10.3389/fncom.2018.00095

18. Yang, M., et al. (2017). Comparative proteomic exploration of whey proteins in human and bovine colostrum and mature milk using iTRAQ-coupled LC–MS/MS. *International Journal of Food Sciences and Nutrition, 68*(6), 671–681. https://doi.org/10.1080/09637486.2017.1279129

19. Moreira, L., et al. (2019). Development of procedure for sample preparation of cashew nuts using mixture design and evaluation of nutrient profiles by Kohonen neural network. *Food Chemistry, 273*, 136–143. https://doi.org/10.1016/j.foodchem.2018.01.050

20. Ciocca, G., Micali, G., & Napoletano, P. (2020). State recognition of food images using deep features. *IEEE Access, 8*, 32003–32017. https://doi.org/10.1109/access.2020.2973704

21. Dubey, A., Lazarus, A., & Mangal, D. (2020). Handwritten digit recognition using image preprocessing and CNN. *International Journal of Scientific Research in Computer Science, Engineering and Information Technology*, 896–902. https://doi.org/10.32628/cseit206396

22. Liu, C., et al. (2018). A new deep learning-based food recognition system for dietary assessment on an edge computing service infrastructure. *IEEE Transactions on Services Computing, 11*(2), 249–261. https://doi.org/10.1109/tsc.2017.2662008

23. Risha, Y., Susevski, V., Hüttmann, N., Poolsup, S., Minic, Z., & Berezovski, M. (2021). Proteome of breast cancer derived microvesicles. *Siberian Medical Review*, (2), 68–71. https://doi.org/10.20333/25000136-2021-2-68-71

24. Guo, J., & Xu, T. (2017). Deep ensemble tracking. *IEEE Signal Processing Letters, 24*(10), 1562–1566. https://doi.org/10.1109/lsp.2017.2749458

Chapter 10
Machine Learning for Individual Performance Analysis and Sports Analytics

10.1 Introduction

People have been playing sports for pleasure and amusement from the earliest civilizations [1]. Games and activities were considered important for kings and civilizations in those days. Although the early Olympics were originally staged in honor of Zeus, they subsequently became a key weapon to maintain control over opponents [2]. Games and activities have been used in recent times to preserve positive relations among nations. Each nation has its favorite sports and activities, such as tennis and cricket in Asia [3], football & rugby in Britain [4], and soccer in Argentina [5]. Activities and sports are further subdivided into net and barrier sports, assault sports, and attacking and defending sports. Individual players compete in net and wall sports such as table tennis, volleyball, and handball [6]. Soccer, hockey, and polo are team sports in which the team competes for possession and attempts to score a goal over the opposition's goal line [7].

Baseball and softball are both hitting and catching sports. All of these activities are rapidly evolving [8]. Athletes have advanced with time, and each sport has grown over the years. Athletes' efficiency in their chosen sport has also increased in recent years. Professional athletes are putting greater emphasis on endurance to guarantee their places [9]. However, whatever game it is, competition is intense [10]. To guarantee a place on a squad, each player strives to enhance their ability level. Advanced technology has a role in many aspects here. Technological change assists coaches and players in improving their overall productivity. In practice sessions, many teams use current approaches to develop their talents rather than traditional ones [11]. To keep track of their statistics, the data are kept, maintained, and updated regularly. These figures aid management in understanding the team's abilities. However, in addition to these figures, it is critical to examine the approach taken by the participants. This is where machine learning (ML) enters the picture [12]. This technique has recently been applied in match assessment, player performance estimation, and strategy formulation.

© The Author(s), under exclusive license to Springer Nature Singapore Pte Ltd. 2023   113
G. Chhabra et al., *Artificial Intelligence to Analyze Psychophysical and Human Lifestyle*,
https://doi.org/10.1007/978-981-99-3039-5_10

Sports scientists have long studied and analyzed data concerning sports [13]. The growing scale and availability of this information has also piqued the interest of researchers in ML, computer vision, and AI [14]. An essential objective in exercise science is to increase understanding of critical execution and team competition achievement. Data-driven solutions can successfully overcome the psychological limits of the game (human assessment) and provide improved outcomes for soccer teams. The mathematical approach may give such information to players and teams by promoting a better game and incident analysis beyond what anecdotal experience can do [15].

Principles of effective evaluation have typically pushed the analysis of one-dimensional and discrete key metrics into stochastic and comparative techniques [16]. This, nevertheless, leads to rather restricted knowledge since it limits comprehension of the participant connections that underpin player activities and the team's overall behavior [17]. It is logical to suppose that an investigation of such one-versus-one dynamics in team sports would be inadequate, given the importance of multiple relationships in deciding between winning and losing [18]. As a result, it has been proposed that the evaluation process in organized sports should also focus on the relationships between individuals that maintain a team's overall behavior to measure and understand success [19].

Recognizing how collaboration originates from the connection between components of a system, that is, participant communication, is the key to successful assessment in stochastic processes [20]. Many multiplayer competitive events, such as football, do not have data visualization methodologies that take into account the relationships of the individuals. Experts have lately created a range of methodologies and concepts to assist us in comprehending player pathways in games, influenced by scientific investigations of multiple systems. The monitoring of object transmission among competitors may be used to build engagement or move systems [21–25]. The ability to use binding interactions to acquire a practical knowledge of the basic team strategies is a fundamental difficulty.

Repetitive transfer patterns, for instance, may be detected and connected to a player's game style by evaluating the structure of interactions [26]. When the focus is on the player level, contact systems are used to measure and rank individuals' efforts in total teamwork. Due to their dissimilarity and variety, there is no general methodology for forecasting sports data [27]. Furthermore, no specific subgroups of findings are commonly acknowledged. Because collaboration networks are extremely subjective and variable structures, determining a good network characterization that regulates team formation can be difficult [28]. In team sports, measuring gamers' communication is critical to understanding the dynamic patterns that result in goal potential [29].

The fitness industry is already creating massive data pools of unprocessed performance information which, if intelligently exploited and captured [30], has the potential to transform the business. The use of technological advances and approaches such as ML, AI, and big data allows athletic organizations to move beyond basic report creation and into an age of actual prediction, different suggestions, and speedier execution initiatives [31]. With the introduction of datasets such as event logs (e.g., date and place of activities), surveillance data (i.e., positioning data), and individual observation, athletics has become an industry involving a huge quantity of data (e.g., bio-sensors, Inertial Measurement Unit, GPS) [32]. These statistics are regularly and extensively gathered across a range of sports, both professional and amateur.

The availability of such information necessitates the use of the gathered information for conceptual (e.g., game modeling) [33] and pragmatic (e.g., instruction in major leagues) purposes [34]. Only cooperation between both computing and ML groups can deliver problem-solving approaches. As it provides unique techniques for thinking logically about the gathered information [35], ML is developing as a formidable paradigm for sports analytics. However, the ML groups have generally been independent with their agendas, though there have been additional in-depth discussions [36], where the five topics were:

- **ML collides with athletics**. The purpose of this workshop was to offer insight into certain ML algorithms (inferential modeling, information retrieval) and how they may be utilized in the domain of athletics [37]. ML may be used to evaluate the behavior of clubs and players, enhance sports coverage, measure fans' responses to policy adjustments, and help to minimize the time load on video analysts, among other things.
- **The purpose of athletic training encounters**. ML was to offer an understanding of basic principles in sports psychology to educate ML practitioners. The fundamental themes were the relationship between competing, preparation, and player talents, the framework of success in specific sports, and the requirement for assistance in sports practice. The architecture of organized sports as variable complex interactions with spontaneous activity was discussed in detail, as this is the most common approach sector for ML in athletics [38].
- **Vision-Based Analysis in Sports**. The session's goal was to introduce learners to the method of acquiring knowledge about organized sports using analysis and visualization [39]. The course gives an outline of generic object recognition for sports practice. Three of the speakers are from the profession, including organizations with a major presence in the process of giving data to analytical providers on professional sports like basketball, rugby, and field hockey. The fourth speaker, an academic, presented equipment design and statistical information and has also been engaged in the medium for transmitting predictive analytic methodologies from athletics. The main objective of enlightening attendees about recognition approaches and methodologies was successfully addressed by the presentations of these investigators.
- **A multidisciplinary perspective on approaches**. The session's goal was to create a shared knowledge of techniques and their use in forecasting analytics. The subject of how to describe the broad long-term strategy in computational models remains unanswered, and several possibilities were covered in the instance summary and additional talks [40].
- **Modeling, analyzing, and displaying data models for sporting events**. The ability to properly communicate the outcomes of ML models to industry professionals is a major difficulty [41], which is exacerbated by the black-box aspect of

many of these algorithms. This seminar addressed some approaches for achieving this goal, with clear examples drawn from practice in games such as figure skating, ping-pong, and volleyball [42]. This is still an ongoing study field, and some learnings and solutions for improving communication among subject matter experts and technical specialists were explored.

10.2 Categorization of Sports

- **Conquest sports**. Soccer, skating, and volleyball are all invading games in which opposing teams play for control of the ball or puck and aim to accumulate points by placing the ball into the goal area [43]. The performance measurement in these sports is considerably more comparable in that indicators such as the number of chances, control of the game, and transfer rate of success of the participants are taken into account [44].
- **Net and wall sports**. Net sports such as table tennis and volleyball, and wall sports such as Squash, are identical in that participants attempt to obtain control by kicking the ball into the opposing goal. Although the awarding differs in terms of goals, the play is quite identical [45]. In these games, measurements such as service smashes, wildcards, confrontations, and court usage are used to analyze a player. The service is seen as more crucial in determining the performance of players. Serve velocity, service position, and studs are regarded as significant measures in assessing a serve. How a player traverses the ground and the sets he or she plays is also a form of professionalism [46].

Hitting and field sports are those contested between two groups in which the participants hit the ball into the available land over a closed environment, and the opposing fielders are situated in a position that can save [47]. Cricket and football are two instances. These games, particularly cricket, offer a plethora of statistics to consider. These activities have various criteria for the many roles they play in the game. For example, while playing, winning percentage, average, stroke variation, moving between the stumps, and stroke precision are all taken into account. When batting, the line, length of the delivery, the velocity of the bat, economics, accuracy, and minutes per catch are all taken into account [48].

In the instance of playing and wicket-keeping, catches taken, run-outs, stump-outs (wicket-keeping) [49], outfield covering, and dive effectiveness are all taken into account. A single individual cannot record all of the technical specifications at once. This is when several innovations enter the picture. With the digital revolution, the evaluation of these games has increased, which helps players and coaches in their growth. Softball has the same rules. Soccer analytics is not that dissimilar to cricket assessment.

10.3 Study Technique

It is necessary to have a testing process of the activities to analyze participants in organized sports. Based on the data and statistics extracted from a game, an example case may vary from other games. In baseball, a sample case is 30 games for a team, or a year in which one may obtain comprehensive information on each player [50]. This will be useful for analyzing player performance and teams, and predicting future performance in matches. The characteristics may be determined automatically by entering the player and team. However, a statistical evaluation of success is meaningless without a subjective appraisal. In statistical analysis, the data to produce a report is gathered, and quality performance readings are derived using visualization tools, which are document processing techniques. Likewise, gathered information for each game, squad, and player is collected and evaluated into statistical information. These data points are grouped and saved. Because the information to be kept is quite extensive, retrieving information may be problematic periodically [51].

10.4 ML in Games

Predictive analysis makes use of trained ML methods such as the naïve Bayes classifier, decision trees, regression methods, and deep learning. Bayesian inference methods such as k-means classification and association rules are also used in analytic techniques [52]. These systems can analyze sports knowledge from a range of factors to support significant insights into player teamwork and leadership productivity. There are several circumstances in which ML might be used in sports.

- **Recognizing Player and Team Success**. ML delivers in-depth market research that assists trainers and experts in understanding the aspects that contribute to a victory or defeat [53]:

  - Team members' long-term performance and player ability;
  - The impact of every player on the result of a game;
  - Activities that influence the player's performance;
  - In particular scenarios, the main player scores and goals.

- **Prediction of Injuries**. Data analysis and AI-powered technologies aid in the prediction of symptoms and results, which may influence income production, hospital expenses, recuperation, partnerships, and event tickets. Prolonged practice sessions by athletes are one of the leading causes of injuries in sports. Convolutional neural networks (CNNs) and deep CNNs are deep learning techniques that can recognize and analyze the effects of coaching, player attitude, and approach variations. A stochastic model that predicts aids in analyzing how the team responds to any provided training stimulus and determining the possibility of injury depending on the training burden, which can then be altered to minimize the likelihood of injuries [54].

- **Influencing Uncontrollable Evaluation Criteria**. Other aspects, in addition to a teammate's athletic strength and competence at the sport, are surely strong methodologically. These encompass the pitch, temperature fluctuations, the nourishment and relaxation of the athletes, the collaborative environment, and competing variables [55]. Experts may establish a team's realistic and measurable athletic strength by using ML for this sort of information, enabling trainers, proprietors, and organizers to make the most effective coaching and decision-making.
- **Selection of Teams**. Statistical analysis and classification are ML strategies that make the selection of participants somewhat more effective as they offer a methodology for determining the appropriate player for the best location. Intelligent video data analysis, in conjunction with strategic and monitoring statistics, aids in the evaluation of athletes' abilities, biometric identification, and health records [56]. These observations help members decide on how much funds to invest in athletes after conducting a cost–benefit evaluation, thus efficaciously allocating their assets to create the best possible team.
- **Estimates of Player Performance Based on Historical Information**. Based on previous data obtained on the athletes, ML estimates their future. It enables the assessment of an individual team's value of the contract using objective ability instead of just emotional perception, and it permits a more efficient deployment of player development assets [57].
- **Recognizing the Target Audience and Their Interactions**. Recognizing sporting viewers and their involvement in the sport is crucial because it makes people pleasant and leads to more season ticket sales and profitability. ML assists in understanding followers and patterns in follower interest and behavior to devise more effective and more focused product offerings, to enhance direct bookings, and to improve fan engagement. Annual sales can be better understood by using attrition forecasts with regression analysis. Hypotheses with two tails offer information on the effectiveness of focused advertising campaigns.

For such a sporting industry, ML is a game changer. The core concern is developing hardware systems that assist in controlling player exhaustion, limiting illness, and offering knowledge for pre-match and post-match assessment, staff development, balance, and training demands. With improved statistics and actionable information supplied at precisely the right moment, today's modern sports teams have become more robust and effective [58].

A statistical method of athletic performance has been discovered to yield insights that trainers may employ to improve performance during the mentoring relationship. The player's characteristics should be unpredictable, with various abilities and a high level of participation. The neural network may have produced seeming miracles, but its sluggish gaining of insights, particularly during the playing of a sport, has raised the desire for some AI technologies to handle these issues. The role of ML in athletics is growing regularly and over time. Trainers have to work so hard to reach the summit of their profession that some are still hesitant to yield positions to analytics and robots. ML is assisting in obtaining complicated insights about player and team achievements and processing them into some important tips for trainers to better their capabilities.

ML is also useful in developing game plans and approaches for the adversary, as well as identifying the opposition's weaknesses and advantages. If we had a content technology, one could easily undertake performance testing because it would include spatial semantics and repeated occurrences with uniform properties. Once technology affects the games and entertainment industries, the level of evaluation and characteristics of analysis will rise as well. By employing visuals, automated systems can precisely categorize a batter's cricket strike for an activity that can take as little as 1.2 s. ML techniques will not only alter the visual experience in cricket, but also that in volleyball and soccer. ML is also assisting in the recognition of different sequences, which will be important in developing strategies and plans of action. Metadata from prior games allows the computers to forecast players' performance with the least amount of error. It is also essential for athletes to stay fit and log their activities.

10.5 Review of Conversations

10.5.1 Automatic Sensing of Sophisticated Special Trends in Football

Modern football is popular, and most judgments are based on instinctive intuition from industry specialists. The athletic training literature frequently emphasizes the necessity of scientific proof for football strategies; nonetheless, experts have been unable to generate valuable insights due to restricted skills in modeling football mechanics. Recent technological advancements have increased the availability and affordability of high-quality football statistics. Strategic knowledge, which provides player and game positions during every incident of a sport, can be linked with datasets that contain spatial characteristics on every occurrence occurring on the field [59].

The implementation of ML approaches to property issues, on the other hand, results in a seismic shift in several sectors, especially games. Numerous scientific papers on football analytics have been inspired by the demand for better-informed judgments as well as the automation of time-consuming operations, which has been expedited by access to data. The sports and data science approaches solve the issues of synchronization of positioning and activity knowledge, scientifically measuring attacking operations, and identifying the synchronization of positional and event data, objectively measuring offensive activities, and identification of strategic trends.

Statistical and incident information is specifically used in ML methods to discover eight defined strategic and operational trends in football: high-/mid-/low-block defensive, build-up/attacking play in the offense, counter-pressing and defense during progressions, as well as designs before protecting corners and free kicks, such as player-/zonal- or post-marking. For every occurrence, the writers collaborate with football specialists to define criteria and physically identify enormous quantities of information using surveillance videos. To guarantee that every structure is good, inter-annotator dependability is applied.

In the future, semi-supervised algorithms will be utilized to decrease the amount of labeling work. How can detecting strategic trends improve existing processes in professional teams while also leveraging the scope of insightful analysis in exercise physiology by acquiring previously undiscovered observations? Furthermore, the ML arena assesses performance tuning in monitored and quasi-ML in difficult and serious challenges.

10.5.2 Utilizing Statistics to Quantify Ability in Major Sports, from Bits to Bytes

The study investigated how athletes succeed on a basketball floor, both as a team and individually [60]. Researchers can grasp player capabilities considerably better than any specific instrument permits by combining powerful spatial frameworks with location-specific custom maps. The findings demonstrated these notions by describing the ability and outcome of professional athletes employing visual location information, including thousands of millions of occurrences.

10.5.3 ML Approaches for Analyzing Women's Football

Women's football has come a long way in recent times. Regardless of its increasing prominence, there has been no sufficient statistical technique for women's sports. This subsection summarizes preliminary work on assessing scientific information gleaned from competitive women's football games. It offers three studies based on data sources from women's sports over several seasons. First, the researchers conducted the investigation by computing many chart analyses (e.g., target striking percentages across the campaign, exchange rates, attack positions) and then comparing and contrasting them to analogous men's league statistics, discovering some noteworthy discrepancies. Second, to investigate whether expected goals (xG) models developed for one gender identity are applicable to data from a specific gender. Third, early studies examining the differences in the locations and timing of various activities between women and men were presented [61].

10.5.4 A Computer Methodology for Measuring Soccer Accessibility

The study proposed a scheduling algorithm for soccer players' accessibility. The possibility that a pass will reach the intended player without being disputed by adversaries is described as accessible. A digital model for this likelihood is based on simulations of ball movements, player motions, and the throw recipient's professional qualities. To estimate a unified connectivity rating, simply combine those values for all potential deliveries to the destination player. Using information across 58 soccer games, the technique surpasses provincial competition statistically. Furthermore, the findings show that the model can outperform soccer trainers in predicting the availability of professional athletes based on static photographs [62].

10.5.5 AI Videography for Competitive Hockey

The majority of computer vision studies for athletics focus on the transmission channels of competitive contests. Nevertheless, for considerations of size and expense, ML and AI could find even bigger uses in individual sports. For every player, there are 1000 recognized professional athletes in the United States, yet minor teams could often afford to engage a team of seasoned videographers for every match. These criteria inspire the creation of inexpensive AI video methods for professional hockey; we have addressed three main research questions crucial to this objective. The first issue is one of selective attention. Although hockey is played on a huge surface area, immediate play is extremely localized, and supporters in the stands employ both focused perception and sensorimotor processes to maintain their focus on the action.

We will detail our attempt to employ geographical awareness to provide an equivalent seeing experience to individuals watching at home in this area. The resultant alert computer vision software constantly monitors the action in an 8 K broad-range image, autonomously producing a variable HD-focused video that is transmitted in real time to spectators. The second issue is one of spatial attentiveness. While most hockey games last 60 min of regular time, interruptions can cause tournaments to last 140 min. The findings describe a behavioral concentration method that utilizes sensory and auditory signals to extract meaningful outdoor game times from a captured movie, permitting the whole gameplay to be experienced remotely in less time. The third issue is the automated tagging of teams based on organization, which is required for generating performance metrics. An unattended learning technique that enables stable team distribution, even for fresh individuals, allows the approach to be utilized widely without training.

10.5.6 AI in Sporting Events and Medicine

Ubiquitous computer devices are becoming more essential in both leisure and competitive athletics. They are divided into two sections. First, instruments for capturing cardiovascular (ECG, EMG, etc.) and biomechanical (motion sensors, odometers, etc.) information are placed in garments and equipment. Second, tiny microcontrollers (such as those found in smartphones) are employed for data analysis and tracking. These tools, when combined, can give actual data and comments for scientific investigations into real-world sporting scenarios. Several problems must be overcome to deploy these technologies. The study focuses on four of the most common of these. (1) Interconnectivity: sensors and embedded processors must be integrated inconspicuously and capture a range of information. (2) Information exchange: devices and microchips must communicate securely, safely, and efficiently in body-area networks. (3) Interpretation: biological and biomechanical data must be analyzed using information based on ML techniques. (4) Simulation and modeling: comprehending sensor readings is required to precisely describe activities in athletics; simulation approaches assist here by providing fundamental knowledge to guide such simulations [63].

Data mining techniques offer methods for assessing the massive amounts of pharmacological and biomechanical information recorded in athletic scientific research. In practice, the number of people participating and the type of measurement values are limitless, particularly when employing smart wearable devices. Conventional regression allows us to think that we are frequently incapable of dealing with this huge amount of information. As a result, the investigation is frequently limited to independent factors instead of multilayer connections, and a significant amount of data is overlooked. Furthermore, the results are usually skewed by the researcher's expectations. Knowledge mining's unbiased statistics can help here by providing beneficial resources for analytical activities. These technologies are capable of dealing with complex datasets, analyzing numerous aspects at the same time, working with statistics instead of research hypotheses, and providing important ideas about training impacts and risk events.

10.5.7 Soccer Predicament Classification

Events in soccer matches are automatically annotated. At first glance, this appears to be a conventional training data issue. In a reinforcement learning scenario, nevertheless, prediction accuracy is anticipated to correlate strongly with the number of labeled situations: more labeled training data simply promises superior efficiency. However, quasi-labeled scenarios in soccer matches are few, costly, and nearly invariably necessitate the use of human specialists; a reinforcement learning solution looks to be impractical. As a result, the researchers classify the issue into two parts and gain knowledge by: (1) relevant visual features on unsupervised learning at massive scales using discretization and unsupervised learning; and (2) a large-margin clustering algorithm supposed to act in this higher dimensional space, even though using only a few (interactively) manually labeled illustrations of the situation of significance.

10.5.8 Soccer Surveillance Data Captured in Real Time

Tracab is a prominent source of soccer measurements, calculating all teams' locations. The study discusses optical embedded sensors, which were initially introduced around 15 years ago and which have experienced ongoing improvements since then. Considering that attendees at the Dagstuhl conference belong to the athletics research community and use center-of-mass optical player tracking software in their research, the researchers put a special focus on the advantages and limits of optical monitoring systems. The objective is to provide those individuals with a more comprehensive understanding of the information they obtain. The researchers emphasize the significance of conventional object recognition approaches as well as how contemporary learning algorithms are used in the design to facilitate reliability and automation [64].

Furthermore, the study illustrates how general intelligence, in the form of software vendors, has been employed to supplement the capabilities of automated systems, as well as how operational burdens have been minimized with improved technology. The researchers present new enhancements to the technology that exceed the center-of-mass estimate. The researchers specifically show how new algorithms using deep learning enable 3D limb scanning and how this may be used to dramatically boost the speed and efficiency of quasi-infraction determination systems to improve the Video Assistant Referee (VAR) process in soccer. Finally, the study explores how ML algorithms may provide a more comprehensive stream of player statistics based on their physical stance. This data collected ought to be useful for quality analysis soon.

10.6   Conclusion

This study represents the very first indication of an ML-enabled technique for segment autonomous prediction analysis and assessment, with the ability to identify regional quantitative indicators of team development. As the technology develops, it is increasingly important to extend it across several domains. Thus, ML, in conjunction with fitness trackers, can have a significant influence on athletes by generating trends, tactics, and scheduling, minimizing the probability of injury and improving process and quality.

Sporting events are the most popular type of entertainment. There are several forms of sports. Some of these are performed solo, while others are performed in groups. Each country strives for worldwide recognition in many activities. Countries invest in sports and entertainment to enhance the capabilities of the athletes and teams to obtain renown. Many individuals are involved with the research of sports achievements, such as: notational analysts, who develop game plans and tactics; biomechanists, who are responsible for the fitness of players and strive for exceptional outcomes; and team managers and coaches. With the emergence of ML in sporting events, there has been a significant advancement in the assessment of accomplishments.

References

1. Titterton, D. H., & Weston, J. L. (2004). *Strapdown inertial navigation technology* (2nd edn). IEEE.
2. Moeslund, T. B., & Granum, E. (2001). A survey of computer vision-based human motion capture. *Computer Vision and Image Understanding, 81*, 231–268.
3. Moeslund, T. B., Hilton, A., & Krüger, V. (2006). A survey of advances in vision-based human motion capture and analysis. *Computer Vision and Image Understanding, 104*, 90–126.
4. Wang, L., Hu, W., & Tan, T. (2003). Recent developments in human motion analysis. *Pattern Recognition, 36*, 585–601.
5. Aggarwal, J. K., & Cai, Q. (1999). Human motion analysis: A review. *Computer Vision and Image Understanding, 73*, 428–440.
6. Bandouch, J., Jenkins, O. C., & Beetz, M. (2012). A self-training approach for visual tracking and recognition of complex human activity patterns. *International Journal of Computer Vision, 99*, 166–189.
7. Turaga, P., Chellappa, R., Subrahmanian, V. S., & Udrea, O. (2008). Machine recognition of human activities: A survey. *IEEE Transactions on Circuits and Systems for Video, 18*, 1473–1488.
8. Luštrek, M., & Kaluža, B. (2009). Fall detection and activity recognition with machine learning. *Informatica, 33*, 205–212.
9. Luštrek, M., Kaluža, B., Dovgan, E., Pogorelc, B., & Gams, M. (2009). Behavior analysis based on coordinates of body tags. In M. Tscheligi, B. de Ruyter, P. Markopoulos, R. Wichert, T. Mirlacher, A. Meschtscherjakov, & W. Reitberger (Eds.), *Ambient intelligence*. Lecture notes in computer science (Vol. 5859, pp. 14–23). Springer.
10. Darby, J., Li, B. H., & Costen, N. (2010). Tracking human pose with multiple activity models. *Pattern Recognition., 43*, 3042–3058.
11. Mayol-Cuevas, W. W., Tordoff, B. J., & Murray, D. W. (2009). On the choice and placement of wearable vision sensors. *IEEE Transactions on Systems, Man, and Cybernetics, 39*, 414–425.
12. Kern, N., Schiele, B., & Schmidt, A. (2003). Multi-sensor activity context detection for wearable computing. In E. Aarts, R. Collier, E. van Loenen, & B. de Ruyter (Eds.), *Ambient intelligence*. Lecture Notes in Computer Science (Vol. 2875, pp. 220–232). Springer.
13. Zijlstra, W., & Aminian, K. (2007). Mobility assessment in older people: New possibilities and challenges. *European Journal of Ageing, 4*, 3–12.
14. Mathie, M. J., Coster, A. C. F., Lovell, N. H., & Celler, B. G. (2004). Accelerometry: Providing an integrated, practical method for long-term, ambulatory monitoring of human movement. *Physiological Measurement, 25*, R1–R20.
15. Wong, W. Y., Wong, M. S., & Lo, K. H. (2007). Clinical applications of sensors for human posture and movement analysis: A review. *Prosthetics and Orthotics International, 31*, 62–75.
16. Altun, K., Barshan, B., & Tunçel, O. (2010). Comparative study on classifying human activities with miniature inertial and magnetic sensors. *Pattern Recognition, 43*, 3605–3620.
17. Patel, S., Park, H., Bonato, P., Chan, L., & Rodgers, M. (2012). A review of wearable sensors and systems with application in rehabilitation. *Journal of NeuroEngineering and Rehabilitation, 9*, Article number 21.

18. Sabatini, A. M. (2006). Inertial sensing in biomechanics: A survey of computational techniques bridging motion analysis and personal navigation. In R. K. Begg & M. Palaniswami (Eds.), *Computational intelligence for movement sciences: Neural networks and other emerging techniques* (pp. 70–100). Idea Group Publishing.

19. Fong, D.T.-P., & Chan, Y.-Y. (2010). The use of wearable inertial motion sensors in human lower limb biomechanics studies: A systematic review. *Sensors, 10*, 11556–11565.

20. Aminian, K., Robert, P., Buchser, E. E., Rutschmann, B., Hayoz, D., & Depairon, M. (1999). Physical activity monitoring based on accelerometry: Validation and comparison with video observation. *Medical & Biological Engineering & Computing, 37*, 304–308.

21. Roetenberg, D., Slycke, P. J., & Veltink, P. H. (2007). Ambulatory position and orientation tracking fusing magnetic and inertial sensing. *IEEE Transactions on Biomedical Engineering, 54*, 883–890.

22. Najafi, B., Aminian, K., Loew, F., Blanc, Y., & Robert, P. (2002). Measurement of stand-sit and sit-stand transitions using a miniature gyroscope and its application in fall risk evaluation in the elderly. *IEEE Transactions on Biomedical Engineering, 49*, 843–851.

23. Najafi, B., Aminian, K., Paraschiv-Ionescu, A., Loew, F., Büla, C. J., & Robert, P. (2003). Ambulatory system for human motion analysis using a kinematic sensor: Monitoring of daily physical activity in the elderly. *IEEE Transactions on Biomedical Engineering, 50*, 711–723.

24. Tao, Y., Hu, H., & Zhou, H. (2007). Integration of vision and inertial sensors for 3D arm motion tracking in home-based rehabilitation. *International Journal of Robotics Research, 26*, 607–624.

25. Viéville, T., & Faugeras, O. D. (1990). Cooperation of the inertial and visual systems. In *Traditional and nontraditional robotic sensors* (59th edn). NATO ASI Series (Vol. F63, pp. 339–350). Springer.

26. *Proceeding of the Workshop on Integration of Vision and Inertial Sensors (InerVis)*, Coimbra, Portugal, June 2003; Barcelona, Spain, April 2005.

27. Special issue on the 2nd workshop on integration of vision and inertial sensors (InerVis05) (2007). *The International Journal of Robotics Research, 26*, 295–302

28. Zhu, R., & Zhou, Z. (2004). A real-time articulated human motion tracking using tri-axis inertial/magnetic sensors package. *IEEE Transactions on Neural Systems and Rehabilitation Engineering, 12*, 295–302.

29. Yun, X., Bachmann, E. R., Moore, H., & Calusdian, J. (2007). Self-contained position tracking of human movement using small inertial/magnetic sensor modules. In *Proceedings of International Conference on Robotics and Automation*, Rome, Italy, April 10–14 (pp. 2526–2533). IEEE.

30. Junker, H., Amft, O., Lukowicz, P., & Tröster, G. (2008). Gesture spotting with body-worn inertial sensors to detect user activities. *Pattern Recognition, 41*, 2010–2024.

31. Bicocchi, N., Mamei, M., & Zambonelli, F. (2010). Detecting activities from body-worn accelerometers via instance-based algorithms. *Pervasive and Mobile Computing, 6*, 482–495.

32. Zappi, P., Lombriser, C., Stiefmeier, T., Farella, E., Roggen, D., Benini, L., & Tröster, G. (2008). Activity recognition from on body sensors: Accuracy-power trade-off by dynamic sensor selection. In R. Verdone (Ed.), *Wireless sensor networks*. Lecture Notes in Computer Science (Vol. 4913, pp. 17–33). Springer.

33. Ghasemzadeh, H., Loseu, V., & Jafari, R. (2010). Collaborative signal processing for action recognition in body sensor networks: A distributed classification algorithm using motion transcripts. In *Proceedings of the 9th ACM/IEEE International Conference on Information Processing in Sensor Networks*, Stockholm, Sweden, April 12–16 (pp. 244–255). ACM.

34. Schwarz, L. A., Mateus, D., & Navab, N. (2012). Recognizing multiple human activities and tracking full-body pose in unconstrained environments. *Pattern Recognition, 45*, 11–23.

35. Ward, J. A., Lukowicz, P., Tröster, G., & Starner, T. E. (2006). Activity recognition of assembly tasks using body-worn microphones and accelerometers. *IEEE Transactions on Pattern Analysis and Machine Intelligence, 28*, 1553–1567.

36. Wang, L., Gu, T., Tao, X. P., Chen, H. H., & Lu, J. (2011). Recognizing multi-user activities using wearable sensors in a smart home. *Pervasive and Mobile Computing, 7*, 287–298.

37. Yurtman, A., & Barshan, B. (2012). Inter- and intra-subject variations in activity recognition using inertial sensors and magnetometers. In *5th International Conference on Cognitive Systems, Collection of Posters*, Vienna, Austria, February 22–23 (p. 8). Technical University of Vienna, Austria.
38. Roggen, D., et al. (2009). Opportunity: Towards opportunistic activity and context recognition systems. In *IEEE International Symposium on a World of Wireless, Mobile and Multimedia Networks & Workshops*, Kos Island, Greece, June 15–19. IEEE.
39. Lukowicz, P., Timm-Giel, A., Lawo, M., & Herzog, O. (2007). WearIT@work: Toward real-world industrial wearable computing. *IEEE Pervasive Computing, 6*, 8–13.
40. Pantelopoulos, A. (2010). A survey on wearable sensor-based systems for health monitoring and prognosis. *IEEE Transactions on Systems, Man, and Cybernetics—Part C, 40*, 1–12.
41. CONFIDENCE: Ubiquitous care system to support independent living, FP7-ICT-214986. http://www.confidence-eu.org/, 01.02.2008–31.07.2011.
42. Preece, S. J., Goulermas, J. Y., Kenney, L. P. J., Howard, D., Meijer, K., & Crompton, R. (2009). Activity identification using body-mounted sensors—a review of classification techniques. *Physiological Measurement, 30*, R1–R33.
43. Mathie, M. J., Celler, B. G., Lovell, N. H., & Coster, A. C. F. (2004). Classification of basic daily movements using a triaxial accelerometer. *Medical & Biological Engineering & Computing, 42*, 679–687.
44. Bao, L., & Intille, S. S. (2004). Activity recognition from user annotated acceleration data. In A. Ferscha & F. Mattern (Eds.), *Pervasive computing*. Lecture Notes in Computer Science (Vol. 3001, pp. 1–17). Springer.
45. Allen, F. R., Ambikairajah, E., Lovell, N. H., & Celler, B. G. (2006). Classification of a known sequence of motions and postures from accelerometry data using adapted Gaussian mixture models. *Physiological Measurement, 27*, 935–951.
46. Pärkkä, J., Ermes, M., Korpipää, P., Mäntyjärvi, J., Peltola, J., & Korhonen, I. (2006). Activity classification using realistic data from wearable sensors. *IEEE Transactions on Information Technology in Biomedicine, 10*, 119–128.
47. Maurer, U., Rowe, A., Smailagic, A., & Siewiorek, D. (2006). Location and activity recognition using eWatch: A wearable sensor platform. In Y. Cai & J. Abascal (Eds.), *Ambient intelligence in everyday life*. Lecture Notes in Computer Science (Vol. 3864, pp. 86–102). Springer.
48. Pirttikangas, P., Fujinami, K., & Nakajima, T. (2006). Feature selection and activity recognition from wearable sensors. In H. Y. Youn, M. Kim, & H. Morikawa (Eds.), *Ubiquitous computing systems*. Lecture Notes in Computer Science (Vol. 4239, pp. 516–527). Springer.
49. Ermes, M., Pärkkä, J., Mäntyjärvi, J., & Korhonen, I. (2008). Detection of daily activities and sports with wearable sensors in controlled and uncontrolled conditions. *IEEE Transactions on Information Technology in Biomedicine, 12*, 20–26.
50. Yang, J.-Y., Wang, J.-S., & Chen, Y.-P. (2008). Using acceleration measurements for activity recognition: An effective learning algorithm for constructing neural classifiers. *Pattern Recognition, 29*, 2213–2220.
51. Tunçel, O., Altun, K., & Barshan, B. (2009). Classifying human leg motions with uniaxial piezoelectric gyroscopes. *Sensors, 9*, 8508–8546.
52. Khan, A. M., Lee, Y. K., Lee, S. Y., & Kim, T. S. (2010). A triaxial accelerometer-based physical-activity recognition via augmented-signal features and a hierarchical recognizer. *IEEE Transactions on Information Technology in Biomedicine, 14*, 1166–1172.
53. Ayrulu-Erdem, B., & Barshan, B. (2011). Leg motion classification with artificial neural networks using wavelet-based features of gyroscope signals. *Sensors, 11*, 1721–1743.
54. Lara, O. D., Pérez, A. J., Labrador, M. A., & Posada, J. D. (2012). Centinela: A human activity recognition system based on acceleration and vital sign data. *Pervasive and Mobile Computing, 8*, 717–729.
55. Aung, M. S. H., Thies, S. B., Kenney, L. P. J., Howard, D., Selles, R. W., Findlow, A. H., & Goulermas, J. Y. (2013). Automated detection of instantaneous gait events using time-frequency analysis and manifold embedding. *IEEE Transactions on Rehabilitation Engineering* [Epub ahead of print].

56. Witten, I. H., & Frank, E. (2005). *Data mining: Practical machine learning tools and techniques* (2nd ed.). Morgan Kaufmann.
57. Hall, M., Frank, E., Holmes, G., Pfahringer, B., Reutemann, P., & Witten, I. H. (2009). The WEKA data mining software: An update. *ACM SIGKDD Explorations Newsletter, 11*, 10–18. http://www.cs.waikato.ac.nz/ml/weka/
58. Duin, R. P. W., Juszczak, P., Paclik, P., Pekalska, E., de Ridder, D., Tax, D. M. J., & Verzakov, S. (2007). *PRTools 4.1, A MATLAB toolbox for pattern recognition*, Delft Univ. of Tech., 2600 AA, Delft, The Netherlands, August, http://www.prtools.org/download.html. version 4.1.
59. Xsens Technologies B. V. (2009). Enschede, The Netherlands, MTi and MTx User Manual and Technical Documentation. http://www.xsens.com
60. Altun, K., & Barshan, B. (2010). Human activity recognition using inertial/magnetic sensor units. In A. A. Salah, T. Gevers, N. Sebe, & A. Vinciarelli (Eds.), *Human behavior understanding*. Lecture Notes in Computer Science (Vol. 6219, pp. 38–51). Springer.
61. Pfister, G. (2015). Assessing the sociology of sport: On women and football. *International review for the sociology of sport, 50*(4–5), 563–569.
62. Zhao, H., Chen, H., Yu, S., & Chen, B. (2021). Multi-objective optimization for football team member selection. *IEEE Access, 9*, 90475–90487.
63. Chidambaram, S., Maheswaran, Y., Patel, K., Sounderajah, V., Hashimoto, D. A., Seastedt, K. P., & Darzi, A. (2022). Using artificial intelligence-enhanced sensing and wearable technology in sports medicine and performance optimisation. *Sensors, 22*(18), 6920.
64. Ren, J., Xu, M., Orwell, J., & Jones, G. A. (2010). Multi-camera video surveillance for real-time analysis and reconstruction of soccer games. *Machine Vision and Applications, 21*, 855–863.

Chapter 11
Predictive and Performance Analytics in Fitness and Sport

11.1 Introduction

Fitness can be broken down into two types: fitness for a healthy body and fitness for athletic competition. The body's capacity for environmental, sports, and life adaptation is known as fitness. The degree of physical fitness a person possesses determines how well their heart, lungs, circulatory system, and muscles can function to carry out everyday chores without being unduly weary, giving them more time to engage in leisure and entertainment pursuits and be ready for emergencies. The five elements of healthy physical fitness—muscle strength, muscle endurance, flexibility, cardiopulmonary endurance, and body composition—are related to the capacity and standard of daily life or physical activity. According to the principle of health promotion, being in good health refers to a person's total degree of satisfaction, balanced health habits, and full lifestyle, rather than merely avoiding illness. In other words, a person's environment has the potential to either improve or worsen their level of health. A health-promoting lifestyle scale with six dimensions—self realization, social support, health responsibility, exercise behavior, nutritional behavior, and stress management—was created by Sousa et al. [1] based on Poder's theory. A health-promoting lifestyle was described by the authors as a multidimensional spontaneous behavior and perception utilized by people to increase or maintain feelings of happiness, self-satisfaction, and self-realization. The link between regular exercise and a healthy lifestyle has long piqued the curiosity of scientists on a national and worldwide scale. The five pillars of health are directly associated with a person's quality of life, capacity for daily tasks, and capacity for physical activity, according to studies. The human body eventually loses the capacity to adjust to activities as the function of its organs and tissues degrades, which results in disease. Healthy physical fitness benefits pupils in the following ways, according to Hammame et al. [2]: to perform daily tasks like working or reading; adequate levels of health promotion encourage healthy habits and a balanced development of every part of the individual. Baginska and others [3] think that the most fundamental requirements for young people to develop a quality life are good health and fitness. Physically active

G. Chhabra et al., *Artificial Intelligence to Analyze Psychophysical and Human Lifestyle*,
https://doi.org/10.1007/978-981-99-3039-5_11

people have greater stamina for completing their daily tasks, feel more invigorated, have more free time for extracurricular activities, and are better equipped to deal with minor diseases [4]. According to a refined version of the theory of health-promoting behavior, personal traits and prior experiences may have had a direct or indirect impact on prior health-promoting conduct, and the degree to which that influence was felt may have an impact on subsequent health-promoting behaviour. People who exhibit particular behavioural patterns may be affected by cognitive and emotional factors that either directly or indirectly influence their behavioural decisions, promoting health through environmental responses and cognitive factors. However, science is clear on whether a person's level of health fitness influences and predicts health-promoting behaviors among the factors described above. In conclusion, leading a healthy lifestyle and maintaining good physical health go hand in hand. However, lifestyle refers to a person's manner of life or attitude toward their everyday activities. Any action can be managed by a person, including risky and arbitrary behaviors that jeopardize health [5]. There is limited research on whether fitness levels may predict a lifestyle that promotes health, and a few authors in the literature articulate a clear connection between the two in China.

11.2 Components of Physical Fitness

Although you may be aware of the numerous advantages of exercise, such as less risk of chronic disease, enhanced mental well-being, and higher standards of living, what does being physically fit actually entail? You can use the five aspects of fitness that are related to your health as a guide to help you get fit and encourage good health. Here are five areas to concentrate on while you pursue fitness. Cardiovascular endurance is one of his five fitness-related health domains [6].

- **Strength**: The amount of power or weight that a muscle can lift.
- **Muscular Endurance**: The capacity of a muscle to continue moving for an extended amount of time.
- **Flexibility**: The capacity to rotate joints and muscles in all directions.
- **Body Composition**: The ratio of skeletal and muscular lean mass to total body fat.
- **Exercise**: Supports good health and has various advantages.

The immediate advantages include better blood pressure, sleep, mood, and insulin sensitivity. According to various studies, it also provides defense against a variety of diseases and health problems, including heart disease, stroke, type 2 diabetes, osteoporosis, depression, dementia, and some types of cancer. It can also promote good aging and extend the amount of years that one spends healthy and active.

11.3   Sport Performance Analysis

Sport performance analytics offer unbiased data that coaches and athletes may use to analyze and enhance team and player performance. Analysts or coaches who watch and "mark" events and actions during competitive games and practice sessions often undertake analysis. You may concentrate on the entire game and analyze your team's performance by using marked events and actions. You could also concentrate on specific players. Sports performance analysis software often uses a timeline with highlighted events and actions to provide detailed statistical data. Statistics that are visually represented in charts and graphs can offer quick and precise feedback. Additionally, video feedback is provided by sports performance analytics so that athletes may see where they can improve [7].

Coaches and athletes can better grasp a team's and a player's strengths and shortcomings with the use of sports performance analysis. Improve player skills, streamline schedules, and empower your team with enhanced knowledge and resources.

To continue to be successful, coaches and players must recognize the strategies, tactics, and adjustments that have worked and failed in previous games. These findings from sports performance analysis are supported by quantifiable numbers as opposed to conjecture or gut feeling. It is simpler to understand what defines a good or terrible performance when sports performance is analyzed. Coaches cannot base their decisions on what they observe throughout a game. According to studies, coaches typically use 40% of the crucial performance variables in a game. Gains in performance are constrained if the observations are very shaky. Sports performance analytics decisions are measurably accurate.

11.4   Predictive Fitness Analytics

Predictive analytics is a key application since it may show how a team should play on game day. Which interns help the team perform better?

We can forecast which players would perform better in which positions on match day using machine learning algorithms. Some approaches are based on game variables like player statistics, how they perform versus rival teams, and where they play: at home or away? Therefore, based on the game's circumstances and your opponents, you can forecast which player will fit in which position [8].

- **Player Analysis**: To enhance each player's on-field performance and level of fitness. Using team statistics, team administrators can determine winning combinations and their probability using cutting-edge machine learning models like deep neural networks and support vector machines (SVMs).
- **Fan Management Analytics**: In order to find trends within the fan base, clustering algorithms, targeted advertising, and social media data can all be used. Club management can concentrate on increasing those components to both draw in

new fans and keep hold of current ones when they are aware of the features that appeal to fans the most.

Data are used in predictive analytics to foretell future trends and occurrences. To assist you in making strategic decisions, use past data to forecast prospective scenarios. The forecast could be for anything short term, like a machine breakdown later in the day, or it could be for something more long term, like the company's cash flow for the next year. You can perform predictive analytics manually or with the aid of machine learning techniques. In either scenario, predictions about the future are based on historical evidence. Regression analysis, which enables you to ascertain the link between two variables (basic linear regression) or three or more variables, is one tool for predictive analysis (multiple regression). Mathematical formulas are used to define relationships between variables in order to predict results when variables change. Predictive models that assess player performance and calculate the probabilities of winning or losing a sporting event have been developed thanks to advances in predictive analytics. The use of these analytics to forecast athlete performance in sports is a well-known success story [9].

The process for which Predictive Fitness has filed a patent application has been the subject of ongoing study and development since 2005. It consists of a high-end, exclusive dataset with biometric and performance data from over 50 million internationally optimized training sessions for athletes. Data mining, machine learning, artificial intelligence, and other advanced analytics are used to collect and analyze data, together with advanced data normalization technologies and a variety of analytical and prescriptive tools.

11.5 Technology and Sports Analytics

For sports teams, IT companies are creating wearable technology. In order to assist coaches and staff in making informed judgments, businesses are changing the landscape by precisely analyzing player performance metrics, health, and safety. Players are more vulnerable to injury as sports require higher levels of performance. Wearable sports technology is used to track injury rehabilitation, prevent illness and injury, and measure performance during practice and competition. There are numerous different sizes and styles of portable workout equipment. The seamless design of the gadget is also used in sportswear materials, sporting equipment like balls and rackets, and small devices worn by athletes that fasten to their bodies in waistbands, skin patches, or shoes. Equipped with Bluetooth and GPS technology, these devices provide coaches with real-time feeds to laptops and other electronic devices for analysis.

Either sports betting companies or clubs that are directly participating in the game commission sports analysts. Any sport or game data can be used to illustrate sports analytics. These data can be utilized to create predictive machine learning models, which can be used by management to make defensible judgments, like player statistics, weather data, and recent team wins and defeats. Sports analytics' major goal is to boost a team's performance and its chances of winning games. The benefit of success is evident in numerous ways, including: seats at stadiums filled with fans, TV deals, souvenirs in fan shops, parking lots, concessions, sponsorships, registrations, fervor, and even community pride.

11.5.1 Injury Prediction

Many athletes and teams know that apprehending situations raising the danger of injury is the most important information. Injuries to teams can have a detrimental impact on income creation through medical expenditures, recovery, sponsorships, and ticket sales as they lose their early competitiveness. Similar to how it can benefit athletes, knowing how to prevent injuries can help them earn more money, lengthen their careers, and maximize their ratings. We must make efforts to balance exertion and stress with appropriate recuperation time, diet, and sleep in order to be more successful in predicting injuries. Increased injury rates may result from overtraining and overuse injuries. A binomial logistic regression model helps predict the likelihood of injuries by identifying how players react to particular training stimuli. Models can be grouped according to the stage of the season (preseason, early competition, late competition). To reduce the chance of injury, you can modify your exercise load accordingly. Neuromuscular data are collected using a strength platform and motion analysis software to analyze how each athlete uses their various body muscles as well as their speed, reaction time, and weak points. Motion capture and high-speed cameras can be used to analyze stances that are dangerous. Convolutional neural network (CNN) models, one type of deep learning technology, can be constructed to better understand changes in athlete posture and technique.

11.5.2 Player Scouts

Teams that invest money in their players use automated video analytics, location, and tracking data for their scouts more and more. When they are virtually evaluating their abilities, biometrics, and medical data, insights like this offer them confidence. Particularly in the post-pandemic age, this technique has proved quite beneficial. Similar to this, using machine learning methods like clustering and statistical analysis greatly simplifies player scouting by giving scouts a data-driven method for choosing the right players. After determining the important metrics that affect the choice of suitable players, clustering can be done. The k-means algorithm can efficiently divide player groups into various clusters, considerably streamlining the process of data presentation. These clusters aid in the discovery of players that have comparable influence but less substantial financial value than well-known players.

11.5.3 Strategy

Finding the best plans for each game situation requires anticipating the strengths, weaknesses, and trends of the opposition's teams and coaching staff. Opposing teams can use GPS monitoring measures to gain insight about player movement patterns. The team is always changing, therefore an individual no longer plays the entire game in the same configuration. The vectors between each player and their remaining teammates during a game were calculated, and the average of the vectors between each pair of players, over predetermined time periods, was used to decide the formation. This provides a precise assessment of relative positions. Teams can alter their tactics by determining the clusters of defensive and attacking formations that are most frequently paired. By offering reliable insight into what might happen after each decision to reach optimal performance, data science in sports can assist in maximizing revenues.

11.5.4 Transition of Commuter Pass

It is less expensive to keep current season ticket holders than to bring in new ones. For a sports organization to forecast its Return on Investment (ROI), predicting customer turnover and determining the causes of client churn are crucial. Poor on-field performance, low game attendance, and low customer engagement can all be contributing factors to turnover. Season ticket holders that are more likely to churn can be identified using a prediction model that employs logistic regression.

11.5.5 Player Evaluation and Growth

Understanding the true value of players and the associated risks to create better rosters can save organizations significant costs. In order to compete in larger leagues, financially weaker teams can now sign the proper players using a data-driven strategy. This gives players time to adjust to a system that supports their growth. Analytics can be utilized to develop training plans and tactics that boost the value of players. Similar to this, you can evaluate a player's strengths and flaws by providing a brief commentary on the player's performance during a game or practice.

11.5.6 Pricing

The primary source of income for every sporting group is ticket sales. By assessing ticket prices in light of past performance data, pricing models aid in maximizing revenue. Organizations can use this data to determine occupancy based on competition and resistance, and change ticket pricing based on the desired income.

11.6 Performance Analysis

Performance analysis is a field of study that offers unbiased data to athletes and coaches to assist them in analyzing their performance. Systematic observations that offer accurate, trustworthy, and comprehensive information regarding performance serve as the foundation for this approach. By offering objective statistical analysis and visible feedback (video analytics), performance analytics enhance the coaching process (data analytics). Video analysis involves real-time feedback to help you better comprehend and execute your strategies and moves [10]. Examples include data analysis. A gap comparison between our performance and that of our competitors is provided by speed split data which is accurate to 1/100th of a second.

Decisions can be made more rationally and less speculatively thanks to objective information. Athletes who receive comments based on data are better able to pinpoint exactly what they did to achieve success or failure. Athletes and coaches can perform consistently by using this knowledge to make the appropriate choices at the right times. Athletes can benefit from improved technical and tactical understanding, better decision-making, and more confidence. Coaches gain from these advantages because they can better identify athletes' strengths and shortcomings and improve their own coaching techniques.

The Sports Institute's Performance Analysis Team goes above and beyond the conventional methods of video analysis; by utilizing cutting-edge performance analysis software, athletes and coaches will have a better understanding of performance and be able to make better decisions regarding their training and interventions [11].

Example 1: Support for Competition

Analysis of performance is used to record the performances of athletes and, when appropriate, their rivals. Analyzing videos of athletes competing provides coaches with quick information for making decisions in the moment. Performance analyzers are aware that coaches have access to precise data and footage of events, allowing the athletes to focus. These records/data are used for purposes other than direct competitive events:

- To encourage strategic thinking, and to provide examples and statistics on your adversary, you have data showing how well athletes perform, and you can create plans to decrease the performance gap between these athletes and the best in the world. You can assess the demands of your rivals using data. Hence, you will gain a deeper comprehension of what it takes to succeed and how to employ the most effective performance tactics available as a result.

• Future training interventions will be informed by data.

11.7   Performance Analysts in Sport

Sports performance is evaluated through the process of performance analysis in order to better comprehend activities that can guide decision-making, improve performance, and assist coaches and players in achieving their goals. This includes tactical scoring, movement analysis, video and statistical databases and modeling, as well as the presentation of coach and player data, in various team sports.

Prior to a few years ago, the sole responsibility of a performance analyst was to record practices and games and produce highlighted videos for coaches and players to watch. The analyst's job entailed a sizable portion of video capturing and editing. The function of a performance analyst has changed now, necessitating them to have greater proficiency in the variety of tracking hardware and software that technology advancements have brought to market. In order to improve data collection, storage, and presentation, coaching is becoming more and more necessary. Professionals studying the enormous volumes of data gathered in the world of sports must analyze, disseminate, and derive insights from that data as the big data phenomenon expands.

Like everyone else, performance analysts are located in a team's locker room. They must record all play during a game, tag it later, and produce a video playlist for each player the following day. The management team then organize one-on-one meetings with the players during which are presented and discussed videos highlighting the game's successes and flaws. In addition, team meetings will be held to go through offensive and defensive formations, tactical analysis, and pertinent actions that coaches should take while watching the video analysis of the game. When they believe it necessary to review a particular area that is pertinent to them in order to improve, players and coaches may also request one-off clips and analysis.

In addition to keeping records and conducting educational activities, a football maximum performance analyst is responsible for a variety of other duties. Pre-match analysis for the team's health assessment, competition evaluation, live-day coding, and editing of player injury photos for the submission of health reports, upkeep of education databases and logs for each session, and updating of statistical and video databases for performance evaluation are some of these duties.

Analyst jobs have become considerably more specialized in a subset of the functions a conventional analyst may have performed in the past. Roles like scouting analyst, tactical analyst, studies analyst, technical scout, education analyst, or goalkeeper analyst are emerging positions within the world of overall performance evaluation. However, while they reflect the importance of such roles in competitive carrying teams, they may also be eroding the formerly more defined role of an overall performance analyst and his or her duties.

11.7.1 Importance of Performance Analysis

Less than half of the significant acts and motions that occur on the field are remembered by coaches and players, according to research, so, like everyone else, other strategic information gained during the game is obscured. The information gathered from matches through video recording aids in eradicating these biases and offers a more impartial account of what transpired during the game. Performance analysts gather data from each on-field activity and generate pertinent analytics, either upon coaches' requests or based on their own assessments, to communicate to players and coaches what went well and what didn't.

11.7.2 The Skillset Required for a Performance Analyst

When compared to other analyst professions in other industries, the performance analyst's nature is athletic. Sports are typically at the extreme end of the spectrum by default, and analysts' daily lives reflect this. In comparison to many other analytical stances, it has greater highs and lows. In a field where every team member, from player to employee, is expected to contribute 110% of his time, long hours, quick turnarounds, last-minute demands, and high standards and expectations have become the norm. To succeed in this industry, a performance analyst must have a few specific qualities and hard skills [12]:

- **Expertise in Sports**: The utilization of contextual information to produce insights is the primary distinction between statisticians and analysts. For the sake of the team's success as well as her own coaching style of team management, she must comprehend what is significant and what is not in the sport she is evaluating. What do players' coaches expect of them? Performance analysts can assist their team to succeed by utilizing players, other coaches, club philosophy, and history in addition to tactical understanding.
- **Establishing Connections with Trainers**: The backroom crew of the team includes analysts. This means that, as with any team, building strong bonds with the coaches and players is essential to gaining their respect and getting credit for a job well done, including listening. In fact, it can take an analyst up to four years to truly adjust to a top-notch team of specialists. Analysts must always be aware of the coach's exact needs and be prepared to offer fast, reliable analysis and information. Today, an analyst's main responsibility is to give the information that his or her coaching staff asks for.
- **Effectively Address Criticism**: The analyst's capacity to adapt the work generated to the requirements and preferences of the staff and players is consistent with developing connections with coaches. To produce extremely deep insights, analysts can dig into detailed data analysis for hours. Trainers and other staff members require knowledge in an easily applied, accessible format for planning and decision-making.

- **Awareness of Data**: For each study or report they produce, analysts must be able to distinguish between data items that are relevant and those that are redundant, and from a variety of sources, both internal and externally gathered. Additionally, they must be able to evaluate the accuracy and dependability of the data used and possess sophisticated knowledge of how it was gathered, kept, or accessed. Mismanagement of records can lead to false reports that mislead coaches and athletes.
- **Presentation of Analytical Reports**: Analysts should give coaches, players, or team managers exceptional interpretations of their findings depending on the club's ideology and the coach's reputation. Analysts have the chance to establish themselves on the coaching staff and gain credibility by being able to explain outcomes to coaches in a clear and concise manner. For analysts to deliver their findings to athletes and coaches, effective communication skills are a necessity.
- **Hard Analytical Skills**: It should go without saying that analysts need to be well-versed in a range of analytical tools and coding languages, from Excel basics to complex SQL, R, or Python coding. To create and comprehend complicated data, it is crucial to have strong math, IT, research, and analysis skills. To present results in an understandable way, skill with tools like Tableau is essential. Data visualization also plays a significant role.
- **Performance Analysis Goals in Sport and Fitness**: To enable coaches to gain quick insights in areas needing their attention, the vast amount of quantitative and qualitative data included in the complex and dynamic conditions in recreation needs to be carefully disseminated and authentically presented. This can be achieved by utilizing clear visual aids such as tables, charts, or specialized diagrams like visual representations of the playing surface. Performance analysis enhances the ability of the teacher to "feed-forward." It aims at identifying a competitor's strengths and weaknesses through presenting a thorough competitor evaluation to provide a learned understanding that enables the team to practice the right performances and enhance the character skills of those individuals who could be a resource for outperforming the immediate competitor.

Coaches can choose a squad and make tactical decisions that will best capitalize on an opponent's vulnerabilities and defeat their strengths with the use of insights obtained from performance analysis work and competition evaluation. Historically, those decisions were made in their entirety after a teacher had gained knowledge from years of participation in the sport, frequently having previously competed at elite levels themselves. However, research has repeatedly demonstrated that teachers recall critical incidents occurring during a sporting event in only a range of 42% to 59% of instances. Furthermore, the events that are remembered are susceptible to incompleteness, emotional bias, inaccuracy, and misinterpretation due to the inherent limitations of human perception and cognitive capacity. Coaches have adapted to technology and analytics to gain instant access to past goal statistics as well as instant video clips so as to review specific events they wish to remember and reassess in order to overcome these barriers in an increasingly competitive environment. For this, the majority of top-level coaches now benefit from their own performance analyst departments, which give them the necessary data collection, data manipulation, analysis, and video evaluation skills to enable them to benefit from the large amounts of data generated from their game while still obtaining those key elements most important to them in a clear, timely, and concise manner.

11.8 Conclusion

By reading this chapter, athletes can improve their technical and tactical understanding of sports as well as their performance. When you are aware of your areas requiring development, you may concentrate your time and efforts there. Players are more prepared to choose wisely when playing the game. Decision-making under duress is made simpler when team members are aware of the analyst's game plans, the best way to carry them out, and an overview of his or her colleagues' performance. All of this helps team members gain confidence and performance in-game. This chapter has pointed out that each player must be treated individually based on their physical, mental, social, and economic status. Common approaches during training/coaching negatively impact player performance. Personalized training/coaching/monitoring is difficult without performance analysis tools. This system helps trainers manage and monitor their training/coaching activities. As part of the future scope, other aspects such as nutrition planning, training sessions, medication, and counseling sessions that may affect an athlete's performance in competition could be integrated.

References

1. Sousa, P., Gaspar, P., Fonseca, H., Hendricks, C., & Murdaugh, C. (2015). Health promoting behaviors in adolescence: Validation of the Portuguese version of the adolescent lifestyle profile. *Journal of Pediatrics, 91*, 358–365. https://doi.org/10.1016/j.jped.2014.09.005
2. Hammami, A., Randers, M. B., Kasmi, S., Razgallah, M., Tabka, Z., Chamari, K., et al. (2017). Effects of soccer training on health-related physical fitness measures in male adolescents. *Journal of Sport and Health Science, 7*, 169–175. https://doi.org/10.1016/j.jshs.2017.10.009
3. Baginska, J., Rodakowska, E., Kobus, A., & Kierklo, A. (2018). The role of Polish school nurses in the oral health promotion for 7–19 year-old children and adolescents. *European Archives of Paediatric Dentistry, 38*, 32–34. https://doi.org/10.1007/s40368-020-00546-6
4. Mooney, B., Timmins, F., Byrne, G., & Corroon, A. M. (2010). Nursing students' attitudes to health promotion to: Implications for teaching practice. *Nurse Education Today, 31*, 841–848. https://doi.org/10.1016/j.nedt.2010.12.004
5. Al-Qahtani, M. F. (2019). Comparison of health-promoting lifestyle behaviours between female students majoring in healthcare and non-healthcare fields in KSA. *Journal of Taibah University Medical Sciences, 4*, 508–514. https://doi.org/10.1016/j.jtumed.2019.10.004
6. Abalo, J., Varela, J., & Manzano, V. (2007). Importance values for importance–performance analysis: A formula for spreading out values derived from preference rankings. *Journal of Business Research, 60*(2), 115–121. ISSN 0148-2963. https://doi.org/10.1016/j.jbusres.2006.10.009

7. Vazou, S., Mischo, A., Ladwig, M. A., Ekkekakis, P., & Welk, G. (2019). Psychologically informed physical fitness practice in schools: A field experiment. *Psychology of Sport and Exercise, 40*, 143–151. https://doi.org/10.1016/j.psychsport.2018.10.008

8. McGarry, T., O'Donoghue, P., & de Eira Sampaio, A. J. (Eds.). (2013). *Routledge handbook of sports performance analysis.* Routledge.

9. Barnekow-Bergkvist, M., Hedberg, G., Janlert, U., & Jansson, E. (1998). Prediction of physical fitness and physical activity level in adulthood by physical performance and physical activity in adolescence–an 18-year follow-up study. *Scandinavian Journal of Medicine and Science in Sports, 8*(5 Pt 1), 299–308. https://doi.org/10.1111/j.1600-0838.1998.tb00486.x. PMID: 9809389.

10. Blanchfield, J. E., et al. (2019). Developing predictive athletic performance models for informative training regimens. *Systems and Information Engineering Design Symposium (SIEDS), 2019*, 1–6. https://doi.org/10.1109/SIEDS.2019.8735633

11. Luo, M., Yu, Y., Xu, W., Zhang, Q., & Xia, J. (2020). Analysis and prediction on sports performance of primary school students. *Chinese Automation Congress (CAC), 2020*, 1041–1045. https://doi.org/10.1109/CAC51589.2020.9327386

12. Liu, H., Liu, Y., & Li, B. (2021). Predictive analysis of health/physical fitness in health-promoting lifestyle of adolescents. *Frontiers in Public Health, 18*(9), 691669. https://doi.org/10.3389/fpubh.2021.691669.PMID:34490182;PMCID:PMC8416607

Chapter 12
Computer Vision for Pose Estimation in Real Time

12.1 Introduction

Pose estimation is a type of computer vision that predicts and tracks the positions of people and other objects. This is done by combining observations of the stance and orientation of the particular person or object. Determining the joint locations of the human body from images and videos is a procedure known as "human posture estimation." A person's actions can be deduced by studying the movements of their body across a series of photographs to identify the storyline. This makes the recognition of actions a natural extension of the evaluative human stance. Over the past ten years, deep neural network developments have significantly improved human posture estimation methods. The subject of human pose estimation and its application to motion detection is not extensively documented, despite studies looking at innovative approaches for motion detection [1, 2]. The fact that action recognition can use human position estimation does not imply that the two tasks are unrelated or that action recognition is a downstream activity. Action recognition might be what keeps human pose estimation from stagnating. For instance, a precise estimate of skeletal joint locations is necessary to detect motor activity. Accurate body joint locations must be taken into account when creating an explainable diving rating system so that it can accurately assess diving performance.

12.2 Human Pose Estimation

Finding, connecting, and following semantically important points is necessary when performing computer vision tasks such as human position estimation and tracking. This alludes to how a subject is posed in a picture or video. Pose estimation, on the other hand, is the challenge of determining where and how to point a camera at a certain person or object. To do this, it is typical to identify, locate, and track a number of important spots on a certain object or person. Corners or other distinctive features

© The Author(s), under exclusive license to Springer Nature Singapore Pte Ltd. 2023
G. Chhabra et al., *Artificial Intelligence to Analyze Psychophysical and Human Lifestyle*,
https://doi.org/10.1007/978-981-99-3039-5_12

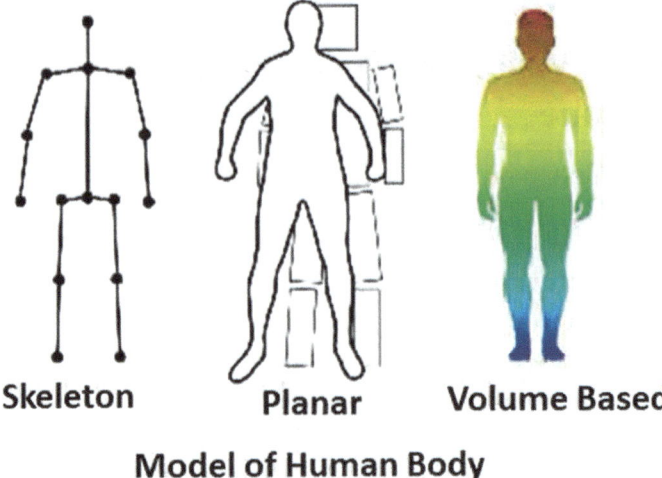

Skeleton   Planar   Volume Based

Model of Human Body

Fig. 12.1 Model of the human body

of an object may be included. The elbow and knee are two important joints in humans that relate to these crucial regions. The purpose of machine learning techniques is to follow these focal points in images and movies [3].

The terms "left knees," "vehicle's left brake lights," and "right shoulders" are examples of semantic key phrases. The substantial processing resources required to carry out semantic keypoint tracking in live video footage have reduced the precision of posture assessment. Recent innovations have made it possible to implement new applications with real-time requirements, such as self-driving cars and robotic last-mile delivery. Convolutional neural networks (CNNs) are the foundation for the best image processing algorithms currently available. Therefore, cutting-edge techniques are frequently built on creating a CNN architecture that is especially suited for human pose inference.

As shown in Fig. 12.1, there are three different methods for modeling the human body.

12.3 Categories of Pose Estimation

These key points serve as the human equivalents of the elbows, knees, wrists, and other major joints. Human pose estimation is the name given to this process. One particular class of flexible objects includes people. When our arms or legs are bent, key points will be positioned differently in relation to one another. Inanimate items tend to be stiff. For instance, regardless of the brick's orientation, the distance between its corners is constant. Rigid posture estimation is the process of predicting where these items will be. Additionally, there is a significant difference between the 2D and 3D posture estimates. The term "2D pose estimate" refers to the straightforward estimation of keypoint locations in 2D space in connection to an image or video frame. For each keypoint, the model predicts an X and Y coordinate. When using a 3D posture estimate, an object in a 2D image appears to be 3D by inserting a z-dimension in the forecast.

To predict where a person or object will be located in space, we can utilize a 3D posture estimation. The development of datasets and algorithms that account for a variety of factors, such as the background environment of an image or video and lighting conditions, is complex, making 3D posture estimation a bigger challenge for machine learning. Discovering one or more objects in a photo or video differs from finding many objects. These two methods, which are essentially self-explanatory, go by the labels "single" and "multipose estimation": single-pose estimation methods only identify and follow one person or object, in contrast to multipose estimation methods [1].

12.3.1 Pose Estimation Matter

In the past, object detection systems have viewed humans as nothing more than a bounding box (a square). By performing stance detection and pose monitoring, computers may train themselves to comprehend human body language. However, conventional pose tracking methods lack the necessary speed and occlusion resistance to be useful. High-performance real-time pose identification and tracking will be the key enabler for some of the most important advancements in computer vision. By following a person's whereabouts in real time, for example, computers will be able to develop a more detailed and logical understanding of human behavior. Many other businesses, including autonomous driving, will be strongly impacted by this. The majority of self-driving car collisions now involve "robotic" driving, in which a human driver collides with a self-driving car that has made an approved but unexpected stop. Using real-time human stance detection and tracking, computers can comprehend and anticipate pedestrian behavior substantially better, enabling more natural driving.

Pose estimation enables us to precisely track an object or person (or a group of people, as we will discuss in a moment) in actual space. There are countless potential applications for this strong attribute.

Pose estimation is also significantly different from other common computer vision problems in a number of important respects. The process of finding things in an image is called object detection. The object is typically contained within a bounding box in this localization, which is usually coarse-grained. By predicting the exact location of the object's keypoints, pose estimation goes one step further.

Pose estimation can be used to automatically follow human movement. It has the potential to result in the creation of a new generation of automated tools designed to evaluate the precision of human movement, ranging from AI-powered personal trainers and virtual coaches for sports to monitoring movements on production floors to ensure worker safety [2]. Pose estimation provides additional possibilities beyond monitoring human motion and activities in a range of areas such as gaming, robotics, animation, and augmented reality.

12.3.2   Working of Pose Estimation

With a fundamental grasp of what pose estimation is, how it varies from other types of pose estimation, and the applications it might serve, let us take a closer look at how it works.

We will look at numerous machine-learning-based methods for pose estimation and assess their advantages and disadvantages, with a focus on neural networks, which have emerged as cutting-edge approaches for pose estimation.

In general, deep learning architectures suitable for pose estimation are built on variations of CNNs. A top-down strategy and a bottom-up strategy are the two main approaches. The model first attempts to arrange clusters of keypoints into skeletons for various objects using a bottom-up approach to find every instance of a particular keypoint (for instance, all left hands) in an image. An object detector is used to crop each instance of an item in a top-down approach, and the network then estimates the keypoints within each cropped region.

Despite the fact that we have already addressed it, it is important to remember the distinction between 2 and 3D posture estimates. The two methods are applied to various kinds of problems and entail different amounts of data (2D pixel values vs. a 3D spatial arrangement).

12.4   Human Pose Estimation Using Machine Learning

The study of pose detection is a current topic in computer vision. There are hundreds of research articles and models that attempt to address the issue of posture detection. The extensive range of applications and practicality of pose estimations are what draw so many machine learning applications to them. Here, we will discuss one such use of pose detection and estimation that makes use of several practical Python tools and machine learning.

Pose estimation is a computer vision technique used to track the motion of an object or person. This is usually done by locating key areas for the products that are provided. By comparing other positions and motions to these fundamentals, we may assess them. Pose estimates are frequently used in the augmented reality, gaming, and robotics industries.

Several different posture estimation approaches have been developed over the past ten years (e.g., DeeperCut [4], DeepPose [5], DeepLabCut [6], OpenPose [7], ArtTrack [8], and AlphaPose [9]). These techniques enable the usage of pretrained networks that are publicly accessible as well as the training of brand-new networks that are specialized for various research or therapeutic needs. A common pretrained network that comprises keypoints of the body, feet, hands, and face is the human pretrained demo of OpenPose, for example. It has been used in a number of recent studies for the quantitative analysis of human movement. It is frequently necessary to use many computer resources to track new films and build new networks. Therefore, using a graphics processing unit (GPU) with the sufficient processing power may be required to ensure processing times stay within reasonable bounds. As observed in some situations, the documentation for many algorithms often contains suggestions for the best hardware to use for this function. For processing more quickly, some computing environments, such as Google Colaboratory, allow users without their own GPUs to access the GPU. However, because the processing is done externally, these settings might not be suitable for applications that hold protected health information. Processing without a GPU may be sufficient while being slower, depending on the user's time constraints and processing needs (e.g., length of videos, the number of people tracked, the number of key points tracked). Pose estimation can be used for real-time movement monitoring as well. Some users may find this capability to be especially helpful because it may be used to give real-time biofeedback for a variety of applications. Other approaches include optimization and filtering methods in addition to these deep learning methods that are growing in popularity for posture estimation.

12.5 Classical and Deep Learning

The main focus of HPE (Human Pose Estimation) techniques is computer vision, which is used to comprehend the complex geometry and kinematic data of the human body.

This section discusses two approaches to HPE: the conventional technique and the deep learning-based approach. We will also discuss how deep learning techniques, such as CNNs, outperform conventional methods for capturing the geometry and motion data of the human body.

12.5.1 Classical Approaches to 2D Human Pose Estimation

Typically, "classical approaches" refers to methods and tactics that use machine learning techniques. For instance, in earlier work, human position was evaluated using random forests within a "pictorial structure framework." This was used to forecast the joints of the human body.

The visual structural framework is one of the common methods for assessing a human Positional Structural Framework (PSF). The PSF was divided into two sections:

1. Discriminator: This calculates the likelihood that a particular component will be found in a particular place. In other words, it identifies the parts of the body.
2. Prior: Modeling the probability distribution over poses using the discriminator's output is the process; the modeled posture needs to be precise.

The primary goal of PSF is to display the human body as a set of coordinates for each body part in a given input image. Nonlinear joint regressors, ideally two-layered regressors from a random forest, are used in PSF. These models work well when there are distinct and visible limbs in the input image, but they are unable to identify and model limbs that are hidden or veiled from a certain angle.

Utilizing feature-building methods such as the histogram-oriented Gaussian (HOG), contours, or histograms these issues were resolved. Despite using these strategies, the classical model lacked accuracy, correlation, and generalization abilities; therefore, transitioning to a more successful tactic was inevitable.

12.5.2   Deep-Learning-Based Approaches to 2D Human Pose Estimation

One of the most important features of deep-learning-based approaches is their ability to generalize any function. For computer vision tasks, deep CNNs outperform all other techniques, and HPE supports this. Because it can extract patterns and representations from an input image more precisely and accurately than any other technique, CNN is a great tool for tasks such as classification, detection, and segmentation.

Contrary to the traditional approach, where the features were manually created, CNN is capable of learning complicated features given enough training validation.

12.6   Human Pose Estimation Applications

Let us take a closer look at some of the most common real-world applications of HPE.

12.6.1   Personal Trainers with AI

Currently, maintaining our physical health has become essential to living a fulfilling life, and working with a qualified trainer can help us get to the fitness level we want. It is not surprising that the industry has been oversaturated with apps that use AI to improve fitness. For instance, the AI-powered yoga app Zenia leverages HPE to direct you toward adopting the ideal posture while doing yoga. Your stance is detected using the camera, and it calculates how accurate it is; if it is accurate, the anticipated pose will be shown in green. Red takes the place of green if the stance is incorrect. In addition to yoga, HPE has also been used in other types of physical activity. For instance, it is now frequently used in weight lifting, where it may instruct app users on how to conduct a proper weight lift by looking for common errors and providing advice on how to correct them to avoid injury.

12.6.2 Robotics

Robots can be created to follow the trajectories of a human posture skeleton that is acting rather than having to be manually programmed to do so. A robot may be efficiently taught specific acts by a human instructor simply by watching them being performed. The robot may then determine the best way to position its articulators to carry out the desired action. One of the development fields with the quickest growth has been robotics.

Deep learning techniques can help, as programming a robot to follow a routine can be laborious and time-consuming. Robots can be successfully trained using methods such as reinforcement learning, which employ a simulated environment to reach the accuracy level necessary to carry out a specific task.

12.6.3 Motion Capture and Augmented Reality

For CGI applications, human pose estimation is a fascinating use case. If the person's human position can be calculated, graphics, styles, extravagant improvements, equipment, and artwork can be superimposed on them. The produced images may "naturally suit" the person as they move by keeping track of the various iterations of this human posture. The film industry, in particular, spends much money on computer-generated visuals to produce special effects, enigmatic creatures, fantastical landscapes, and much more.

Because it takes so much work—such as wearing specialized clothing and masks to capture motion, producing surface-level effects in the approximated position, processing power, and significant time commitments on top of that—CGI is expensive. HPE can build a 3D rendering of a 2D input by automatically extracting important points, which may then be used to add effects, animations, and other things.

12.6.4 Detection of Athletes' Poses

Currently, data analysis plays a significant role in practically all sports. Pose recognition can assist players in honing their technique and obtaining better outcomes. Pose detection also enables analysis and understanding of the strengths and weaknesses of the adversary, which is crucial for professional athletes and their coaches.

12.6.5   Gaming with Motion Tracking

Pose estimation has another intriguing usage in in-game applications, where users can add poses to the gaming environment by using HPE's motion-capturing technology. The objective is to develop an interactive game environment. For instance, Microsoft's Kinect tracks player movements and employs 3D pose estimation (using data from IR sensors) to render character actions digitally in the gaming world.

HPE is another tool that can be utilized to analyze newborn movements. This is highly useful for examining the baby's behavior as it develops, especially for determining the pace of its physical growth. When cerebral palsy, movement difficulties, or traumatic injuries are to blame, infants may be born with major health problems affecting their muscles, joints, and neurological system.

Motion analysis can be used to pinpoint which muscles or joints need to be adjusted. Pose estimates can identify minute irregularities in the infant's movement, which doctors can examine and treat appropriately. Additionally, HPE can be used as a tool for advice on how to help children with their physical abilities so that they can be as independent as possible.

12.6.6   Recognition of Activities

Activity, gesture, and gait identification can all be performed by tracking a person's changes in position over time. The same has a variety of applications, such as programs that can tell if a person has fallen or is ill:

- Software that can teach suitable exercise routines, sports techniques, and dance moves on its own;
- Software programs that can comprehend full-body sign language (e.g., traffic signals, runway signals at airports);
- Programs that can improve surveillance and security.

12.7   Problems with Pose Detection in Humans

Due to dynamic variations in the body's appearance brought on by various kinds of garments, arbitrary occlusions, occlusions produced by viewing angles, and surrounding contexts, pose estimation is a challenging problem. Pose estimation needs to be resistant to challenging real-world variations such as light and weather. The challenge for image processing models is to recognize the fine-grained joint coordinates. Finding tiny, scarcely noticeable joints to follow is very difficult. The estimation of a person's head posture is a common computer vision challenge. Estimating head posture can be used for a variety of tasks, such as face alignment, 3D model fitting to movies, and modeling attention. Traditionally, the target face's keypoints are employed to compute the head position and solve the 2D to 3D correspondence problem using a mean human head model. The 3D posture of the head can be recovered as a result of keypoint-based facial expression analysis, which is based on the extraction of 2D facial keypoints using deep learning techniques. These techniques can withstand obstructions and drastic pose changes.

The majority of cutting-edge techniques concentrate on tracking and detecting human body poses. However, some models were created to work with both cars and animals (object pose estimation). Additional difficulties with animal posture estimation include a dearth of labeled data and a high frequency of self-occlusions. As a result, animal databases are often tiny and comprise a small number of animal species. A difficult computer vision problem is estimating the pose of many animals because of the frequent interactions that lead to occlusions and make it difficult to attribute important locations to the appropriate animal. It can be difficult for animals to interact with each other more closely than people would normally. Techniques called transfer learning have been developed to reapply human solutions to animal issues. The tracking and estimation of various animal positions using DeepLabCut, a state-of-the-art, well-liked, open-source posture estimation toolkit for both animals and people, is one example.

12.8 Conclusion

The fascinating possibility exists for making quantitative investigations of human movement kinematics substantially more approachable with the rise and continued development of HPE approaches. Pose estimation algorithms quickly address the important and widespread demand for low-cost, user-friendly, and accessible technology that enables the tracking of human movement in virtually any setting, including the home, clinic, classroom, playing field, and other "in the wild" circumstances. We think that these technologies are still in their infancy in terms of their potential for use in both research and therapeutic contexts, although applications for human performance and health have begun to surface in the literature. Users must be aware of the limitations that still exist and adjust their expectations accordingly. We believe that pose estimation applications in human health and performance will continue to advance in the coming years, although these technologies will provide powerful tools for capturing significant human movement features that have been difficult to record with conventional methods.

References

1. Siddiqui, M., & Medioni, G. (2010). Human pose estimation from a single view point, real-time range sensor. *IEEE Computer Society Conference on Computer Vision and Pattern Recognition - Workshops, 2010*, 1–8. https://doi.org/10.1109/CVPRW.2010.5543618
2. Changotra, R., et al. (2022). A comparative study of pose estimation. In *2022 2nd International Conference on Innovative Practices in Technology and Management (ICIPTM)* (pp. 210–216). https://doi.org/10.1109/ICIPTM54933.2022.9754071
3. Bakken, R. H., & Eliassen, L. M. (2012). Real-time 3D skeletonization in computer vision-based human pose estimation using GPGPU. In *2012 3rd International Conference on Image Processing Theory, Tools and Applications (IPTA)* (pp. 61–67). https://doi.org/10.1109/IPTA.2012.6469538
4. Insafutdinov, E., Pishchulin, L., Andres, B., Andriluka, M., & Schiele, B. (2016). DeeperCut: A deeper, stronger, and faster multiperson pose estimation model. In B. Leibe, J. Matas, N. Sebe, & M. Welling (Eds.), *Computer vision – ECCV 2016*. ECCV 2016. Lecture Notes in Computer Science (Vol. 9910). Springer. https://doi.org/10.1007/978-3-319-46466-4_3
5. Toshev, A., & Szegedy, C. (2014). DeepPose: Human pose estimation via deep neural networks. In *Proceedings of the IEEE Computer Society Conference on Computer Vision and Pattern Recognition, Columbus, OH, USA*, 23–28 June 2014 (pp. 1653–1660).
6. Mathis, A., Mamidanna, P., Cury, K. M., Abe, T., Murthy, V. N., Mathis, M. W., & Bethge, M. (2018). DeepLabCut: Markerless pose estimation of user-defined body parts with deep learning. *Nature Neuroscience, 21*, 1281–1289.
7. Cao, Z., Simon, T., Wei, S. E., & Sheikh, Y. (2017). Realtime multi-person 2D pose estimation using part affinity fields. In *Proceedings of the 30th IEEE Conference on Computer Vision and Pattern Recognition, Honolulu, HI, USA*, 21–26 July 2017 (pp. 1302–1310).
8. Insafutdinov, E., Andriluka, M., Pishchulin, L., Tang, S., Levinkov, E., Andres, B., & Schiele, B. (2017). ArtTrack: Articulated multiperson tracking in the wild. In *Proceedings of the 30th IEEE Conference on Computer Vision and Pattern Recognition, Honolulu, HI, USA*, 21–26 July 2017 (pp. 6457–6465)
9. Fang, H., Xie, S., & Lu, C. (2018). RMPE: Regional multi-person pose estimation. arXiv:1612.0017373

Studies in European Economic Law and Regulation

Volume 11

Series editors
Kai Purnhagen
Law and Governance Group, Wageningen University, Wageningen

Josephine van Zeben
Worcester College, University of Oxford

This series is devoted to the analysis of European Economic Law. The series' scope covers a broad range of topics within economics law including, but not limited to, the relationship between EU law and WTO law; free movement under EU law and its impact on fundamental rights; antitrust law; trade law; unfair competition law; financial market law; consumer law; food law; and health law. These subjects are approached both from doctrinal and interdisciplinary perspectives.

The series accepts monographs focusing on a specific topic, as well as edited collections of articles covering a specific theme or collections of articles. All contributions are subject to rigorous double-blind peer-review.

More information about this series at http://www.springer.com/series/11710

Irena Georgieva

Using Transparency Against Corruption in Public Procurement

A Comparative Analysis of the Transparency
Rules and their Failure to Combat Corruption

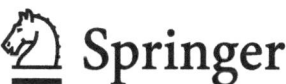 Springer

Irena Georgieva
PPG Lawyers
Sofia, Bulgaria

ISSN 2214-2037   ISSN 2214-2045   (electronic)
Studies in European Economic Law and Regulation
ISBN 978-3-319-51303-4   ISBN 978-3-319-51304-1   (eBook)
DOI 10.1007/978-3-319-51304-1

Library of Congress Control Number: 2017933696

Printed on acid-free paper

This Springer imprint is published by Springer Nature
The registered company is Springer International Publishing AG
The registered company address is: Gewerbestrasse 11, 6330 Cham, Switzerland

Foreword

This is a most timely and most welcome work. It is timely because it arrives just as the new procurement directives package of 2014 has come into force; it is most welcome because it addresses the very serious matter of corruption in public procurement with a comparative law perspective. The author has a mission – an ambitious and exciting one – to contribute to the awareness of the part that corruption still plays in procurement. It is one thing to have paperwork in order, to tick the boxes, as it were, but it is quite another thing to establish that there is no elephant in the room. Appearances can be deceptive, and the field of procurement is certainly no exception.

Working from the experience and practice in Bulgaria, with comparators in the German and Austrian systems, Dr Georgieva offers the reader a clear and surprising insight into just how what might look above board is in fact decidedly underhand. The importance of transparency in procurement cannot be overestimated, although of course there are many aspects to compliance and successful high-quality procurement and procurement processes. The attractiveness of Dr Georgieva's work lies in the systematic and almost enchanting way in which she peels back the veils of corruption, like a magician removing layer after layer of covers to reveal the hidden jack-in-the-box. This is a work with a pan-European message and imagery.

While in some countries people think that procurement is straightforward, there is no Member State that is free from some form of diversion from the yellow brick road: a meeting here or there, a favour to someone's family, a holiday or two in an agreeable location or even a straightforward brown envelope with some enriching contents. Corruption in procurement is not, thankfully, endemic, but it is more prevalent than many would like to admit.

European Union law has sought to coordinate national rules relating to procurement, so that above the thresholds a clear systematic approach will apply, albeit with some options available for the Member States. Often, contracting authorities find the European rules irritating, even burdensome, but that is to misunderstand why the rules are there and how they operate to promote a level playing field characterised by undistorted competition, transparency and open access to market participants within the internal market that is at the heart of the European Union's structure. The new rules have given much – perhaps even too much – room for social and other certain policy objectives to play a role. These objectives are laudable and may indeed be essential (in particular as regards the environment); however, they can also be abused to disguise the desire of local politicians and others to promote their hobbyhorses and the interests of their friends and allies. Corruption may also be intellectual and not just financial in nature.

The general criterion of MEAT (the most economically advantageous tender) is certainly better than simply looking at the lowest price, which may well not always be the best value for money. In applying MEAT contracting authorities must remain within the legitimate bounds of their discretion and stay on the yellow brick road. Dr Georgieva's work should assist those who wish to ensure that contracting authorities succeed in doing so. Her book deserves a wide and interested readership, and I wish her and it success.

University of Groningen   Prof. Laurence W. Gormley
Groningen, Netherlands

Preface

Writing about corruption is not particularly easy. Writing about corruption in your own country – even less so. However, the effort is worth it if the problematic issues revealed and the suggestions provided bear fruit and change the status quo for the better. Performing the process of awarding public procurements correctly and in the interest of all stakeholders, especially a country's taxpayers, is of extreme significance as well as a very challenging topic, and the search for the right path continues.

This book is aimed at all those who sooner or later face a public procurement award due to the nature of their business or because they have to apply the regulations in their capacity as a contracting authority, as well as to the academics who continue to study this vast subject. Procurements themselves represent an artificial mechanism which seek to protect public resources by creating much stricter rules for spending 'common funds' than are usually found in the relations governing ordinary traders. When a resource is shared, however, determining responsibility for it is often more complex. Who owns the resource actually, who is liable for its distribution and what rules should regulate the transaction can be hard to determine and difficult to oversee. Finally, it is much more challenging to prove theft from the state than from a particular person. That is why in this atypical 'vacuum' of rules and procedures, corrupt practices emerge much more frequently, and because the appetites are much larger, corruption in this sector flourishes abundantly.

Procurement rules will continue to have its ups and downs, and their adaptation to real life will continue much longer. It is for this reason that I hope my work on this book, and the contrast that is made between the different countries, will be taken into account in the implementation of the new procurement rules at European level. Indeed, EU is a community of countries that have agreed to profess the same values, but to be successful the eyes of this alliance must be focused precisely on the 'individual cases'. This is especially true for public procurements and the many corruption opportunities they create.

I would like to thank all who have contributed to bringing this book into being and to helping my analysis of the three Member States researched here acquire meaning and completion.

I express my special gratitude to Prof. Laurence W. Gormley (University of Groningen, Netherlands) for the enormous dedication, guidance and support. Further, many thanks to Prof. Georgi Dimitrov (Bulgarian Academy of Sciences, Bulgaria) for his assistance and belief in his former student; to Prof. Elisabetta Manunza (University of Utrecht, Netherlands), Prof. Huib van Romburgh (University of Groningen, Netherlands) and Prof. Gert-Wim van de Meent (University of Amsterdam, Netherlands) for sharing their valuable opinions on my work; and, last but not least, to the public procurement legal expert Johannes Stalzer for taking the time to consult me on my work on the analysis of Austria.

Thanks to all my friends and especially my family, for having supported me throughout and for having always stood by my side.

Sofia, Bulgaria   Irena Georgieva
October 2016

Contents

About the Author

Dr Irena Georgieva is a Bulgarian attorney and expert in public procurement law with over 15 years of practice. Currently, she works as a legal advisor and manager of her own niche law office in Sofia focused on public procurement and data protection matters. Dr Georgieva has graduated in law from Sofia University (master in law 2003) and has also a postgraduate qualification in accountancy from the University of National and World Economy, Sofia (2005). She obtained her doctoral degree in the University of Groningen, Netherlands (PhD 2015), with dissertation thesis on public procurement law. She takes part in many undertakings related to public procurement matters – round tables, open discussions and seminars – and is also a regular author of public procurement articles published in domestic and international law and business magazines. She is a member of the Sofia Bar Association.

Abbreviations

ANAO	Bulgarian National Audit Office Act (*Закон за сметната палата*), S. 12/12.2.2015, as amended
AO	Austrian Audit Office (Rechnungshof)
APCA	First Bulgarian Award of Procurement Contracts Act, SG 9/3.1.1997, repealed SG 56/22.6.1999
APFIA	Bulgaria Public Financial Inspection Act (*Закон за държавната финансова инспекция*), SG 33/21.4.2006, as amended
BAK	Austrian Federal Bureau of Anti-Corruption (*Bundesamt zur Korruptionsprävention und Korruptionsbekämpfung*)
BAKG	Austrian Federal Law on the Establishment and Organisation of the Federal Bureau of Anti-Corruption (*Bundesgesetz über die Einrichtung und Organisation des Bundesamts zur Korruptionsprävention und Korruptions-bekämpfung*), BGBl. I No. 72/2009, as amended
BBG	Austrian Federal Public Procurement Agency (*Bundesbeschaffung GmbH*)
BHO	German Federal Budget Code (*Bundeshaushaltsordnung*), BGBl. I S. 1284/19.8.1969, as amended
BIAC to OECD	Business and Industry Advisory Committee to the OECD
BKMS	German Business Keeper Monitoring System
BORKOR	Bulgarian project BORKOR (*БОРКОР*), launched under the aegis of the Minister of Interior and the Deputy Prime Minister in 2009
BVergG	Austrian Federal Procurement Act (*Bundesvergabegesetz*), BGBl. No. 17/2006, as amended
CM	Council of Ministers of Bulgaria (*Министерски Съвет*)
CMS	Bulgarian Corruption Monitoring System of the Center for the Study of Democracy

Civil and Criminal Law Conventions against Corruption	Civil Law Convention on Corruption (adopted 4 November 1999) CETS 174 and Criminal Law Convention on Corruption (adopted 27 January 1999) CETS 173
CPB	Central Purchasing Body, as defined Article 2(16) Directive 2014/24/EU
CPC	Bulgarian Commission for Protection of Competition (*Комисия за защита на конкуренцията*)
CPCCOC	Bulgarian Center for Prevention and Countering Corruption and Organised Crime (*Център за превенция и противодействие на корупцията и организираната престъпност*), established by decree of the Council of Ministers on 29 July 2010
CPI	Corruption Perceptions Index of Transparency International
CPV	Common Procurement Vocabulary, provided for in Regulation (EC) No. 2195/2002 of the European Parliament and of the Council as the reference nomenclature for public contracts
CSD	Center for the Study of Democracy (*Център за Изследване на Демокрацията*), founded 1989 in Sofia, Bulgaria, as an interdisciplinary public policy institute dedicated to the values of democracy and market economics
Directive 2004/17/EC	Directive 2004/17/EC of the European Parliament and of the Council coordinating the procurement procedures of entities operating in the water, energy, transport and postal services sectors OJ L134/1
Directive 2004/18/EC	Directive 2004/18/EC of the European Parliament and of the Council on the coordination of procedures for the award of public works contracts, public supply contracts and public service contracts OJ L134/114
Directive 2014/24/EU	Directive 2014/24/EU of the European Parliament and of the Council on public procurement and repealing Directive 2004/18/EC OJ L94/65
Directive 2014/25/EU	Directive 2014/25/EU of the European Parliament and of the Council on procurement by entities operating in the water, energy, transport and postal services sectors and repealing Directive 2004/17/EC OJ L94/243
ECJ	European Court of Justice
ESPD	European Single Procurement Document under Article 59 of Directive 2014/24/EU
EU	European Union
EU Commission	European Commission

First PPA	First Bulgarian Public Procurement Act, SG 56/22.6.1999, repealed SG 28/2004
GATT	General Agreement on Tariffs and Trade, signed in Geneva on 30 October 1947
GDP	Gross domestic product
GRECO	Group of States against Corruption, established in 1999 by the Council of Europe to monitor states' compliance with the organisation's anti-corruption standards
GWB	German Act against Restraints of Competition (*Gesetz gegen Wettbewerbsbeschränkungen*), Federal Gazette I, p. 2546, of 26 August 1998, as amended
GWB (VergRModG)	GWB after the transposition of the New Procurement Directives and the amendments made with VergRModG
IACA	International Anti-Corruption Academy, initiated by UNODC, OLAF and the Republic of Austria in 2010
IMK	Standing Conference of the Ministers and Senators of the Interior of the *Länder* in the Federal Republic of Germany
MEET	Bulgarian Minister of Economy, Energy and Tourism (*Министър на икономиката, енергетиката и туризма*)
Member State(s)	Current state(s), which is/are member(s) of the EU
NAO	Bulgarian National Audit Office (*Сметни палата*)
New PPA	Now applicable Bulgarian Public Procurement Act (*Закон за обществените поръчки*), transposing of the New Procurement Directives, SG 13/16.2.2016, effective as of 15 April 2016
New Procurement Directives	Collective reference to Directive 2014/24/EU and Directive 2014/25/EU
OECD	Organisation for Economic Co-operation and Development, founded in 1961 to promote economic progress and world trade
OECD Anti-Bribery Convention	Convention on Combating Bribery of Foreign Public Officials in International Business Transactions (1997) adopted by the OECD Negotiating Conference
OJEU	Official Journal of the European Union

OLAF	European Anti-Fraud Office (*Office européen de lutte antifraude*), charged by EU to protect its financial interests, established 1999
Pact	Integrity Pact created by TI as tool for monitoring procurement projects in Bulgaria
PFIA	Bulgarian Public Financial Inspection Agency (*Агенция за държавна финансова инспекция*)
PPA	Bulgarian Public Procurement Act (*Закон за обществените поръчки*), applicable before the transposition of the New Procurement Directives, SG 28/06.4.2004
PPAgency	Bulgarian Public Procurement Agency (*Агенция по обществени поръчки*)
Procurement Directives	Collective reference to Directive 2004/17/EC and Directive 2004/18/EC
Remedies Directive	Directive 2007/66/EC of the European Parliament and of the Council amending Council Directives 89/665/EEC and 92/13/EEC with regard to improving the effectiveness of review procedures concerning the award of public contracts [2007] OJ L335/31, as amended
SAC	Bulgarian Supreme Administrative Court (*Върховен Административен Съд*)
SektVO	German Ordinance on the Award of Public Contracts by Utilities (*Verordnung über die Vergabe von Aufträgen im Bereich des Verkehrs, der Trinkwasserversorgung und der Energieversorgung*), BGBl. I S. 3110/23.9.2009, as amended
SGB	Austrian Criminal Code (*Strafgesetzbuch*), BGBl. I S. 3322/13.11.1998, as amended
SME	Small and medium enterprises
Solution Model	Solution Model in the Area of Public Procurement, launched on 21 February 2012 by CPCCOC
StGB	German Criminal Code (Strafgesetzbuch), Federal Gazette I, p. 945, p. 3322, of 13 November 1998, as amended
TEU	Treaty on European Union, signed in Maastricht in 1992
TFEU	Treaty on the Functioning of the European Union, consolidated version OJEU C326/47, 30 October 2012
TI	Transparency International, founded in 1993 as a non-governmental organisation that monitors and publicises corporate and political corruption in international development

TIBG	Bulgarian branch of Transparency International (*Прозрачност без Граници България*), founded in 1998
Treaties	Collective reference to TEU and TFEU
TUAC to OECD	Trade Union Advisory Committee to the OECD
UNCAC	United Nations Convention Against Corruption, signed 9 December 2003 in Merida, New York
UNODC	United Nations Office on Drugs and Crime, founded in 1997
VergRModG	German Act for the Modernisation of Public Procurement Law (Gesetz zur Modernisierung des Vergaberechts), BGBl. I S. 203/23.2.2016, Federal Gazette I, p. 2546, of 26 August 1998, as amended
VergRModVo	German Regulation for an Act for the Modernisation of Public Procurement Law (Verordnung zur Modernisierung des Vergaberechts), 18 March 2016
VgV	German Ordinance on the Award of Public Contracts (Vergabeverordnung), BGBl. I S. 321/22.02.1994, as amended
VOB/A	German Procurement Regulation for Public Works (Vergabe– und Vertragsordnung für Bauleistungen), 20.9.2009, BAnz. 196a/29.12.1997, as amended
VOF	German Procurement Regulations for the Award of Independent Contractor Services (*Verdingungsordnung für freiberufliche Leistungen*), 12.05.1997, BAnz. 164a/03.09.1997, as amended
VOL/A	German Procurement Regulation for Public Supplies and Services (*Vergabe– und Vertragsordnung für Leistungen*), 31.7.2009, BAnz. 155a/15.11.2009, as amended
WIN	Whistleblowing International Network
WKStA	Austrian Public Prosecutor's Office for *White-Collar Crime* and Corruption (*Zentrale Staatsanwaltschaft zur Verfolgung von Wirtschaftsstrafsachen und Korruption*)
WTO	World Trade Organisation, formed on 1 January 1995 under the Marrakesh Agreement, the successor to the GATT

Table of Cases of the European Court of Justice and the General Court (in chronological order)

Chapter 1
Introduction

1.1 Aspects Analysed

The book scrutinises the transparency obligations, the procurement rules, and the participants and responsible control institutions in procurement award in three Member States. It seeks to prove that obedience to the transparency principle is not an essential element of the proper response to corruption in the spending of public funds. The comparison between the Bulgarian public procurement system and the German and Austrian systems is performed through detailed research not only as regards adherence to the transparency principle, but also as to the use of other mechanisms to limit corruption, insofar as they are appropriate and could be adapted in other countries which lack sufficient anticorruption measures. The broad-spectrum analysis of these Member States' anticorruption rules in the procurement process also refers to the new procurement package and the new national legislation. The book contains a strong critical line on the broadened (with the new rules) discretion of the contracting authorities, the new legal solutions that could actually expand the corruption in the sector, as well as the separate national solutions designed with the transposition of the new rules.

The types of infringements involving corruption typical of the different phases of the award process are classified and discussed in additional detail, as is their link to violations of the transparency principle. The following methodology is used in this part of the work: (i) description of the EU law provisions breached[1]; (ii) description of the infringement itself; (iii) violation of transparency rules, if any; and (iv) types of corruption loopholes opened. Structured in this manner, the method I have applied not only helps prove that in most cases manifestations of corruption and infringements do not depend on the level of publicity of the process and often do not

---

[1] And, where applicable, also national legislative provisions. Some infringements have already been overcome in some Member States, but in others (like Bulgaria) they remain an issue.

© Springer International Publishing AG 2017
I. Georgieva, *Using Transparency Against Corruption in Public Procurement*,
Studies in European Economic Law and Regulation 11,
DOI 10.1007/978-3-319-51304-1_1

even violate transparency, but also identifies the weak points in the award process which still need treatment and future legislative solutions.

The systems of control and appeal against the contracting authority's actions within the various legislative schemes are reviewed and compared, and the legislative weaknesses which fail to reduce corruption are highlighted. The functions of the control and appellate authorities of the three Member States are examined so that the ineffectiveness of some of the institutions (ie in Bulgaria) is clearly revealed, along with their lack of awareness of the process participants' actual activities, tending mainly to monitor the legal compliance of the award process and the observation of procedural requirements.

By way of background and thus to achieve all the above, I also introduce a brief historical overview of the Bulgarian legislation in the field of public procurement and corruption. This serves both to illustrate the trend towards the constant increase in transparency rules and to highlight the individual social and economic specificities of corruption in this Member State. A proper understanding of the 'national identification' of corruption in a given country and its origins is extremely important if the most common manifestations of corruption are to be identified, as well as properly to analyse the options available to deal with corruption and limit its occurrence to a minimum. In this light, some of the conclusions drawn in this book can be viewed as general conclusions regarding how corruption should be prevented in procurement, but others need to be considered through the prism of the national characteristics and specificity of one Member State to achieve an appropriate level of objectivity.

1.2 Benchmarking

The benchmarking presented in this book aims to reveal that the legislation of the countries which succeed in combating corruption does not focus on cumbersome imperative rules making procurements public knowledge, and does not rely so much on transparency in the fight against corruption. Although all the countries examined are Member States of the EU and base their legislation on European directives, they achieve a balance between the amount of transparency rules and the quality of prevention of corruption in entirely different manners.

Comparison between these Member States is important for the development in the regulation of public procurement towards clearer and simpler procedural rules and towards meaningful anticorruption measures. It exposes the main weaknesses in a legislative system which over the last decade has undergone endless amendments and supplements, but has not yet succeeded in limiting corruption and the resulting considerable loss of public funds. The goal of the work is to 'debunk' the unconditional policy to pursue transparency as the key way to combat corrupt procurement participants and pre-allocation of public funds. Although this policy is in fact dictated by the EU, in the example of Bulgaria the attempts to overcome criticism against widespread corruption in public contracts have been manifested solely through legislative changes targeting at the monitoring and publicity of procedures, but not through efficient rules aimed at enhancing the competence of control bodies and/or strengthening the sanctioning mechanism against corruption.

Various criteria have determined the selection of the countries with which the procurement system of Bulgaria is compared so that the contrast between the legislative solutions can be discerned. The goal was to select those examples whose good practices could actually be implemented in countries with similar issues to Bulgaria, practices which do not appear outlandish or impossible to apply to this legal system, or diametrically opposite to the economic and social situation of the country. This is of utmost importance in ensuring that the conclusions highlighted from this comparative work are reliable and applicable to other countries with similar concerns within the EU. The Member States were examined in view of the following characteristics: (i) corruption levels, (ii) procurement system efficiency, and (iii) historical, substantive and economic similarities. Precisely from this perspective, Germany and Austria turned out to be a logical choice for benchmarking, given that a good proportion of the above criteria were met, along with proximity of legislative systems and deep existing economic relations between the three countries.

Germany and Austria are reviewed on the basis of their main legislative rules regulating public procurement and the transparency rules applicable to procurement awards. Their main legislative and institutional solutions for combating corruption are reviewed. Positive practices which could be adopted by other countries with less success in this sphere have been identified, as have such which yield good results in Germany and/or Austria (and/or are EU based legal solutions) but cannot be regarded as suitable to other Member States.

The book presents an in-depth review of three different legislative solutions regulating public procurement which focus (each employing its own means) on the fight against and the prevention of corruption in the selection of contractors. The parallels drawn between those Member States provide findings which could contribute both to combating corruption at the national level and to the creation of more appropriate and effective anticorruption measures at the EU level. For this reason the works' contribution is relevant not only to the particular legal systems reviewed in detail but also to other Member States in which public spending is systematically threatened by corruption. The distinguishing angle taken by the research in this respect makes the work particularly useful – good EU legislative solutions are not just extracted and identified as such, but account is taken of the possible applicability of the measures and how they can be approached practically in countries which still do not fit within the definition of an average Member State.

Chapter 2
The EU Principles in Public Procurement. Transparency – Origin and Main Characteristics

> 'Cellophane, Mister Cellophane
> Should have been my name
> Mister Cellophane
> 'Cause you can look right through me
> Walk right by me
> And never know I'm there!'
> (Fred Ebb 'Mister Cellophane', 'Chicago' musical)

2.1 The Procurement Principles. The Concept of Transparency

Transparency is an important element in public procurement policy and law. Particularly given the socially significant nature of the complex system needed for the proper use of public money by all those institutions and commercial companies defined as 'contracting authorities', the basic principles governing such spending should be well defined, and a central plank of these principles is transparency. In all aspects of public procurement the public sector can influence the market structure, affect the competitive process between the market participants, and affect significantly the economic behaviour of the participants in procurement processes. As a rule, contracting authorities rely on the competitive environment in public procurement to achieve the most efficient use of their budgets. They are interested in buying products at low prices and of high quality, since their resources are usually more constrained than the needs to be met. In a market economy, an effective competitive process can lead to lower prices or higher quality, or more innovation in the goods or services offered.

Based in particular on these needs of contracting authorities and the market, European legislation outlines the basic principles, rules and procedures for procurement, the control of the expenditure of public funds, and the provision of information relevant to the award of public contracts. This approach restricts (from accession to the European Union) individual Member States from defining their procurement

© Springer International Publishing AG 2017
I. Georgieva, *Using Transparency Against Corruption in Public Procurement*,
Studies in European Economic Law and Regulation 11,
DOI 10.1007/978-3-319-51304-1_2

rules freely and at their own discretion. Public procurement contracts have to be awarded based on the procedures laid down in EU legislation and transposed into Member State's national law, and in accordance with the following basic principles: equal treatment, non-discrimination, proportionality and transparency. These principles are interrelated and often overlap in their key functions to ensure competitive, fair and incorruptible procedures.

Article 18(1) Directive 2014/24/EU[1] establishes the following principles as the fundamental basis on which all procurement rules are implemented:

> Contracting authorities shall treat economic operators equally and without discrimination and shall act in a transparent and proportionate manner.

The principle of equality ensures that all candidates in public procurement processes are subject to exactly the same conditions for submission and evaluation of tenders and are treated in exactly the same way. This includes ensuring that they receive equal and satisfactory information about the object of a contract. Accordingly, this principle often incorporates the main elements of the principle of transparency. Equality requires identical situations to be treated equally for all participants in a process and equal opportunity to compete to be ensured, regardless of differences between the candidates as to their commercial organisation, nationality,[2] etc. This principle thus also covers the requirement of non-discrimination against any candidate who is knowingly deprived of legal rights in participating in a process or of sufficient information to present an adequate and satisfactory offer.

> In the European context, the concept of equal treatment requires yet another definition since, in this context, the concept of equality is, in addition, based on nationality or on the origin of goods, such that all economic operators of Community nationality and all bids including goods of Community origin must be treated equally (this is the principle of non-discrimination). This is more than simply an extension of the concept of equal treatment. It implies that any condition of eligibility or origin (based on nationality or local provenance) will automatically give rise to unequal treatment, since those conditions will, by definition, discriminate against a certain group of (foreign) economic operators or favour another. However, whilst discrimination in a given context will produce unequal treatment, unequal treatment does not always give rise to discrimination.[3]

The principle of non-discrimination prohibits discrimination based on preferences due to nationality of the suppliers and producers – eg local tenderers at the

---

[1] Directive 2014/24/EU of the European Parliament and of the Council on public procurement and repealing Directive 2004/18/EC OJ L94/65; The general principles of procurement are inherited by the provisions of European Parliament and Council Directive 2004/18/EC on procedures in public works contracts, public supply contracts and public service contracts, OJ L 134, 30.4.2004 and slightly amended. These principles comply with the principles of the Treaty on the Functioning of the European Union (TFEU) and in particular the free movement of goods, freedom of establishment and the freedom to provide services, as well as the principles deriving therefrom - equal treatment, non-discrimination, mutual recognition, proportionality and transparency.

[2] See Case 31/87 *Gebroeders Beentjes BV v Netherlands* [1988] ECR 4635.

[3] OECD, 'Public Procurement in the EU: Legislative Framework, Basic Principles and Institutions' (2011) Sigma Brief 1, accessed 20 April 2016 <www.sigmaweb.org/publications/Public_Procurement_EU_2011.pdf>.

expense of foreign ones. Accordingly, this principle represents a real division of the principle of equality, and is therefore also defined in the already replaced Directive 2004/18/EC: Recital 9 of the Preamble refers to 'the principle of equal treatment, of which the principle of non-discrimination is no more than a specific expression'. This principle is also inextricably linked to the principle of transparency, which is responsible therefore for ensuring maximum information to be available on a contract, so that every entity can participate in a tender, regardless of its country of registration.

The principle of proportionality expresses the expectation that the required award criteria are proportional and appropriate to the objective of the procurement. It is strictly linked to the other principles. The principle of proportionality requires inquiry into whether the selected measure is appropriate to meet the objective pursued, but also whether the measure exceeds what is necessary to achieve that end. In cases where a contracting authority's requirements go beyond what is necessary for a particular procurement, the principles of non-discrimination and equal treatment are also automatically infringed, since competitive participants are restricted from taking part in the procedure due to these overweening requirements.

The principle of transparency is mainly to do with the amount of information to be provided on orders and procedures, and the publicity of the actions/inactions of the contracting authorities on selection of a contractor. Some perceptions of this principle are too narrow in defining it and limited only to the advertising of the notice of public instruction and ensuring the necessary minimum level of publicity with regard to procedures. Transparency is generally viewed as the concept of ensuring openness and publicity at the various stages in a process, to enable participants and supervisory authorities to observe its progress and ascertain that the contract has been awarded and be satisfied (or not) that the process was conducted legitimately and fairly. Other concepts of transparency expand the functions of the principle so as to ensure a competitive environment, the ability to monitor the implementation of procurement, and also view the principle as an anticorruption measure. The 'public's right to know'[4] is perceived to be a successful response to the needs for fair and less corrupt disbursement of public funds, and has been recognised at Treaty level, with transparency of proceedings being an essential obligation incumbent on the EU institutions: Article 15(1) of the Treaty on the Functioning of the European Union (TFEU) requires that they must conduct their work as openly as possible in order to promote good governance and ensure the participation of civil society. Curtin (1999) has drawn attention to the vertical aspects of transparency within the European Institutions (now reflected in Article 15(3) TFEU), as well as transparency's place in the pantheon of more horizontal principles (such as the protection of fundamental rights; the objective legal basis of legislation; effective judicial protection, and decisions being taken as openly as possible).[5] In the context of

---

[4] R Oliver, *What is transparency?* (New York: McGraw-Hill, 2004) ix.

[5] D Curtin, 'The Fundamental Principle of Open Decision-making and EU (Political) Citizenship', in D O'Keeffe and P Twomey (eds), *Legal Issues of the Amsterdam Treaty* (Oxford: Hart, 1999) 71, 72–73.

procurement legislation and case law, transparency unsurprisingly plays a key role, essentially facilitating the proper conduct of, and confidence in the procurement process.

Some writers, however, still criticise the 'prominent place'[6] of transparency in public procurement claiming that this 'gives rise for concern not only because of its questionable foundation but also because it may lead to unexpected and certainly unwanted results and deprive the [European Union] procurement regime of the legal certainty it requires'.[7]

There is indeed not much theoretical consensus on what transparency in procurement actually means in practice, as a consequence of the lack of a unanimous definition of the general term 'transparency', as reviewed below.

Authors usually define the transparency principle in government procurement using two separate approaches: (i) strictly describing its main purposes to ensure non-discriminatory and open treatment in proceedings,[8] or (ii) describing the obligations which should be imposed on participants in the proceedings to ensure a proper level of transparency.[9]

The arguable meaning of transparency reflects the volume and the onus of the obligations imposed on the parties involved in procurement, which vary considerably across national legal frameworks. This uncertainty also creates a 'fundamental obstacle to progress on [the] questions' towards multilateral agreements on transparency in government procurement and the reasonable need for such agreements, as Arrowsmith (2003) observed.[10] Finally, as a consequence of these different approaches to defining the essence and applicability of transparency, the principle of publicity and information openness also leads to different (positive, neutral or even negative) results in its main purpose to combat corruption and its implications, as will be analysed in the later chapters of this work.

In any event, all four basic principles of public procurement – equality, non-discrimination, proportionality and transparency, convergent in some characteristics – should be considered through the prism of the provision of the minimum ethical standards to be respected for the process of allocation of taxpayers' money in a Member State. These principles demonstrate the will of the legislator to ensure fair competition and economically advantageous products and services; they ensure the procedures to be conducted in the most honest way and finally, they guarantee that public money is not spent for corrupt personal gain.

---

[6] P Trepte, *Public procurement in the EU* (Oxford: Oxford University Press, 2007) 16.

[7] Ibid.

[8] See eg S Schooner, 'Desiderata: Objectives for a System of Government Contract Law' (2002) 11 *Public Procurement Law Review* 103; M Krivachka, M Markov, E Dimova. and Z Lilyan, *The new aspects in the Public Procurement Act* (Sofia: IK Trud i Pravo, 2006) 33.

[9] See eg S Arrowsmith, *The law of public and utilities procurement* (London, Sweet & Maxwell, 2005); Trepte (n 6).

[10] See S Arrowsmith, 'Transparency in Government Procurement: The Objectives of Regulation and the Boundaries of the WTO' 37 (2003) *Journal of World Trade* 283; and S Arrowsmith, 'Towards a multilateral agreement on transparency in government procurement' (1998) 47 *International and Comparative Law Quarterly* 793–816.

The objective of this book is primarily focused on the role of transparency as a principle of public procurement and mostly in terms of its anticorruption function. That is why in this chapter the elements and the formation of the principle, and its controversial nature are scrutinised, as well as its place in the European procurement legislation. The functions of transparency are highlighted and discussed below (separating the general functions of this principle and the role it plays as a principle in the procurement process), where their development, evolution and the shift of priorities in terms of their use are further commented on. The book provides a detailed analysis of transparency and its link to anticorruption politics by comparing the transparency rules in the procurement systems of three Member States and by opposing the two contrasting approaches observable in the EU of (a) 'overkill' in the enactment of imperative rules to ensure transparency in the procurement process, aiming at limiting corruption (which is an apparently dysfunctional model, as evidenced by the legal system in Bulgaria); or (b) enacting moderate transparency rules, treating the principle rather as a moral obligation, and providing other methods for dealing with corrupt behaviour (as found in countries such as Germany and Austria). This is why this chapter also includes a description of the Bulgarian approach to transparency and points the way to deeper reflection on the negative aspects of laws which inherently provide for maximum transparency of procedures for the awarding of contracts, but fail to reduce the prevalence of corruption, often providing more opportunities for the circumvention of fair competition rules.

2.2 Transparency – How Does it Start?

The connection between transparency and the award of public procurement contracts is essential for the present book, which seeks to compare and pinpoint the manifestations and various applications of this principle in a number of EU Member States. That is why the core of the transparency principle, its 'history', basic elements, as well as the objectives it aims to achieve in various spheres of life are structured and summarised as a part of this chapter. In order for the nature and the positive and negative consequences of the presence of the transparency principle in public procurement to be analysed, its origin in a global sense and its meaning, as elaborated in theory, should be considered. The establishment of the principle and its evolution, as well as the problems related to its definition, will provide a clearer view and understanding of the issues that this principle emerged in response of in the field of public procurement.

During times of definite distrust of government policies, frequent market instability and increasing corruption in the late 1990s, society seemed to stumble upon a panacea to combat virtually every sin – the transparency principle. In every state and at every institutional level, transparency is on the lookout for irregularities. But what exactly this principle entails, what its actual content is, how it should be applied and whether it is indeed the best instrument to combat corruption are questions which cannot be answered with any level of certainty.

Dynamic inter-state integration increases the risk of a nation's actions in politics or economics negatively affecting other nations and international organisations. On the other hand, integration enables successful government practices to serve as examples for others. Therefore, the experience of one nation becomes valuable for another. At some point (ie the last decade of the twentieth century, being the point at which society awoke to the concept of transparency), countries started to unmask governments and to legislate to require publicity and openness at all levels of institutional activities.

As the veil concealing corruption, money laundering, non-competition, discrimination and all the other complaints of the global community began slowly to be drawn open, society matured to respect information and to protect the right to receive it. The simple desire to be socially informed started to transform into encoded rules and obligations aimed at ensuring the availability and accessibility of proper information as well as the supervision and exposure of the actions of the authorities at international, domestic and regional levels. The aim of these rules and obligations was called 'transparency', or in other words, creating the possibility that government policy would become transparent, see through.

Slowly but surely 'transparency [...] has taken on a life of its own'.[11] It crystallises in international law as one of the recognisable and general principles of a democratic, legitimate and social state. The principle creates different obligations for governments and government institutions to ensure publicity of their actions. Transparency is associated more often with a reliable instrument: 'Greater transparency reduces uncertainty'[12] and 'decentralizes global power by breaking governments' monopoly over information and by empowering Nongovernmental Organizations (NGO's) and citizens'.[13]

The growing significance of the transparency principle appears in international economic law, commercial relations between state institutions and private entrepreneurs, anti-bribery policies, environmental protection, counterterrorism, and many different areas of life. In Europe the European Union (the EU) began to prescribe different practices and requirements in numerous areas in order to guarantee proper levels of transparency and information, as well as the diligent implementation of government procedures and regulatory regimes. National legislation remains free to require a greater degree of transparency and to provide supervisory powers to different authorities, wherever Member States consider it effective and in conformity with the specificities of the relevant legal regime.

---

[11] Above (n 4).

[12] K Lord, *The perils and promise of global transparency* (Albany: State University of New York Press, 2006) 2.

[13] Ibid.

2.2.1   The Meaning of Transparency

Despite the 'trend towards greater transparency'[14] and the significance and applicability of the transparency principle, which is widely discussed and questioned in academic literature, there is as yet no common definition of the term. The more 'fancy' and discussed transparency has become, the vaguer and more diluted its definition has become.

While the discussion which follows does not attempt to cover all the variations of the concept of transparency or definitions of transparency, or even to determine which is the most appropriate, several completely distinct approaches are examined considering various perspectives. The discussion proposes a summary of all the elements of transparency, which describes this universal principal in the most comprehensive way.

In order to introduce a single common, practically orientated and not strictly legal example of a definition of the transparency principle (or, more accurately, an explanation of it in its essence), it is convenient to focus on some simple propositions from Oliver's (2004) book 'What is transparency?'.[15] Authors like Oliver (2004) tried to cover the more functional aspects of transparency by claiming that this principle 'is taking a whole new meaning: "active disclosure"'. His explanation of the increasing role of transparency in our century is that it serves the most cherished right of the (international) public – to know and to be aware of the facts and the circumstances which influence those facts. Oliver's (2004) view about the new 'watchword', as he qualifies transparency, focuses on these elements of the principle which regard access to information as the right of society actively to receive comprehensible, complete and indisputable information on every aspect of life and thus to defend its (legal) rights and interests.[16] Oliver's (2004) methodology, although suffering a lack of specificity, could be accepted as a simplified and general explanation of transparency – and could be used to assist in reaching a definition of the principle from a legal perspective.

An example of a more theoretical and sophisticated attitude, defining transparency as a legal instrument and not generally as a public right (as in Oliver's (2004) approach) is presented by Chayes and Chayes (1995).[17] Although starting from a brief and concrete meaning of the term simply by defining it as 'the availability of and access to information', in the course of their description they further supplement this definition by identifying transparency as:

---

[14] Ibid.

[15] Above (n 4).

[16] Oliver (2004) (n 4), commented that 'being transparent is 'table stake' for politicians around the world [...]. Government transparency extends from the local town council to the federal government in each action'.

[17] A Chayes and A Chayes, *The new sovereignty* (Cambridge, Mass., Harvard University Press, 1995), 135.

The availability and accessibility of knowledge and information about: (1) the meaning of norms, rules, and procedures established by the treaty and practice of the regime, and (2) the policies and activities of parties to the treaty and of any central organs of the regime as to matters of relevant to treaty compliance and regime efficacy.[18]

Chayes and Chayes's (1995) analysis identifies three main operations for transparency:

(i) facilitating coordination converging on a treaty norm;
(ii) reassurance of no advantage by similar actions and compliance with norms, and
(iii) deterrence against 'actors contemplating non-compliance'.[19]

This definition offers one academic approach by describing transparency as an informational tool for the observance of deviations among 'regime participants', where transparency could and should be used in order to penalise participants in such deviations. Further, the perception of Chayes and Chayes (1994) leans towards the 'self-reporting of parties, subject to evaluation'.[20]

Finally, dictionary definitions are also useful to clarify the term 'transparency' by aiding comprehension of its main characteristics and how it is generally perceived. Two useful descriptions of transparency are: 'Minimum degree of disclosure to which agreements, dealings, practices, and transactions are open to all for verifications'[21]; and 'Essential condition for a free and open exchange whereby the rules and reasons behind regulatory measures are fair and clear to all participants'.[22]

The spotlight in these definitions falls elsewhere from the one presented above and is not on the quantity of and/or accessibility of available information, but rather on the possibility for verification and on the regulatory measures. However, these are other significant features of transparency which also clarify why this principle is considered so valuable for society and how it is used to defend people's rights, and which are obviously the most recognisable for observers.

To conclude, the main characteristics of transparency, detected in the different approaches to the definition of the principle can be conveniently summarised as follows:

---

[18] Ibid.

[19] Ibid.

[20] JE Nolan (ed), A. Chayes. and A Chayes, *Regime Architecture: Elements and Principals* in *Global Engagement: Cooperation and Security in the 21st Century* (Washington DC: Brookings Institution, 1994) 66–67. Although quite comprehensive, the definition of Chayes and Chayes (1995) and the analysis of the transparency principle lead to some conclusions of the authors which could not be completely shared. The idea that transparency is an instrument which enhances the compliance with treaty norms by imposing on participants the (passive) obligations to report and to inform about a particular regime and its practices is only the best case scenario in which access to and the availability of information leads necessarily to the positive effect of obedience to the regime.

[21] BusinessDictionary.com, 'What is transparency? definition and meaning' <www.businessdictionary.com/definition/transparency.html> accessed 20 April 2016.

[22] Ibid.

A concept, used in national and international legal systems to ensure the public's right to the availability and accessibility of a certain level of information about (institutional) norms, rules, procedures and regimes, and the actions of participants; where the information provided should be presented in an understandable and clear manner and should always be sufficient to facilitate monitoring, verification and assessment.

2.2.2 Features and Functions of Transparency

Just as transparency has no single definition accepted in theory and practice, its inherent features and functions are understood and complemented differently in time. The reason for this is again the ambiguity regarding its role in the government of each state as well as in the various spheres of state activity. On the other hand, as demonstrated by the various methods writers have adopted to define transparency, some have assigned more moderate expectations about its positive impact on civil society to the principle, while others seriously expand its scope.

Of course, as noted above, transparency is not and could not be associated with the simple provision of information for a particular process led by a public institution, even though this is a basic and integral part of its essence. The main features of transparency can be classified into two streams to which its most recognisable functions belong:

(i) *Representative features* – information provision; legitimacy of state institutions, demonstrating the political will for openness in governance; strengthening the relationship between state institutions and the public; and

(ii) *Control features* – enabling the monitoring of the actions of all government bodies; clarity regarding the rights and obligations of individual institutions; allowing the public to take part in the decision making of the government bodies; anticorruption tools against backroom manipulation to the detriment of society.

These main features of transparency also serve to measure the level of democracy in a society. It is often believed that the more developed a government's publicity institutions are, the more developed the society is too. Transparency is dictated by the public interest, that the activities of all state bodies be performed for the public good – effectively and economically sustainably.

The work classifies the functions of transparency based on these two fundamental features. Due to the complexity of transparency and the fact that it covers different types of activities, the functions are grouped into five separate groups, which nevertheless constantly condition and depend on each other.

Providing the Right Amount of Information

As reviewed in the discussion of the various definitions of 'transparency', the information provided must be accessible to the public and easy to assimilate in order for the whole range of this principle's functions to be deployed. The provision of all or any information is not a characteristic of transparency in its true sense. The provision of the *right* amount of information is the correct and expected expression of transparency. The information must be (a) in an exact quantity, (b) relevant to the respective action, (c) not misleading, (d) presented timely and, last but not least, (e) available to a broad group of people.

Given these additional features, which define an activity as transparent and public, the pursuit of transparency must be conditioned and regulated so as to make 'transparent' those specific elements of an activity to provide sufficiently effective control, but not those which would actually enable its manipulation. Therefore, if the balance in the function of transparency to inform the public about the actions of government institutions (in general) is disturbed, the principle itself becomes meaningless, since it causes more damage to a state government than good. The anticorruption drive is choked ab initio as the provision of too much information opens scope for various manipulations.

With respect to the above, it should always be borne in mind that ensuring transparency entails direct costs to the states. Governments usually seek an appropriate balance between the task of ensuring transparency and efficiency. Therefore, if the level of transparency (awareness) is properly defined, the benefits will outweigh the costs, especially when comparing the initial cost for ensuring transparency with any potential negative consequences of corruption and their impact on public confidence. European countries are gradually requiring the disclosure of more information in an effort to ensure the publicity of their actions. However, they tend to define what information should *not* be disclosed at any stage of the process and to whom to prevent the principle of transparency turning against them.

It could moreover be harmful if the information is not disclosed consistently and in a timely manner (eg the disclosure of information about other procurement contracts awarded in the context of a limited competition, which is the focus of this book) as this increases the possibility of collusion between stakeholders who can identify their competitors and contact them. This would impact directly on the market and the various competing bids offered and, in public procurement, respectively, this means concerted practice (bid rigging) to the detriment of the proper allocation of budgetary resources.

Last but not least, the obligation to provide information (even in terms of the purely technical and practical organisation of this activity) should in no case affect the task carried out by the institution subject to transparency. If the obligations are excessive and actually obstruct the actions of the administrative apparatus, the provision of information switches from 'concomitant activity' into a priority activity for civil servants. The internal control and the efficiency of the performance of the actual task set of the institution thus suffers. A brilliant example of this is Bulgaria, which is examined in this work.

Increase of Competition

By providing the right amount of information on the subject matter and the characteristics of public activities, transparency helps expand the circle of participants in such activities and thus increases competition in the relevant sector. The higher the level of competition the better the market efficiency, pricing and fair market conditions.

In fact, one of the preconditions for the deployment of effective competition is the presence of opportunity for consumers (even a closed group of consumers, as is the case for public procurement) to compare prices and the commercial conditions of the various undertakings, eg suppliers of goods or services. The availability of this option demands a certain level of transparency, which in turn appears to be an invariably necessary precondition for the deployment of the competitive process. If transparency is not ascertained 'open competition cannot prevail, corrupt dealings can proliferate, and other failings in the procurement process may be covered up, so weakening accountability'.[23]

Further, the increased level of competition not only literally extends the range of participants in an activity of public importance, but also offers an opportunity for SMEs to participate in the market, where through operation of the principle of transparency they will receive adequate and sufficient information on the needs of a given sector and thus be prepared to meet them. Transparency in fact therefore aims to decrease the levels of discretion and discrimination towards the various market stakeholders.

The exchange of information which enhances transparency is useful for effective competition as far as it does not create conditions for concerted or coordinated practices (as discussed in the course of the book). There are certain types of information however, which, if exchanged and made available to the stakeholders, would lead to exceeding the favourable level of transparency and would actually limit the competition between the stakeholders involved. In this sense, the exchange of information should not lead to a reduction of incentives for the stakeholders to follow competitive behaviour in the relevant sector and to remove or significantly reduce the business risk coming from obscurity on the current or future market behaviour of competitors and their planned marketing strategies to attract more users.

Ultimately, the functions of providing optimal level of information and increasing competition should achieve three main objectives:

(a) reduction of prices of basic goods and services to their actual market level (which highly refers to the public procurement procedures),
(b) increase of the innovative proposals in a given sector (as the higher level of competition leads directly proportional to increase of the level of the innovative proposals), and

---

[23] D Jones, 'Competition and Transparency in Government Procurement in Southeast Asia', in C Wescott, B Bowornwathana and LR Jones (eds), *The Many Faces of Public Management Reform in the Asia-Pacific Region* (Research in Public Policy Analysis and Management, Volume 18) (Bingley: Emerald Group Publishing Limited, 2010) 97–121.

(c) reduction of corruption pressure from participants in various activities affecting the entire society (which is displayed as a separate function of the transparency below).

These objectives, however, are sporadic in the individual sectors and the balance between the functions of transparency is often disturbed, as is clear from the analysis performed in this work. Very often, the transparency about actions of public significance is used to meet the 'representative goals' of the political class and its role shifts from positive to negative in terms of the levels of competition (eg, Increased transparency in a market with high concentration is likely to lead to elimination of competition. The exchange of information significantly increases the barriers to entry in the market because it allows the established market players immediately to notice any new market penetration and react to protect their market position).[24]

Control, Collaboration and Participation in Government Policies

If transparency is an integral part of good governance, it is an inevitable condition for integrity in performing any activities of public importance in a Member State.

> Transparency can be regarded as a sort of layman's basic map of an organisation and reveals the depth of access it allows, the depths of knowledge about processes it is capable of revealing, and the level of attention to citizen response it provides (Welch and Hinnant, 2002).[25] In a sense we can say that the more transparent an organisation is (via its website or otherwise), the more it is willing to permit citizens to monitor its performance and to participate in its policy processes.[26]

This principle thus acquires its other main function – to represent an opportunity for society to exert control over the public authorities and to participate actively in their decision-making process. Transparency is one of the qualities of publicity and, along with that, a principle which is fundamental in the work of the various state institutions, as the institutions and the public receive various benefits by relying on transparency.

It has until recently been actually unthinkable for society to review the public performance of the control bodies, their structure, goals and objectives. From this angle, it is felt that the lack of transparency and publicity disturbs the relationship between the controlling and the controlled party. Today there has been a novelty in the control practice, there is a new trend changing the role of the controlled and the controlling bodies. The publicity of the work of the controlling bodies permits society also to monitor the state institutions.

---

[24] CPC Decision 1778–2011.

[25] EW Welch, CC Hinnant, *Internet Use, Transparency, and Interactivity Effects on Trust in Government* (2003) Proceedings of the 36th Hawaii International Conference on System Sciences.

[26] D Curtin, *Executive power of the European Union: Law, Practices and the living Constitution* (New York: Oxford University Press, 2009), 219.

The state represents the public power, but the 'public opinion' of it should also be added to this power. Public opinion is formed by the perceptions of the public and civil society. The control over state institutions is thus not only expressed in the controlling function which a particular state organisation may have (eg Audit office). The control of the civil society, provided by the transparency of the activities of state institutions, is sometimes a much more powerful guardian and corrective of the legitimate use of the representative power. On its own, the publicity results from the interaction of public authorities and civil society, and vice versa – this function of transparency is the result of the interaction between the public authorities and civil society.

The opportunity for monitoring and controlling the governmental institutions broadens the scope of this function of transparency by allowing the public to be in actual collaboration with these state structures. Providing information, thus not only helps to evaluate the work of the government and its management, but also actively involves the public, the citizens of the state concerned, who become complicit in its management. Transparency becomes part of a 'much larger project [...] that allows widespread *participation* in policy-making processes',[27] as Curtin (1999) evaluates. This function of citizen participation in the governance of their own country is particularly in evidence when it comes to the allocation of general government funds through procurement procedures.

Gasco (2017), tracks the relationship between transparent management and the active participation of citizens in decision-making very systematically, making the following interrelated definitions part of the concept of an 'open government':

> A transparent government, that is, a government that is accountable and that delivers information to citizens about its strategies, plans, and performance.

> A collaborative government, that is, a government that involves citizens and other external and internal actors in the design, delivery and evaluation of public services.

> A participative government, that is, a government that promotes citizens engagement in political processes, and, particularly, in the design of public policies.

> A government that prioritizes the use of two key tools: open data [...] and open action [...].[28]

Thus transparency provides added benefits, such as (i) increasing trust between the parties, (ii) increasing communication between the parties, (iii) enhancing the reputations of public organisations, and (iv) greater objectivity etc.

Of course, these benefits grow on condition that transparency is used to the right extent and in timely fashion, as discussed above, and one is always obliged to search for 'the opposite side of the coin' when it comes to possibilities. Therefore, along with the variety of formal information channels available and the variety of regulated mechanisms for public access to the process of government, it should be born in mind that these mechanisms very often fail to mobilise more active citizenship. Weak public interest is relied on by the local authorities to underplay the participation

---

[27] See above (n 5), 86.

[28] CE Jimenez-Gomez and M Gasco-Hernandes, *Achieving Open Justice through Citizen Participation and Transparency*, (Hershey: IGI Global, 2017), 158.

of citizens. At the same time, the more unfamiliar and unengaged the public remains the more their suspicions of the opacity and unaccountability of the actions of the state authorities grow. Citizens thus lose their desire to participate in the government of their own country and/or to be part of making collective decisions in the interest of the whole society and, as consequence, this feature of transparency can remain 'stillborn'.

The aspects underestimated by local government (such as public awareness, participation and contribution in the decision-making process) emerges as a very serious deficit in their activities. The attention of the governance is often focused mainly on the budget winning projects and the other administrative activities. Thus, the local authorities proceed from the assumption that this in itself would provide civil support. The attention being paid to citizen participation is low and in many cases the authorities are also openly discouraged due the low social interest.

Anticorruption Instrument

The relationship between transparency and corruption has become axiomatic over the years and the two terms become almost inseparable from one another. Their influence is evident in most political and social statements by the ruling elites in every state as well as at an international level.

Naturally and logically, if transparency performs the three functions discussed so far – to disclose optimal quantity of information, to increase competition and to create a basis for thorough monitoring and control – it should also be a very successful tool to combat manipulation and other corrupt practices which permit the unjust enrichment of private individuals and groups from state budgets.

> The idea that transparency diminishes corruption is well-established and uncontroversial, and was coined over 200 years ago. According to Bentham, exposure to public scrutiny promotes virtue in public officials, and diminishes the chance of dishonest behaviour. 'Sunlight is the best disinfectant,' as Supreme Court Justice Brandeis held in 1913. Transparency is often introduced as a tool to fight corruption, and is prominently featured in chapter 5 of the UN Convention against corruption, which deals with the prevention of corruption. The international financial institutions also promote transparency as a tool to fight corruption.[29]

However, the set of functions, and mostly the anticorruption function, of a principle whose definition continues to challenge theoreticians and practitioners should not be exaggerated to such an extent that it does not consider its negative features and/or weaknesses.

As the focus of this work, through the examples and the comprehensive comparative analysis provided, is to assess the anticorruption function of transparency in the sphere of public procurement in particular, the evolution of this principle as a bulwark against corruption is discussed separately in 2.5 below.

---

[29] A Buijze, *'The Principle of Transparency in EU Law'* (Den Bosch: BOXPress, 2013), 47–48.

A Moral Postulate

As a summary of the existence of all basic features of transparency, systematised in this part of the chapter and related almost homogeneously with each another, one more function which goes well with the others should inevitably be added – transparency sets moral standards. Looking a little beyond the focus of this work, this function is fundamental to the principle, since if transparency is not perceived as a moral standard, it will lose all its other functions and their value for society. In contrast, as demonstrated in the following chapters, and especially in Chap. 5, transparency and the rules it imposes are very often used as 'iron cover' for what is happening beyond the scope of the public monitoring.

> In fact, transparency should be regarded more as a symbol – a symbol of the will of the legislator and the market to ensure fair competition and economic procurement, a symbol of a moral standard known for centuries, but not recognisable in today's bids; a symbol and a promise that the allocation of public funds will not entail theft.[30]

That is why it is extremely important that the perception of transparency as a set of components and features does not merely provide ready-positives and access to information on the management of a Member State (which in itself means that the very existence of transparency already solves pressing problems of the modern democratic society). Quite the opposite - transparency is expected to provide actual opportunities for the public to be actively involved in management: sufficient information for decisions to be properly assimilated and, ultimately, for the public to feel the need, the moral obligation, to observe and monitor compliance with European values in government.

This aspect of transparency is likely to be assessed and met relatively rarely in theory, but the legal and regulatory framework cannot exist in isolation from the 'natural rules' of behaviour and outside the historical and socioeconomic conditioning of how a country is run. This additional function should therefore stand alongside all the other features of transparency listed above. The comparative analysis performed in this book also definitely supports this view.

2.3   Transparency in the EU Public Procurement Legislation and the Work of International Organisations. Evolution of the Principle

Having systematised transparency in terms of its definition (in general), and its main features and functions, the discussion here focuses again on transparency in the field of public procurement. Due to the marked lack of unanimous opinion about

---

[30] I Georgieva, 'The miracle of transparency' (2015) *'Capital' newspaper* <http://www.capital.bg/biznes/vunshni_analizi/2015/09/27/2616907_chudoto_na_prozrachnostta/>, accessed 2 October 2016.

the role of transparency in public procurement, it is necessary first to discuss how this principle is codified in the EU legislation, and its specific nature in the award process to be elucidated. Therefore the systematisation of the material acts and practice within the EU and the work of the main international organisations towards expanding the scope of transparency are a milestone for this chapter. The 'character' of transparency in public procurement will thus be built consistently, along with its specific elements, as a common understanding of this principle to be achieved.

2.3.1 The Treaties and the European Court of Justice

The Treaty on European Union (TEU) and the TFEU, collectively referred to as the Treaties,[31] do not specifically regulate any issues concerning the award of public procurement contracts, except through the normal internal market provisions.[32] The transparency principle is not explicitly regulated by the Treaties.

However, the European Court of Justice (ECJ) deliberately addresses this problem in the *Telaustria* case[33] in 1998. This judgment practically imposes an additional element to the principle of free movement in the EC Treaty in the context of public procurement, namely the obligation of transparency. According to the ECJ '[t]hat obligation of transparency which is imposed on the contracting authority consists in ensuring, for the benefit of the potential tenderer, a degree of advertising sufficient to enable the services market to be opened up to competition and the impartiality of procurement procedures to be reviewed'.[34]

The transparency principle in the public procurement regime finds its origins in the provisions of the Treaties through the *Telaustria* case.[35] This means that the transparency obligations become applicable to all procurement procedures irrespective of their value, ie whether they are below or above the EU thresholds. This general application of the principle has been widely criticised as creating confusion and

---

[31] The current consolidated version of these Treaties can be found in OJ 2016 C202, p. 13 and 47 respectively.

[32] The main relevant provisions are Arts 34–36 TFEU on the free movements of goods, Arts 49–55 TFEU on the freedom of establishment, Arts 55–62 TFEU on services and Art 106 TFEU on special or exclusive rights on public undertakings and entities.

[33] C-324/98 *Telaustria Verlags GmbH and Telefonadress GmbH v Telekom Austria AG* [2000] ECR I-10745.

[34] In light of the discussion of the lack of any unanimous definition of transparency, Arrowsmith (n 9) 191–199, discusses whether the conception of transparency provided by the ECJ in *Telaustria* is indeed clear and comprehensive and whether transparency involve requirements other than advertising.

[35] Historically, the first case which considered the principle of transparency is Case C-87/94 *Commission v. Belgium (Walloon Buses)* [1996] ECR I-02043. Case C-275/98 *Unitron Scandinavia A/S* [1999] ECR I-8305 then added that transparency should always apply, even when no tendering requirements are under consideration. However, *Telaustria* had the most definitive impact on the implementation of this principle in public procurement procedures.

undermining clarity in the procurement process, rendering unclear which particular obligations and rules should be complied with. Arrowsmith's (2005) view that 'the Treaty's transparency principle should be fashioned to apply only when there are no [...] alternatives in place'[36] seems to be a rather better approach than the uncertainty created by the *Telaustria* case.

Further, Trepte (2007)[37] explains in detail why the *Telaustria* conclusions are open to criticism, by discussing three main issues:

(a) advertising below the threshold might contradict national policies with respect to when the value for money principle applies (advertising below a certain value of contract could be considered not cost efficient);
(b) the imposition of thresholds for contracts of higher value, which are most likely to affect competition seriously reflects the desire of the legislator that such procurements be treated more strictly and follow a chain of rules which are considered unnecessary for contracts under a certain value (this is in effect a *de minimis* principle);
(c) the imposition of a general transparency requirement implies that an advertising obligation would apply even to those numerous specific contracts excluded from the scope of the applicable procurement legislation, which 'cannot be what was intended'.[38]

Following *Telaustria*, these issues have arisen in numerous subsequent cases,[39] as well as in *Coname*,[40] where, however, the scope of application of the common Treaty rules, and in particular transparency, was limited to contracts which are of interest to bidders from other Member States (even if below the thresholds).

Finally, in 2007, Advocate General Sharpston clarified to the greatest extent so far the uncertainty regarding the application of the transparency rules to contracts below the threshold in *Commission v Finland*.[41] She adopted a much more liberal approach to below-threshold contracts, concluding that the degree of publicity for low value contracts should be determined by national law (meaning that the general rules of the Treaties could not apply sufficiently to such contracts).[42] She opined that the imposition of detailed publicity requirements for these contracts would lead to legal uncertainty.

---

[36] Arrowsmith (n 9) 197.

[37] Trepte (n 6) 19–22.

[38] Ibid 22.

[39] See Case C-59/00, *Bent Mousten Vestergaad v Spottrup Boligselkab* [2001] ECR I-9095; Case C-264/03 *Commission v France* [2005], ECR I-8831; Case C-458/03 *Parking Brixen GmbH v Gemainde Brixen, Stadtwerke Brixen AG* [2005], ECR I-8612 – which reiterate to a great extent the conclusions in *Telaustria* and discuss again the applicability of the general rules of the Treaties to below-threshold contracts.

[40] Case C-231/03 *Consorzio Aziednde Metano ('Coname') v Padania Acque SpA* [2005] ECR I-7287.

[41] Case C-195/04, *Commission v Finland* [2007] ECR I-3351, 3353.

[42] See paras 79 to 98 of the Opinion of Advocate General Sharpston in that case.

As will be seen in this book, it is not always the case that, where European legislation or ECJ decisions provide Member States with greater freedom of action in the application or regulation of a certain element of public procurement procedure, this freedom finds expression in a successful and practical legal rule. In many cases, eg in Bulgaria, the legislator tends to 'play it safe' and attempts to secure its work against possible criticism by the EU and so, despite the availability of an option of a lighter regime, chooses to regulate procedures in such a way as to make them far more complicated and difficult to apply than necessary. In this specific case, however, it is possible to draw the general conclusion that the opinion of Advocate General Sharpston in *Commission v Finland* puts a stop, at the very least, to the issue of the endlessly widened application of the general Treaty rules[43] following *Telaustria* and subsequent cases, and the uncertainty as to how and to what extent below-threshold contracts should be advertised and publicised.[44]

2.3.2   The Directives

Council Directive 71/304/EEC and Council Directive 71/305/EEC[45] were the first European measures which introduced the basic principles of public procurement conduct – non-discrimination, equal treatment and transparency. However, the original texts of these directives[46] did not mention the term 'transparency' explicitly but rather implied the need for such a rule and some of its elements.

Further, the four directives[47] which regulated public procurement procedures before the current EU public procurement legislation were also concise as to matters

---

[43] See also paras 27 to 32 of the judgment in *Commission v Finland* (n 41).

[44] See also D McGowan, 'Clarity at Last? Low value Contracts and the Transparency Obligations' (2007) 4 *Public Procurement Law Review* 274–283.; T Kotsonis, 'The Extent of the Transparency Obligation Imposed on a Contracting Authority Awarding a Contract Whose Value Falls Below the Relevant Value Threshold: Case C-195/04, *Commission v Finland*, 26.4.2007' (2007) 5 *Public Procurement Law Review* NA119–NA122.

[45] Council Directive 71/304/EEC of 26.7.1971 concerning the abolition of restrictions on freedom to provide services in respect of public works contracts and on the award of public works contracts to contractors acting through agencies or branches [1971] OJ L185; and Council Directive 71/305/EEC of 26.7.1971 concerning the coordination of procedures for the award of public works contracts [1971] OJ L185/5.

[46] The preamble to Directive 89/440/EEC [1989] OJ L210, amending Directive 71/305/EEC, discusses the need for increased transparency in the procedures to improve monitoring of the compliance with the prohibition of restrictions to the Treaties freedom of establishment and the freedom to provide services.

[47] ie Council Directive 92/50/EEC relating to the coordinating of procedures for the award of public work contracts [1992] OJ L209/1; Council Directive 93/36/EEC co-ordinating procedures for the award of public supply contracts [1993] OJ L199; Council Directive 93/37/EEC concerning the co-ordination of procedures for the award of public works contracts [1993] OJ L199; and Council Directive 93/38/EEC co-ordinating the procurement procedures of entities operating in the water, energy, transport and telecommunications sectors [1993] OJ L199.

of concrete transparency rulings. By way of exception, Council Directive 93/38/EEC[48] discussed in its preamble the need to ensure a 'minimum level of transparency [...] for monitoring the application of this Directive'.

However, based on the requirements and restrictions of these four directives, Arrowsmith (2005)[49] determines quite comprehensively the four basic aspects of the transparency principle in government procurement and the corresponding obligations of the parties involved in procurement which reflect these elements. She distinguishes six explicit transparency rules, which require that entities:

1. advertise contracts Europe-wide through the European Commission,
2. hold a competition between interested firms. Entities may dispense with an advertisement and competition only in exceptional and specific cases, such as extreme urgency.
3. exclude firms from the competition only for justified reasons specified in the directives, mainly concerned with the firm's lack of financial or technical capacity.
4. respect minimum time-limits for important phases of the procedure, to ensure that all firms have time to participate.
5. award the contract based on the results of the competition, on the basis of criteria specified in the directives and notified in advance.
6. provide information on decisions to interested parties, including tenderers.[50]

The four aspects of transparency which Arrowsmith (2005) sees as directly linked to these obligations are:

(a) publicity for all contract opportunities;
(b) publicity for the rules governing each procedure;
(c) limitation of discretion, particularly relevant to preventing concealed discrimination and
(d) opportunities for verification and enforcement.[51]

The first EU procurement legislative measures that explicitly set out rules and concrete provisions on how transparency should be secured in the conduct of any public procurement procedure were Directive 2004/17/EC and Directive 2004/18/EC[52] (collectively referred to as the Procurement Directives). While these Procurement Directives and their current replacements – Directive 2014/24/EU and

---

[48] Council Directive 93/38/EEC co-ordinating the procurement procedures of entities operating in the water, energy, transport and telecommunications sectors [1993] OJ L199.

[49] Arrowsmith (n 9) and S Arrowsmith, *The law of public and utilities procurement. Vol. 1* (London: Sweet & Maxwell, 2014).

[50] Ibid 155 and 164–166 and Arrowsmith (n 9) 127–128.

[51] Although Arrowsmith (n 9) does indeed provide the most detailed explanation of the transparency principle, covering all its possible features and characteristics, I remain unsure whether transparency in procurement must be such an overly meaningfully loaded idea.

[52] Directive 2004/17/EC of the European Parliament and of the Council coordinating the procurement procedures of entities operating in the water, energy, transport and postal services sectors OJ L134/1; and Directive 2004/18/EC of the European Parliament and of the Council on the coordina-

Directive 2014/25/EU[53] (collectively referred to as the New Procurement Directives) – will be discussed as appropriate in this work, it is worth noting at this stage that none of these directives contain a definition of the term 'transparency'. Although the new procurement package, which should have been transposed in all Member States by April 2016, contributes to the expansion of transparency to some extent (eg by promoting e-procurement), the focus of the changes is elsewhere: facilitating procedures, supporting small and medium enterprises, fighting corruption and regulating social and economic goals in procurement.[54]

2.3.3 The Work of International Organisations[55] Towards Transparency in Public Procurement Procedures

In the light of the growing importance of transparency as a tool to combat corruption in public procurement, some international organisations have prepared guidance on this principle and have researched into good practice in transparency in government policy as a priority. The role of the World Trade Organisation (WTO), the Organisation for Economic Co-operation and Development (OECD) and Transparency International (TI) are of particular importance in this respect.[56]

---

tion of procedures for the award of public works contracts, public supply contracts and public service contracts OJ L134/114.

[53] Directive 2014/24/EU of the European Parliament and of the Council on public procurement and repealing Directive 2004/18/EC OJ L94/65; and Directive 2014/25/EU of the European Parliament and of the Council of on procurement by entities operating in the water, energy, transport and postal services sectors and repealing Directive 2004/17/EC OJ L94/243 (both directives to be transposed by 18 April 2016).

[54] The mechanism provided by all these European directives in the field of the public procurement, past and present shows that the European legislator has rejected full harmonisation of all public procurement procedures, with the idea of 'general harmonisation' being perceived as sufficient. Individual Member States have thus preserved some differences in their legislative schemes, which also affects the transparency rules.

[55] Not exhaustively enumerated and reviewed.

[56] The EU and the United Nations have also developed specific anticorruption policies and endorse transparency programmes and instruments as the fundamental instruments to combat corruption. See also the 2011 Uncitral Model Law on Public Procurement, (Uncitral.org 2011) <www.uncitral. org/uncitral/en/uncitral_texts/procurement_infrastructure/2011Model.html> accessed 20 April 2016.

WTO

The WTO started operation in 1995 as the successor of the General Agreement on Tariffs and Trade (GATT).[57] The WTO is an international organisation created to act as a supervisor of international trade and its work is directed towards regulating trade between different countries and to providing framework trade agreements.

One of the major achievements of the WTO in public procurement regulation is the Agreement on Government Procurement (GPA).[58] The GPA covers matters such as public works, supplies and other services contracts, the principles which should be observed and dispute resolutions. It also sets out sample transparency obligation provisions. Although the GPA remains an optional agreement for WTO members and could not become an obligatory measure, it is a positive step towards the concretisation of a procurement regulatory scheme at an international level.

After the good example of the GPA another creative initiative of the WTO was the unsuccessful attempt to establish a multilateral agreement for transparency in procurement. In 1996 the Singapore Ministerial Conference set up a WTO Working Group on Transparency in Public Procurement to 'conduct a study on transparency'[59] in different countries' government procurement by reviewing national policies. At the Doha WTO Ministerial Conference, held in November 2001, the need for a multilateral agreement on transparency in government procurement was broadly discussed. The delegates agreed to negotiate further[60] and decided that the 'negotiations shall be limited to the transparency aspects and therefore will not restrict the scope for countries to give preferences to domestic supplies and suppliers'.[61]

However, the lack of clarity about the main purposes of transparency and its regulation and the delegates' differing views resulted in a decision on the future of the transparency agreement only in 2004. The WTO General Council adopted a decision,[62] which included determining that the issue of transparency in government procurement 'will not form part of the Doha Work Programme and therefore no work towards negotiations [...] will take place within the WTO during the Doha

---

[57] An international organisation established in 1947.

[58] The *Agreement on Government Procurement* entered into force 1981, and was renegotiated in 1994 (entered into force 1996). The GPA was further revised in 2012, which entered into force on 6 April 2014.

[59] Singapore WTO Ministerial 1996 (Ministerial Declaration) 13 December 1996 WT/MIN(96)/DEC, <www.wto.org/english/thewto_e/minist_e/min96_e/wtodec_e.htm> accessed 20 April 2016.

[60] The agreement of the delegates was for these negotiations to be conducted at the Fifth Ministerial Conference in Cancun, 2003. However, no such negotiations were launched at this Conference and the agenda was referred to the General Council of the WTO.

[61] Doha WTO Ministerial 2001 (Ministerial Declaration) 14 November 2001 WT/MIN(01)/DEC/1 <www.wto.org/english/thewto_e/minist_e/min01_e/mindecl_e.htm> accessed 20 April 2016.

[62] WTO 'Doha Agenda Work Programme' (General Council Decision) 1 August 2004 WT/L./579 <www.wto.org/english/tratop_e/dda_e/draft_text_gc_dg_31july04_e.htm> accessed 20 April 2016.

Round'.[63] This decision discontinued the activity of the Working Group on Transparency in Government Procurement.

OECD

The OECD is an international economic organisation established in 1961 and dedicated to improving democracy, identifying good practices, coordinating domestic and international policies in economic, environmental and social issues. The risk of corruption and the lack of transparency in public procurement is an issue largely covered by the activities of OECD. In 1997 OECD members and associated non-members signed the 'Convention on Combating Bribery of Foreign Public Officials', known as the Anti-Bribery Convention. One of the main recommendations in that text is that member countries should work on increasing transparency levels in public procurement. The OECD Working Group on Bribery undertakes various kinds of activities and publications to promote transparency and accountability. The elements of the transparency principle which ensure integrity in public procurement were described by the OECD as:

> Ensuring a sufficient degree of transparency to promote fair and equitable treatment in the whole procurement cycle (eg record management, e-procurement); Shedding light on non-competitive procurement to enhance integrity (eg specific reporting, rotation, random audits).[64]

As another endorsement, the OECD Revised Recommendation on Combating Bribery in International Business Transactions[65] pledges to support the WTO in their efforts for promoting transparency in public procurements.

Transparency International

Transparency International (TI) is an international non-governmental organisation founded in 1993. It describes itself as a 'global civil society organization leading the fight against corruption'.[66] Its network consists of more than 90 locally established national agencies. The main activity of this organisation is to promote transparency at each level of political and economic behaviour and, in particular, in public procurement. TI approaches other organisations, including the OECD and encourages joint activities and lobbying government to enact and apply anticorruption measures

---

[63] Ibid.

[64] OECD/DAC Joint Venture on Procurement, 'Integrity and transparency in public procurement – from good practice to the OECD Checklist' (Presentation) (2007) Copenhagen, 6.

[65] OECD 'Revised Recommendation of the Council on Combating Bribery in International Business Transactions' (adopted by the Council at its 901st session on 23 May 1997) C/M(97)12/PROV 4.

[66] Transparency International, 'The Global Anticorruption Coalition' <www.transparency.org> accessed 20 April 2016.

and to increase transparency in the international legal framework. In this respect TI is often portrayed as the great supporter and promoter of the OECD Anti-Bribery Convention. TI's policy is to investigate instances of corruption from multiple angles and to support studies, research and reports on corruption.

Currently, the best known of TI's activities is its Corruption Perceptions Index (CPI), which annually ranks all countries according to their degree of perceived corruption. The CPI was developed by TI and was first published as an annual index in 1995. It illustrates (based on subjective principles) the corruption levels in more than 170 countries worldwide. The index is based on studies conducted among representatives of business and analysts from each country considered. The CPI puts particular emphasis on corruption in the public sector and defines it as 'abuse of public status for personal benefit'.[67]

2.3.4 Evolution of the Transparency Principle in the Field of Public Procurement

The aspects of how the transparency principle manifests itself in the process of awarding procurement contracts overlap to some extent with the functions and features of transparency, as a main democratic principle (see Sect. 2.2.2), but they also have their own specific features which are analysed here.

The development of the legal framework governing the transparency rules in awarding public contracts reviewed above clearly demonstrates the evolutionary path that this principle has followed and the functions attributed to it today. A certain ambiguity regarding this principle's definition and content is reflected in its existence in the public procurement system. Along with the purely theoretical differences that burden transparency in this specific area, however, there are other factors which affect the understanding, sense and application of this principle.

Traditional Perception

By way of a summary, the initial attempts to codify this principle in the procurement legislation, the academic attitude towards it (eg the four aspects of transparency in procurement, as observed by Arrowsmith (2005)), and even the OECD's attempts to delineate transparency depict the application of transparency in the award of public procurements as significant in two main respects, which form the traditional perception of the functions of this procurement principle:

(A) Expanding competition between the candidates by providing appropriate amounts of information about the award

---

[67] Transparency International, 'Corruption Perception Index – Transparency International Bulgaria' <www.transparency.bg/en/research/corruption-perception-index> accessed 20 April 2016.

First, transparency in public procurement is perceived mainly as a tool for providing the requisite level of awareness/information for all stakeholders in the award process. Transparency thus becomes a major element of the rules on public procurement due to the very nature of this specific and artificial mechanism for spending the resources of a Member State in the public interest (eg rules on advertising the procurement, publishing the award criteria and its overall documentation etc). This in turn enables society to track compliance with the procedural rules smoothly, and to actually participate in the process of the allocation of its funds, as further discussed below.

Second, transparency is an essential tool for supporting the wider range of competitors and defining the choices faced by citizens. In public procurement the freedom to negotiate is generally exceptional, and the basic idea of this mechanism is to create competition among manufacturers and/or suppliers in a given area, so that the state can take advantage of the most economically advantageous offer on the market.

Transparency, thus, contributes to the expansion of competition in two ways:

(i) Advertisement of the procurement – the notification of each new procurement procedure at local and EU level enables a significant niche market at a European level to take part in public procurement procedures. The common publication requirements imposed by the EU's Procurement Directives, mean that transparency plays a central and irreplaceable role in removing the boundaries and limits for the potential tenderers who are not locally-based. The circle of the competitors increases markedly, which in turn gives a serious impulse to innovation, the demand for goods and services that have proved their quality in different European markets, and the emergence of leaders in presenting the best offers in terms of value for money.

The Procurement Directive sets out step-by-step procedures related to the notice and advertisement of tenders, leaving little choice as to when, where, and how to advertise procurement events. However, fulfilling the obligation of transparency requires the use of transparent language.[68]

(ii) Information regarding the requirements of the award and the parameters of the procurement contract – the specific documentation on the award and the technical requirements for it are also public and transparent, which enables competitors to evaluate the feasibility of concluding the procurement contract. The detailed specifics helps bring in further, SME competitors to orient themselves to the needs and requirements of the contracting authorities and to prove their reliability, and thus to participate equally in the procedures alongside the 'big players'. The participation of SMEs widens the competition and provides the contracting authorities basis for sufficient price and quality comparison.

---

[68] *Briefing No. 3: The guiding principles of public procurement transparency, equal treatment and proportionality* <http://www.clientearth.org/reports/procurement-briefing-no-3-guiding-principles-equal-treatment-transparency-proportionality.pdf> accessed 20 October 2016.

In addition to the publication (advertising) of the subject of the procurement contract and the rules for winning the bid, transparency achieved a reduction in the possibility of subjective discrimination of participants (thus expanding the circle of candidates and the competition further) and also provides an opportunity for control over the application of such rules, as discussed further below. The circle of all the required elements needed to achieve integrity in public procurement closes with transparency, applied in absolute symbiosis with the other principles of the award. Of course, as already commented above, i) and ii) can only survive and develop their potential if the information provided is balanced and optimal in its extent, and does not enable concerted practices and/or manipulation of the procurement procedure.

(B) Enabling the public to participate in the award process, made accessible to the widest possible range of individuals (including but not limited to the stakeholders).

The EU legal framework ensures transparency so that the general public may have full access to the process of public expenditure by providing a wide range of interested parties the right to appeal and/or to interact in the procedure. Interested parties can thus affect the stages of the procurement procedure as well as the enforcement of the contract. They often serve not only their own interest but also the interest of all taxpayers. An interested party can draw the bottlenecks in a procurement tender to the attention of the competent authorities. Therefore, if a discriminatory and/or illegal thread in the procedure or its documentation is established, its correction or cancelation would be of interest to the whole public and not just to the complaining party. Therefore Bovis (2016) reviews this proactive role even as a 'second objective' of transparency, which aims to ensure that this principle 'represents a substantial basis for a system of best practice for both parts of the equation'.[69]

If the view, advanced earlier in this chapter, that society does not always show the necessary trust in government, and often loses the desire to take advantage of the benefits of transparency by gathering information and by direct involvement in the government process, is true for transparency in general, for transparency in the process of procurement the public interest rarely drops due to the clear financial issues involved. Sometimes a narrow range of stakeholders can act as decision-changers, changing the original intention of the contracting authority, doggedly trying to amend the parameters or even annul the entire tender. In general, though, the public interest in an honest allocation of public money matches that of the separate groups of stakeholders (at least when it comes to preliminary documentation and notification). Therefore, active participation in the whole process of procurement would be not possible without openness and publicity of the awards (applying the de minimis principle strictly, however).

In a different perspective the disclosure of the procurement process not only enables public participation in the distribution of public funds, it also forms the overall opinion and satisfaction of the level of accountability of the government.

---

[69] C Bovis (ed), *Research Handbook on EU Public Procurement Law* (Cheltenham: Edward Elgar, 2016), 35.

Transparency in public procurement is critical. The manner in which government conducts itself in its business transactions immediately affects public opinion and the public's trust in good government. In addition to encouraging the public's good will and strengthened trust, the more practical business benefits of transparency are increased competition and better value for goods, services, and construction.[70]

On this basis however, the role of transparency in public procurement in some Member States tends to be exaggerated, and it becomes a true benchmark for a democratic and accountable governance, in line with the European values. The questions whether the transparency principle can actually be trusted to such an extent and whether procurement practice strains the principle with too many expectations are addressed in this book.

Anticorruption Aspect. Shift of Priorities

So far the role of the transparency principle in public procurement has been described mainly as a link between the other principles of the process that provides good level of competition and the possibility of co-participation of the society. Attention now turns to the development of this principle and its targeting in a different direction than originally perceived.

Analysis of the various aspects and nuances of this multilayered principle suggests a secondary conclusion regarding the differences in its content. Apparently, the problem is not only in the theoretical approaches towards transparency, but also in its evolution with a view to the ongoing dynamic changes at EU level. The review of the European legislation governing transparency in public procurement in the last nearly five decades, and the work of the international organisations in this field clearly demonstrates the development in the attitude of the European legislator to this principle. In particular, the legislative framework of public procurement has been amended severely in recent decades, which is a function firstly of the regular post-legislative monitoring processes and the incidental identification of various issues in the process, and secondly the considerable extension of the EU's borders in recent years.

As became clear from the classification of the main functions and features of transparency, when regarded as a basic principle of a state government, it certainly possesses the qualities to serve as an anticorruption tool. Further, expanding the circle of competitors by providing enough information about the process of the award, as well as enabling the community to take direct part in this process facilitates this anti-corruption aspect in the award procedures. It turns out that transparency can help the fight against corruption in public procurement by highlighting the actions of all stakeholders; there is confidence that it will produce results. The procurement principle thus slowly develops from being an information pillar for the

---

[70] *Public Procurement Practice: Transparency in Public Procurement* <https://www.nigp.org/docs/default-source/New-Site/global-best-practices/transparency.pdf?sfvrsn=2> accessed 20 October 2016.

nationwide distribution of resources into a serious anti-corruption tool. From this perspective, the original meaning of transparency shifts to being a useful mechanism for determining the basic and most common corruption scenarios to select a contractor in violation of procurement rules. This anticorruption function of transparency gradually began to outpace the two traditionally perceived aspects of transparency in procurement so far described, and even turns out to be its main characteristic in the award procedure. But why has this shift taken place?

On the one hand, the rising levels of corruption in the sector are a major incentive to refocus the role of transparency in public procurement. This is clearly visible in the discussions depicted in the following chapters of this book. The artificial environment for implementing the exchange of goods and services for state institutions and utilities, regulated strictly, and with (usually) no direct negotiations between traders, leads to serious increase in the attempts to manipulate the process. The limitations in the choice of a procurement contractor and the spending of public money (or spending of money in the public interest) are a driving force for the private sector to overcome the legal barriers to accessing public funds. This creates scope for various corruption schemes, and also challenges for the European legislator seeking to reduce corruption in the procurement sector.

The academic perspective on the legislative changes to the EU directives governing public procurement shows that in recent years corruption in this sector is in the focus of the rules, and in the latest legislative framework the EU is clearly seeking to strengthen the anticorruption measures.[71]

> The ongoing EU legislative reform is meant to facilitate cross-border joint procurement by providing uniformity and avoid the legal and procedural hurdles created by national law conflicts. Its second purpose is to minimize if not eradicate corruption from public procurement process by bringing transparency, integrity and accountability. Solutions and good practices exist and most EU members have taken steps in the right direction but sometimes too small and/or too few. It is true that public procurement corruption still strives in Eastern European EU countries compared to its Western ones. Too often, interests groups are acting on behalf of the citizens on false pretences, spending public money to serve their own interest and living the community with the false impression of progress.[72]

This process of minimising 'corruption from public procurement process by bringing transparency'[73] creates a whole new era in the existence and use of the rules of transparency in public procurement. Moreover, the anticorruption hopes about the power of transparency have gradually reached their zenith. The two terms (corruption and transparency) are almost inextricably linked now. From this point of view a retreat to other aspects of transparency in public procurement is even observed (as already discussed) at the expense of the anti-corruption aspect.

---

[71] See eg Art 35(5), Art 57, Art 83(3) Directive 2014/24/EU.

[72] A Popescu, 'Public Procurement Corruption in the European Union' (2014) Journal of Public Administration, Finance and Law, issue 1/2014 <http://www.jopafl.com/uploads/special-issue-1-2014/PUBLIC_PROCUREMENT_CORRUPTION_IN_THE_EUROPEAN_UNION.pdf> accessed 24 October 2016, 15.

[73] Ibid.

[T]ransparency may facilitate collusion, leading to a conflict between the desire to promote competition and the desire to prevent corruption and favouritism. Rules which limit the pool of potential suppliers (for, say, industrial policy objectives) may have an important effect on the level of competition and on the efficiency of the procurement. Where procurement is used as a tool for the pursuit of such other public policy objectives, the benefits should be carefully weighed against the effects on competition.[74]

On the other hand, the rampant corruption in the allocation of budgetary resources in the EU is not just about the temptations that this artificial mechanism creates itself for the private sector. The growth of corruption in recent years is also a result of the EU's expansion, to embrace now countries which have very different socio-economic status from each other.

The largest EU expansion, which happened to Central and Eastern Europe (CEE), Malta and Cyprus, and saw no fewer than 10 countries become new members in 2004, followed by two more in 2007, did not hamper the overall efficiency of EU decision-making either, not even during the five years in which it functioned on the basis of the Nice Treaty; […]. Nonetheless, 'enlargement fatigue' has become a scapegoat for a range of deeper problems and stumbling blocks in the EU, giving a new understanding to the 'widening versus deepening' dichotomy which characterised the debate prior to the 2004 enlargement round.[75]

As TI has put it: 'EU accession countries often face considerable systemic corruption problems in their public institutions. The scale of the problem has forced the EU to tackle corruption seriously in the accession process. Across the countries concerned, a major weakness of anticorruption reforms undertaken so far has been the significant gap between reforms on paper and their real implementation in practice'.[76]

Against this background, the legislative framework, not only at European but also at local level, began to suffer serious adjustments in the attempt to tackle corruption in public procurement in all (and the new) Member States. As discussed, it is very tempting for civil servants to allow manipulation in the allocation of resources other than own resources, in public procurement procedures. This applies fully to the recent Member States of Eastern Europe and the Balkans:

The accession of Bulgaria and Romania in 2007 is widely perceived as having been carried out too quickly and not preceded by adequate preparation, especially with regard to justice reforms and anticorruption policies. […] To date, recurrent problems with corruption, organised crime and the functioning of democratic institutions in Bulgaria and Romania fuel the EU's 'enlargement blues' but increasingly also mistrust among member states […].[77]

Since Bulgaria is one of the focuses of this book – as an example of a Member State which remains unable to curb corruption in public spending – and its procure-

---

[74] OECD *Competition and Procurement (Key Findings)* (2011) Competition Committee <https://www.oecd.org/daf/competition/sectors/48315205.pdf> accessed 24 October 2016, 56.

[75] R Balfour and C Stratulat *The enlargement of the European Union* (2014) Discussion Paper <http://www.epc.eu/documents/uploads/pub_3176_enlargement_of_the_eu.pdf> accessed 24 October 2016, 1.

[76] Transparency International <http://www.transparencyinternational.eu/focus_areas/enlargement/> accessed 24 October 2016.

[77] See above (n 75), 2.

ment system is part of the comparative analysis performed between three Member States, the attitude towards corruption in that country and the measures taken against this negative phenomenon offer a solid basis for significant conclusions regarding the evolution of the principle of transparency in public procurement and the development of its anticorruption aspect into a substantial third aspect of the principle.

Moreover, the evolution of the meaning and function of transparency in EU legislation and the evaluation of this principle as an anticorruption tool after EU enlargement not only displaces the concept of transparency in public procurement. It crystallises the fact that the anticorruption essence of this procurement principle could complement the other aspects of transparency. The access to information, the level of competition achieved and the participation of society in the award process interact with each other to achieve the best possible results when choosing a contractor in a public procurement, as reviewed above. However, when transparency serves its purpose of limiting the distortions corruption in an otherwise strictly regulated sphere, it could also increase competition among the participants, ie a positive interaction with the anticorruption aspect of transparency also exists. If the information released, being public, useful and accessible to a wide range of individuals, contributes to the increase of competition in the award process, the existence of a corrupt environment has the reverse effect – it reduces serious competition in the sector. Therefore, assuming that transparency has an anticorruption impact on procurements, it certainly helps to ensure its other immanent feature – competition among the stakeholders.

The above discussion shows that the change in the attitude towards transparency as a fundamental principle in procurement does indeed highlight its anticorruption aspects. This arises from the main factors described – the increasing corruption in the sector caused by (but not limited to) the enlargement of EU. That 'priority shift' does not affect the essence of this principle, however, which also remains a main pillar of the competition between the participants and openness of all contracting authorities' actions. On the contrary – it adds value.

Undoubtedly, when the actions of public institutions focused on spending public funds in the interest of all society are as transparent as possible, a major proportion of existing corruption schemes become much more difficult to do, if not impossible. The anticorruption function of transparency is thus justified and its positive impact is undeniable.

By studying corruption in public procurement, however, there are some critical aspects of the correlation between transparency and corruption which become apparent. The anticorruption aspect of transparency in public procurement turns out to be an especially convenient tool for the authorities to demonstrate activity in the fight against corruption. Therefore the actual limitations of transparency as a tool against corruption as well as the assessment of the effectiveness of this principle still remain a grey zone.

These issues in terms of the anticorruption aspect of the transparency principle are at the heart of this book. Numerous issues arise. Can a Member State's legal system which proclaims transparency as its creed rely on transparency to deal with rampant corruption in spending public funds? What kinds of schemes remain hidden from transparency? Can this otherwise proven fundamental principle of modern society sometimes obstruct the efficient operation of state institutions, and even be turned to contribute to the concealment of corrupt machinations? Or, in the words of Lindstedt and Naurin (2010), 'we find that looking only at average effects gives a misleading picture of the significance of transparency for corruption. Just making information available will not prevent corruption'.[78]

That is why the book presents a comparative analysis between the three Member States that demonstrate a radically different attitude to the principle of transparency in the fight against corruption in public procurement, thereby achieving the contrast conclusions on whether the evolution of this principle goes in the right direction.

2.4   Progress and Degradation of the Principle of Transparency. The Example of Bulgaria

2.4.1   Historical Predisposition

A comparative analysis of the laws of different countries is successful and has achieved its objectives only if it considers the historical and/or social basis of the differences in the legislative decisions. It is not possible to arrive at a correct theoretical conclusion without looking at the root of the problem and determining why the tendency to create norms which do not produce results was born. Therefore, this part of the chapter offers a brief historical 'tour' of Bulgarian procurement legislation (as an example of a Member State which mainly relies on transparency to cure corruption in procurement), which sets the background for examining subsequent proposals for changes in legislation, because as useful as the benchmarking with Germany and Austria may be, the individual characteristics of the countries compared is needed for final conclusions not to seem more desirable than applicable in practice.

Bulgarian legislation and Bulgarian legal theory engage with the principle of transparency in public procurement with the typical attitude of a post-communist country attempting to become a reliable EU Member State. At the beginning of its harmonisation process as an associated EU partner (after February 1995)[79] Bulgaria recognised the need to increase the transparency rules in its legislation as the 'inevitable evil' which would somehow persuade EU that the fight against corruption at a domestic level had unequivocally commenced. However, no reliable sanctions were

---

[78] C Lindstedt, D Naurin, *Transparency is not Enough: Making Transparency Effective in Reducing Corruption*, International Political Science Review Vol. 31, No. 3 (London: Sage Publications, Ltd., 2010), 301.

[79] The European Community Association Treaty came into effect on 1 February 1995 for Bulgaria.

proposed against participants in a particular regime for the consequences of infringing the obligations of transparency.[80]

However, after a series of EU Commission reports criticising the high level of corruption and discrimination in the country, and strongly recommending legislative changes to ensure transparency at different institutional levels and in public procurement procedures in particular, Bulgarian members of Parliament began to realise the unavoidable need for fundamental change in the legal *status quo*.

Karadjova (2008)[81] describes the Bulgarian attitude towards the European legislation regulating public procurement and the new principles which Bulgaria has to honour very perceptively:

> The relations between the administration and the private business were built for the West-European countries. This leads to the implementation of a commonly accepted borderline of tolerance by the interference between public and private, reflected in the legislative acts, as well as in unwritten, but approved in time and observed ethical norms. Probably this is one of the reasons for the relatively easy establishment of common regulations for the public procurements by the founders of EEC. As part of the European market since 2007, Bulgaria is obliged not only to accept, but also to adequately apply this legislation. It is a huge challenge, that it should apply not only the Community directives, but also its ethical standards. Because of a number of historical, social and national psychology factors this turns out to be difficult to achieve.[82]

The challenging change expected to happen in the Bulgarian mentality as well as the respect owed to the European principles on a domestic level, started to affect primarily academic theory, where some Bulgarian authors described the principle of 'publicity and transparency' (as it is known in Bulgarian legislation) as 'an important guarantee for the legal assignment, the functioning of the rest of the principles, as well as for the performing of public control over the procedures'.[83]

However, the meaning of the transparency principle is neither clarified in current legislation in Bulgaria, nor studied in theory, with the simple exception that transparency is defined as a principle of public procurement.[84]

Pressed by the EU and the reports of the EU Commission (before and after Bulgaria's accession to the EU), the Bulgarian legislator started a series of amendments and supplements to the existing legislative framework regulating public procurement which demonstrate, one after the other, a huge level of inconsistency in drafting and no reflection in practice.

In order to discuss the Bulgarian legislative approach to public procurement and to highlight the numerous negative changes which Bulgarian legislation has suf-

---

[80] As a consequence of the above, the Bulgarian legal scholarship has not specifically explained and analysed the transparency principle.

[81] M Karadjova, 'Legal mechanisms for decreasing the conflict of interest by the assignment of public procurements' (2008) *Yearbook of New Bulgarian University* <www.nbu.bg/PUBLIC/IMAGES/File/CPA/Godishnik_2008/MilenaKaradjova.pdf> accessed 20 April 2016.

[82] Ibid 3.

[83] M Markov and M Krivachka, *The new aspects in the Public Procurement Act* (Sofia: IK Trud i Pravo, 2006).

[84] Art 2(4) New PPA.

fered, it is useful to investigate in chronological order the various public procurement laws, up to the one currently in force, discussing where appropriate the existence or absence of any transparency requirements.

The first Bulgarian legislation dealing with public procurement was drafted soon after the establishment of the third Bulgarian state.[85] The Ministry of Public Buildings at that time proposed the Public Tenders Act (*Закон за публичните търгове*), which entered into force in 1882. This Act did not formulate any principles for the performance of public tenders. However, some provisions stipulate the need for specific written evidence of the moral qualities of the candidates.[86]

The first Bulgarian act which heralded what might be called a 'transparency principle' as a condition for fair and non-discriminatory procurement awards was drafted in 1906 – the Act on the Public Enterprises (*Закон за публичните предприятия*). The requirements related to transparency obligations were presented in detail. The provisions elaborated the strict order in which the contracting authorities should provide particular information about forthcoming tenders, so that all interested parties might be informed. Further, each tender had to be published in the State Gazette and tender announcements had to be posted in the cities and villages.

Later on, in 1921 the Public Enterprises Act was amended and supplemented. The new act, called The Budget, Accountancy and Enterprises Act (*Закон за бюджета, отчетността и предприятията*), further improved public procurement regulation and was an example of high quality, valuable legislation which guaranteed the implementation of fair and transparent procedures. Unfortunately, the communist regime after 1945 repealed all legal acts which regulated private property and the commercial activities of private enterprises.

The era of the communist regime in Bulgaria was later defined by history and the commentators as a period of flourishing 'organised and official'[87] corruption. Even the communist dictator Todor Jivkov exclaimed: 'Corruption has taken a permanent place in our lives and causes heavy moral and material damages […] sometimes the interests of the state, evaluated in thousands and millions of Levas[88] and Dollars, are sacrificed just for a trivial bribe'.[89] At that time, public procurement no longer existed due to the fact that each property and/or service was distributed directly by the state and the government, and private property was prohibited.

As a symbol of post-communist Bulgaria, Ordinance No 2 of 1991 of the Ministry of Architecture and Construction for conducting tenders in the field of construction (*Наредба No 2 от 1991 г. на Министъра на строителството и архитектурата*

---

[85] After Bulgaria ceases to be part of the Ottoman Empire and regained its independence after five centuries lack of statehood in 1878.

[86] Art 6 Public Tenders Act 1882 stated that 'No one could participate in the tender if he/she does not present a certificate of honesty taken from the local municipality'.

[87] R Avramov, *The communal capitalism – among the Bulgarian economical past* (vol III, Sofia: Centre for Liberal Strategies, 2007).

[88] ie the Bulgarian currency, the Lev, internationally abbreviated as BGN or Lv.

[89] M Ivanov, *Reformation without reforms. Political economy of the Bulgarian communism 1963–1989* (Sofia: Open Society Institute and Ciela 2008).

за провеждане на търгове в областта на строителството) was a first but poor attempt to regulate procurement in the field of construction works. This piece of legislation did not deal with any determination of the principles of the tender procedures whatsoever, although some transparency rules and obligations could be distinguished in some of its provisions. For example, Article 13 required that each tender be announced in advance through the mass media, and Article 14 set out the minimum requirements and information which a call for competition should contain. Even though this system was a step in the right direction, it was nevertheless a vague attempt to structure and regulate the tender procedures for construction works.

In 1995 Bulgaria entered into the Europe Agreement Establishing an Association with the European Communities and their Member States (signed 8 March 1993, entered into force 1 February 1995).[90] Article 68 of this Agreement stated that 'The Parties consider the opening up of the award of public contracts on the basis of the principles of non-discrimination and reciprocity, in particular in the GATT context, to be a desirable objective'.

As a logical continuation of the undertakings from this agreement as well as of the development process in Bulgarian public procurement legislation, 1997 saw the adoption of the first Bulgarian Award of Procurement Contracts Act (*Закон за възлагане на държавни и общински поръчки*, APCA).[91] This was the first attempt to codify public procurement procedures. Far from being a masterpiece, it was widely criticised for being incompatible with the Procurement Directives (despite the ongoing process of harmonisation). The APCA did not create any productive opportunities for promoting and practically enforcing transparency or any other procurement principles. It did not provide any definition of transparency but it did, however, contain some worthy provisions viewed in the light of the transparency requirements, such as:

(a) a call for competition should be promulgated in the State Gazette and in at least two national daily newspapers;
(b) a call for competition for major construction projects should be published at a certain period prior to the tender;
(c) the tender documentation and conditions had to be described in detail;
(d) the criteria for evaluation of the candidates had to be announced in advance etc.

After the APCA, the first Public Procurement Act (*Закон за обществените поръчки*, the First PPA)[92] was enacted as an attempt to harmonise domestic and European legislation. Its main goal was stated to be 'increase of effectiveness in the use of the budget and public funds through: 1. determination of transparency [...]'.[93]

---

[90] OJ 1995 L358/3.
[91] As promulgated SG 9/3.1.1997; repealed by SG 56/22.6.1999.
[92] As promulgated SG 56/22.6.1999; repealed by SG 28/2004.
[93] Art 2 First PPA.

The four principles of the award of public procurement contracts were explicitly set out in Article 9:

1. guaranteed publicity of the procedure and transparency
2. free and fair competition
3. ascertained equal opportunities for participation of all candidates
4. guaranteed protection of the commercial secrets of the candidates and their offers.

The First PPA saw the creation of the first Bulgarian Public Procurement Register. An obligation for contracting authorities to publish in the State Gazette all planned procurement calls of over BGN 1 million (approx. EUR 511,273) by 31 March each year, was also envisaged. However, the information published had the simple purpose of attracting more candidates. Contracting authorities were still not obliged to announce the procurement procedure itself.

This First PPA could be regarded as a positive step towards the harmonisation of the Bulgarian procurement legislation with the Procurement Directives. However, one of its major failings was that it did not stipulate the establishment of a centralised supervisory authority to monitor the accurate application of the law and to control and sanction contracting authorities. The early years of the application of this act thus failed to achieve the desired clearer regulation, transparent actions by the participants in the procedure, and less corruption.

As a consequence of the EU Commission's Regular Report in 2003[94] and its harsh criticism of the state of the public procurement regime in Bulgaria, in 2004 the Bulgarian legislator decided to repeal the First PPA and to start tackling public procurement all over again with a brand new Public Procurement Act (*Закон за обществените поръчки*, the PPA).[95]

A positive outcome of the PPA was the establishment of the Bulgarian public procurement Agency (the PPAgency) as a centralised controlling body specialised only in public procurement. The establishment of the Court of Arbitration by the PPAgency has been a further step towards the recognition of the transparency principle by contracting authorities as one of their ultimate obligations in the award of public procurement contracts.

In 2006 the Procurement Directives were transposed into the PPA which required so many amendments to the PPA and the whole package of applicable secondary legislation that in reality it became an almost entirely new law. Though criticised, the amendments of 2006 were a major step towards a modern, communicable and open regime.

---

[94] In its '*Regular Report on Bulgaria's progress towards accession*' (2003) the European Commission found that: 'As to public procurement, further efforts are necessary to align with the *acquis* and to build up the necessary administrative capacity', 24, and concluded that Bulgaria needs to address urgently the delays incurred in aligning with EU public procurement rules. (European Commission report <http://ec.europa.eu/enlargement/archives/pdf/key_documents/2003/rr_bg_final_en.pdf> accessed 20 April 2016).

[95] SG 28/6.4.2004, as amended.

An additional reason for the radical redrafting of the PPA in 2006 was the monitoring report of the European Commission (EU Commission) of 25 October 2005. The conclusions of the EU Commission were:

Surveys and assessment conducted by both national and international organization confirm that widespread corruption remains a cause for concern and affects many aspects of society. There is a positive downward trend as far as administrative corruption is concerned, but the overall enforcement record in the field of corruption remains very week [...] Some areas of public administration remain particularly vulnerable to corruption. This is the case for those engaged in public works contracting [...] There have been several exemptions already from the new law on public procurement [...] Claims of non-transparent procedures for procurement [...] are continuing.[96]

As a consequence, the amended PPA provided some reasonable measures on how Bulgarian procurement administration could become more effective and transparent (although the corruption levels remain the same). The electronic format of the public procurement register was introduced and helped increase access to applicable procedures and planned procurements. Another positive effect of the amendments was the alignment of domestic law with the changes required by Procurement Directives and the obligation on contracting authorities to publish public procurement calls for competition at the European level as well.

For almost a decade, the PPA has undergone more than thirty amendments and supplements, most of them dictated by negative reports from the EU Commission commenting on the flourishing of corruption and the lack of transparency in the management of public and EU funds in Bulgaria. The EU Commission evaluated the lack of transparency and accountability in the area of public procurement as a 'grave problem' and recommended that urgent action be taken so that Bulgaria could 'improve the supervision and transparency of public procurement procedures at central, regional and local level in strict conformity with the applicable EU rules'.[97]

However, despite the various amendments over the years and the increase in legislative rules which require publicity and transparency in the conduct of award procedures, Bulgarian contracting authorities regarded most of the amendments as obstructive to the procurement process rather than limiting corruption. Practice shows that in some cases the legislative rules made the situation even worse: contracting authorities misinterpreted the new rules and justified their actions on the basis of ambiguity in the applicable legal norms and have thus opened the doors to even greater administrative abuse and corruption.

As of 15 April 2016 a brand new piece of legislation comes into force and replaces the until recently applicable PPA. The new Bulgarian public procurement

---

[96] Commission (EU), 'Comprehensive monitoring report on the state of preparedness for EU membership of Bulgaria and Romania' (Communication) COM (2005) 534 final, 25 October 2005.

[97] Commission (EC), 'On the Management of EU-funds in Bulgaria' (Report from the European Commission to the European Parliament and the European Council) COM (2008) 496 final, 23 July 2008.

act (*Закон за обществените поръчки*, the New PPA)[98] transposes the New
Procurement Directives into national legislation. While still too early to draw general conclusions about its effects in the absence of sufficient practice in its application, quite a large part of the clauses of the New PPA already suggest that it will
follow the fate of its recent predecessor and be subject to many amendments and
supplements. What is immediately noticeable is that the law is definitely not easier
to implement than the previous (which was the main hope of all procurement practitioners). Further, 'despite the respectable volume of the new law there were too
many […] outstanding hypotheses [….] Whether under time pressure and the large
volume of euro-provisions [...] or for some purely national reason it came to the
paradoxical situation the law to refer to the Regulation[99] on substantive aspects'.[100]
The policy of chiefly deploying transparency measures is still evident (albeit with
some slight adjustments, as discussed below). Some problematic aspects of the previous legislation which had left the door open to corruption have been solved, but at
the expense of others which now loom on the horizon (which is not only because of
national decisions, but because of the too liberal approach of the new procurement
package). The law and its provisions is subject to a critical analysis in the following
chapters of this book, along with the laws of the other two Member States considered here.

2.4.2   *Transparency in the Bulgarian Procurement Legislation*

As revealed by the brief historical chronology the system of procurement in Bulgaria
has been caught in an upward spiral of increased transparency rules which continues
to the present day with the now in force (since mid-2016) New PPA, reflecting the
new European legal framework.

One of the substantial amendments to the PPA of 2014[101] and the applicable secondary legislation, before the transposition of the New Procurement Directives into
the New PPA, was dictated by yet another fit of 'ostentatious transparency' on the
part of the Bulgarian legislator, and by the desire to transpose part of the rules under
the New Procurement Directives into Bulgarian legislation (before the transposition
of the rest of the EU rules, for no apparent reason).

Oliver's (2004) words on transparency apply in fully to the PPA in its current
version: '[transparency] has moved […] to center stage in a drama being played out
[…] in many forms and functions. […] It blossomed from a simple ideal to a complex set of expectations and regulations. […] [It] spawned a growing horde of gov-

---

[98] SG 13/16.2.2016, effective as of 15 April 2016.

[99] ie Regulation for Implementation of the New PPA (SG 28/08.04.2016, in force as of 15 April
2016).

[100] I Stoyanov, 'Analytical overview of the main points in the draft Regulation for Implementation
of the PPA' (2016) 3 ZOP+ 7–8.

[101] SG 40/13.5.2014, effective as of 1 July 2014 and 1 October 2014 respectively.

ernment and non-government organizations [...] and created an entire legion of transparency hiders and seekers'.[102]

These changes to the PPA were introduced at a time of severe political instability, which additionally affected the adopted texts, effectively reducing the PPA to a 'patchwork' of endless rules and obligations for publication and promulgation of each and every act and action of the contracting authorities, without, however, protecting the interest of candidates.

The material changes to the legislation were connected to:

(a) *Excessively enhanced importance of the use of the buyer's profile*[103] – The contracting authority publishes the procurement notice (and its main procurement decisions) on the internet portal of the PPAgency, on the buyer's profile on its official webpage and sends it to the Official Journal of the EU (OJEU), where applicable, and to the local media. Further, the contracting authority is obliged to make publicly available almost the whole procurement file[104] on the buyer's profile in brief terms. It is threatened by administrative fines if it does not comply with these obligations.

The Explanatory Memorandum on the amendment to the PPA[105] justifies this superimposition and overlapping of information submitted to the PPAgency and the OJEU and information uploaded on the buyer's profile as working precisely towards enhanced public control of procurement. This effort of the contracting authorities, however, serves to deprive them of the opportunity to exercise *ex ante* and ongoing control over their own procurement procedures (due to lack of nay sufficient time) rather than achieve any other purpose. Such excessive information (although somewhat limited by the New PPA rules, as discussed below) will be of little interest to anyone other than the parties concerned, who will have access to this information anyway, as well as the opportunity to appeal it. Also – the *ex ante* control carried out by the Executive Director of the PPAgency covers an explicitly defined set of documents related to a limited scope of procurement procedures: hence, this largely overlapping information will not be of much use for more efficient control.

---

[102] See above (n 4) ix.

[103] Introduced as an additional but non-mandatory option for ensuring procurement publicity under Art 35 Directive 2004/18/EC (also mirrored in Directive 2004/17/EC). The New Procurement Directives (eg Art 48 Directive 2014/24/EU) also refer to the 'buyer's profile', without adding additional content on the previous rules or making its use obligatory.

[104] ie prior notices, decisions on the launch of procedures, the relevant participation documentation and any supplementary documents and explanations thereto and any other documents containing important information for interested parties and candidates. Further, commission's protocols and reports on procedures; concluded public procurement contracts; subcontracting agreements and information on payments made under those agreements; the date, grounds and amount of each payment made under public procurement contracts and subcontracting agreements including advance payments, if any; and the date and grounds for the release, claim or retention of performance guarantees for each contract are also to be published.

[105] Explanatory Memorandum to the draft Bill amending and supplementing the Public Procurement Act 2013 (2015) <www.government.bg/cgi-bin/e-cms/vis/vis.pl?s=001&p=0211&n=73&g> accessed 28 May 2015.

(b) *Other platforms* – The contracting authority publishes its decisions for the initiation of contracting procedures, for any changes to or termination of procedures, any notices of contracts tendered above a relevant threshold,[106] information on awarded and implemented contracts, information on the progress of procedures in the event of appeal proceedings and any other relevant information in the public procurements register by the PPAgency. Where a procurement exceeds European thresholds, in addition to promulgation in the public procurement register, the contracting authority must advertise in the OJEU all decisions regarding the launching, change and termination of public procurement procedures as well as notices which need to be entered into the register; information on awarded procurements and implemented contracts, information on the progress of procedures in the event of appeal proceedings etc.

(c) *Archive obligations* – All the documents uploaded on the buyer's profile (including any sensitive information and/or commercial secret, if applicable, deleted in advance) must be retained there for a period of 1 year starting from the time of their promulgation or amendment, while the statements of the Executive Director of the PPAgency and any other documents relating to the internal rules of the contracting body and participant contact information must be retained for an indefinite period.

(d) *Tender opening is public* and may be attended by participants or authorised representatives, as well as media representatives and other individuals in accordance with the access regime for the site in which the tender opening will take place. Given that this access regime usually involves a simple ID check, the law actually admits anybody to a tender opening.

(e) *Voluntary transparency* – Separately from all the above, the Bulgarian legislation also regulates the rules on the use of voluntary transparency in compliance with the options provided by Article 37 Directive 2004/18/EC.

This list is not exhaustive but even this abbreviated form is quite sufficient to illustrate the information flow and the numerous obligations of the contracting body intended to ensure transparency throughout the award process. Of course, some of the examples above correspond to the requirements of the Procurement Directives and the New Procurement Directives,[107] but a critical observer will not fail to notice the numerous additional publications that have been layered on the European requirements (as mandatory obligations and not options) and the superfluous overlapping of information thus achieved.

Given that one of the reasons for the EU taking action to replace the prior Procurement Directives with the New Procurement Directives was precisely the

---

[106] The mechanism for award under Bulgarian law is divided on (i) procurements below the thresholds; (ii) procurements above certain national thresholds as determined by the national legislation and (iii) procurements above the EU thresholds as defined by the EU legislation.

[107] It is not clear why the legislator has chosen to transpose some of the rules of the New Procurement Directives into the PPA so early, given the clear intention that the whole package should be transposed at the same.

desire to simplify rules and procedures, the legislative decision to saddle participants with so many additional obligations obviously runs contrary to that desire. As
pointed out in the EU country report for 2014: 'The amendment to the Public
Procurement Act of May 2014 has further aggravated the situation, with different
commencement dates for its specific parts, while a number of weaknesses in the
legal framework remain unaddressed [...] At the same time, however, many procurement procedures are subject to overlapping *ex post* controls, sometimes resulting in
divergent findings'.[108]

The Bulgarian legislator has listened to this legitimate criticism and understands
that developers are bewildered by this sea of obligations to ensure transparency and
took this into account when drafting the New PPA. In the New PPA at least the
information to be uploaded to the buyer's profile is limited and somehow reduced:
this will positively affect the contracting authorities. Overall, however it has so far
proved unable to conclude that the New PPA is an effective legislative solution that
renounces transparency as its main corrective method.[109] On the contrary, the new
rules neither provide for lighter procedures, nor are more flexible. They do not add
any material or substantially different methods for dealing with corruption than
before. Ultimately, the task of ensuring publicity and transparency and prohibiting
the provision of advantages or unreasonable restriction of participation in the procedure on behalf of potential bidders has been supplanted by some inconsistent com-
pilation of documentation and the introduction of restrictive conditions in some of
the procedures. It appears that there is no mechanism for protection against these
actions.

The problems in the above concept of increasing transparency provisions
(although slightly more adequate with the New PPA) are several:

 (i) Against the background of the multitude of procedural and administrative obli-
     gations on the contracting authority, the focus of the latter is shifted. There is
     no time for sufficient quality, ongoing internal control nor the possibility to
     detect serious (fraudulent) infringements;
(ii) To comply with the requirement to maintain an official website of sufficient
     quality and the necessary storage capacity to upload and retain hundreds of
     documents, a contracting authority requires financial means which are unavail-
     able to a great many contracting authorities (eg small municipalities);
(iii) In order to observe all deadlines and upload the documents on the buyer's pro-
     file in the required manner, some contracting bodies need to hire additional
     staff, which will again require financial resources which are simply not
     available;

---

[108] Commission (EC) 'Country Report Bulgaria 2015 including an In-Depth Review on the prevention and correction of macroeconomic imbalances' (Staff Working Document) SWD(2015) 22
final, 26 February 2015, 57.

[109] There is a separate Chapter 5 of the New PPA, as well as Chapter 4 of the Regulation for
Implementation of the PPA, dedicated to publicity and transparency, providing rules for exchange
of information

(iv) Work on the organisation of procurement competitions is still too complicated and burdensome and the aim at combating corruption (by means of the transparency achieved thereby) is completely lost.[110]

In addition to the above, all other characteristics of the transparency principle itself have been pushed far into the background of the Bulgarian procurement legislation. The analysis in terms of how the legislator has opted to ensure transparency in the award process shows that the letter of the law focuses mainly on *publicity* (through the requirements for 'advertisement of the procurement' and 'provision of sufficient information', as highlighted by Arrowsmith (2005)).[111] The remaining aspects of this principle, relating to *limitation of discretion*, *preventing discrimination* and *provision of opportunities for verification and enforcement*, are indeed reflected in the national legislation (based on the requirements of the EU rules), but have failed to achieve the desired result, as is evident in the subsequent chapters of this book as well. It is precisely for this reason that Bulgaria has arrived at the absurd situation – much to the public's perplexity – where EU reports (year on year) continue to demand increased transparency in public procurement regardless the 'efforts' of the legislators to this exact end.

The conclusion which emerged in the course of writing this book and the analysis of the most common violations and models of corruption in public procurement it entailed, is that for as long as the other elements[112] required to achieve sustainability and integrity in public procurement are missing, any elaboration of the transparency principle as a means in itself will serve no purpose; or as Lord (2006) warns: '[g]reater transparency will not necessarily promote democracy and good governance'.[113]

2.5   Concluding Observations

This chapter introduces transparency and its place among the other main principles in the process of procurement – equality, non-discrimination and proportionality. Except in terms of public procurement, the analysis here follows the origin and development of this institution and its main elements and functions.

The global establishment of the principle and its incorporation into the general legislation governing public procurement in EU Member States as a guarantee for fair distribution of budget funds demonstrates the essence of this principle and how

---

[110] See also my comments on these legislative amendments: I Georgieva, 'Bulgarian Procurement: The Old Razzle-Dazzle' (2014) *CEE Legal Matters* <www.ceelegalmatters.com/index.php/component/content/article?id=358:bulgarian-procurement-the-old-razzle-dazzle> accessed 20 April 2016.

[111] See above (n 9).

[112] (a) elements (features) of transparency, as a multi-layered concept, but also (b) elements of the control and prevention system for violations in public procurement (eg the judiciary, the executive power etc).

[113] See above (n 12) 3.

it can function as an anticorruption weapon. The transparency principle is a major feature of the public procurement regime, where it has taken on certain specific characteristics. Secondary EU legislation stipulates requirements and restrictions on the parties involved in procurement procedures, aiming to ensure that the procedures are conducted openly and fairly. National legislation supplements these rules in compliance with the requirements of the Procurement Directives and now – the New Procurement Directives.

But what is transparency and how has it come to be such an important feature not only for the quality award of procurement contracts, but also in all other spheres of public interest? As reviewed, transparency emerged in response to society's need to combat corruption, discrimination and the abuse of government control in different spheres of life. It has crystallised into a public right to the availability and accessibility of a certain level of information, presented clearly and understandably, about the norms, rules, procedures and regimes in procurement, and the actions of the participants. The significance of this principle and the achievement of its objectives has become a priority for a number of international institutions and organisations. It has become clear that transparency in a democratic society is a synonym of legitimacy and trust in the public power and quality of governance.

Over the past 20 years, the EU has implemented multifaceted transparency policies. Starting from a situation of no formal provisions before 1992, pro-transparent Member States succeeded between 1992 and 2006 in bringing about considerable change in the direction of more openness. In the subsequent period, particularly after the EU Commission presented a proposal for a renewal of the access to documents legislation, a deadlock has resulted over the right implementation of transparency since 2012.[114]

Nevertheless, despite all the positive features of transparency enumerated above, an unresolved issue concerning this institution is, paradoxically, the lack of a common definition and the notably varying positions of the Member States regarding the values embraced by this principle. Some authors are very concise in their analysis of this principle and limit it only to the advertising and provision of the minimum necessary level of publicity regarding the work of the public institutions. Others expand the functions of transparency by adding complementary features such as the assurance of a competitive environment or the ability to monitor. One of the most discussed functions of transparency is the possibility the bribery attempts to be limited since it provides public access to all state activities. For this reason, the Bulgarian legislator, for example, (as seen from the comparative analysis between several Member States made in this book) has found an easy way to advertise a somewhat moral principle as a method to combat corruption and to simulate political desire to limit corruption. This leads to impressive levels of obligations to provide information not known in any other state – duties which only hamper the already complex administrative procedures and provide for additional administrative hurdles.

---

[114] MZ Hillebrandt, D Curtin, A Meijer, 'Transparency in the EU Council of Ministers: An Institutional Analysis'   <http://www.clientearth.org/reports/aarhus-centre-resources-library/scholarly-articles/Transparency%20in%20EU%20Council,%20Curtin.pdf>, accessed 2 October 2016, 18.

The functions and elements of transparency – as well as the positives its implementation in state government achieves – are further diluted and often stretched like chewing gum, depending on the angle of review of the principle in the academic researches, the interests of the governing body, the public sphere in which transparency is used etc. It was also shown that the main functions of transparency are intrinsically linked to each other and could be grouped into: (i) provision of the right amount of information, (ii) increase of competition, (iii) provision of control opportunities, (iv) anticorruption functions and, last but not least, (v) ethical functions. All these features build the 'halo' of transparency as a completely irreplaceable part of modern democratic governance.

Apart from the main features and functions of the principle of transparency in general, this chapter discussed transparency in the process of awarding public contracts, as well as the specifics of transparency in that field. The analysis of the regulatory framework at European level shows that transparency in public procurement is perceived mainly as (a) a tool to increase competition by providing the necessary level of information for participation in procedures and (b) a technique for promoting active social participation (ie interested parties) in decision making for the distribution of budgetary resources for the needs of the Member States. In recent years, however, due to the growing levels of corruption in the sector, caused in part but not exclusively by the substantial expansion of the EU by states having divergent socioeconomic statuses, the legislators have given priority to another aspect of the function of transparency (not traditionally perceived until recently), namely its role in combating bribed tenders. Obviously, the information for and elucidation of the award process helps not only to expand the circle of competitors but also to limit the possibilities of secret manipulations and distortion of the choice of contractor. The role of transparency in this respect is indispensable. Therefore, this anticorruption aspect of transparency in the procurement award process has gained serious value in recent decades and has almost superseded the other aspects of the principle. Nevertheless, this aspect of transparency offers considerable cause for doubt as to whether it can indeed be one of its strongest features.

Although the importance of the principle is not disputed here, its implementation (in some cases excessive and wrong) and its use as an antibribery instrument in the public procurement systems of several Member States is subject to testing and is the focus of this work. The conflict between transparency and anti-corruption policies is a major theme throughout the book. The comparison between the three different methods of awarding contracts reveals (a) how this aspect of transparency is achieved (or not) in the laws of those states, (b) what procurement rules have been upgraded over the European legal framework to ensure transparency of procedures and (c) whether indeed this aspect of transparency occurs as expected and limits the corrupt choice of a contractor.

In particular, the example of the Bulgarian approach of transposing transparency rules reveals a failure in comprehension as well as a failure in the numerous attempts to put this principle in motion. Furthermore, despite the continuous increase in transparency rules and ever more complicated legislative bases, the EU continues to claim that corruption in Bulgaria has increased[115] and the heavy transparency obligations imposed on the contracting authorities remain merely a burden on the public procurement award process. 'The result is a ritualistic struggle over openness and privilege, with grave consequences'.[116]

As part of the European market since 2007, Bulgaria is obliged not only to accept but also to adequately implement the European legislation. This was a huge challenge for this post-communist country required to follow the EU directives as well as its ethical standards. For this reason, this chapter also presents a brief historical overview of the legislative framework governing public procurement in Bulgaria, which clarified the legislator's understanding of the principles and rules for distribution of public funds long before that country became an EU member.

The comparative analysis of several Member States and their modes of procurement is especially important for the conclusions in this book and the proper demarcation of the possibilities of transparency to tackle corruption. It shows again that not only the perception and understanding of transparency in each state is different but the approach to it is too. Some countries exercise their endless stream of rulemaking talent on transparency to create an infinite number of obligations and rules to ensure publicity and openness. This approach, however, as is clear from the book, actually stifles the positive influence of transparency over the actions of the state institutions and creates obstacles during the whole working process. In other countries, transparency is expressed as underlying principle of procurement regulation, with which the stakeholders (in the procurement process) conform and comply without delaying or stopping their actions.

Discovering the gaps in this puzzle of transparency features in Member States such as Bulgaria and how the transparency principle can be harnessed as a useful tool in combating the rampant corruption in public procurement are precisely the questions that this work seeks to answer.

From this perspective, this chapter is useful for the analysis throughout the rest of the book, as it not only describes the principle of transparency, set against and understood alongside the other main principles ensuring the lawful progress of public procurement procedures, but it also reveals the main field for discussion in this work. Can it be so reliable a principle to be a trustworthy source of anticorruption tools, when its definition, basic functions and positives are so hazily interpreted, and when each author assigns a different meaning to it? Could it be the case that, despite transparency's indisputable role in increasing the flow of information from the state

---

[115] eg Commission (EU), 'Report from the Commission to the European Parliament and the Council on Progress in Bulgaria under the Co-operation and Verification mechanism' SWD (2016) 15 final; Commission (EU) 'Annex Bulgaria to the EU Anticorruption Report' (The First EU Anticorruption Report) 3 February 2014, <http://ec.europa.eu/dgs/home-affairs/what-we-do/policies/organized-crime-and-human-trafficking/corruption/anticorruption-report/docs/2014_acr_bulgaria_chapter_en.pdf> accessed 20 April 2016.

[116] M Fenster, The Opacity of Transparency (2006) 91 *Iowa Law Review* 893.

to society, it is in essence a 'pervasive cliché'?[117] How and to what extent can it really be used by any or all of the Member States in the fight against corruption in public procurement?

The following chapters and their symbiosis with this initial part of the book will help find the correct perspective for the development of the principle of transparency in the context of the process of procurement award. Some unambiguous conclusions will crystallise as to where to locate the full stop in the determination of the compliance obligations assuring publicity and transparency in order for this principle actually to remain a symbol of the Rule of Law, and not become a meaningless statutory cover for the abuse of public funds.

Bibliography

A Buijze, 'The Principle of Transparency in EU Law' (Den Bosch: BOXPress, 2013)

A Popescu *Public Procurement Corruption in the European Union*, Journal of Public Administration (2014) Finance and Law, issue 1/2014 <http://www.jopafl.com/uploads/special-issue-1-2014/PUBLIC_PROCUREMENT_CORRUPTION_IN_THE_EUROPEAN_UNION.pdf> accessed 24 October 2016

A Chayes and A Chayes, *The new sovereignty* (Cambridge, Mass.: Harvard University Press, 1995)

C Bovis (ed), *Research Handbook on EU Public Procurement Law* (Cheltenham: Edward Elgar, 2016)

C Hood, 'Transparency in Historical Perspective', in C Hood and D Heald (eds), Transparency, the Key to Better Governance? (Oxford, New York: Oxford University Press, 2006)

C Lindstedt and D Naurin, 'Transparency is not Enough: Making Transparency Effective in Reducing Corruption' (2010) 31(3) *International Political Science Review*

CE Jimenez-Gomez and M Gasco-Hernandes, Achieving Open Justice through Citizen Participation and Transparency, (Hershey: IGI Global, 2017)

D Curtin, 'The Fundamental Principle of Open Decision-making and EU (Political) Citizenship', in D O'Keeffe and P Twomey (eds), Legal Issues of the Amsterdam Treaty (Oxford: Hart, 1999)

D Curtin, Executive power of the European Union: Law, Practices and the living Constitution (New York: Oxford University Press, 2009)

D Jones, 'Competition and Transparency in Government Procurement in Southeast Asia', in C Wescott, B Bowornwathana and LR Jones (eds), *The Many Faces of Public Management Reform in the Asia-Pacific Region* (Research in Public Policy Analysis and Management, Volume 18) (Bingley: Emerald Group Publishing Limited, 2010)

D McGowan, 'Clarity at Last? Low value Contracts and the Transparency Obligations' (2007) 4 *Public Procurement Law Review*

EW Welch, CC Hinnant, *Internet Use, Transparency, and Interactivity Effects on Trust in Government*, (2003) Proceedings of the 36th Hawaii International Conference on System Sciences

I Georgieva, 'Bulgarian Procurement: The Old Razzle-Dazzle' (2014) *CEE Legal Matters* <www.ceelegalmatters.com/index.php/component/content/article?id=358:bulgarian-procurement-the-old-razzle-dazzle> accessed 20 April 2016

---

[117] C Hood, 'Transparency in Historical Perspective,' in C Hood and D Heald (eds), *Transparency, the Key to Better Governance*? (Oxford, New York: Oxford University Press, 2006), 3.

I Georgieva, 'The miracle of transparency' (2015) *'Capital' newspaper* <http://www.capital.bg/biznes/vunshni_analizi/2015/09/27/2616907_chudoto_na_prozrachnostta/>, accessed 2 October 2016

I Stoyanov 'Analytical overview of the main points in the draft Regulation for Implementation of the PPA' (2016) 3 *ZOP+*

JE Nolan (ed), A Chayes and A Chayes, *Regime Architecture: Elements and Principals* in *Global Engagement: Cooperation and Security in the 21st Century* (Washington DC: Brookings Institution, 1994)

K Lord, The perils and promise of global transparency (Albany: State University of New York Press, 2006)

M Fenster, The Opacity of Transparency (2006) 91 *Iowa Law Review*

M Ivanov, *Reformation without reforms. Political economy of the Bulgarian communism 1963–1989* (Sofia: Open Society Institute and Ciela, 2008)

M Karadjova, 'Legal mechanisms for decreasing the conflict of interest by the assignment of public procurements' (2008) Yearbook of New Bulgarian University <www.nbu.bg/PUBLIC/IMAGES/File/CPA/Godishnik_2008/MilenaKaradjova.pdf> accessed 20 April 2016

M Markov and M Krivachka, *The new aspects in the Public Procurement Act* (Sofia: IK Trud i Pravo, 2006)

M Krivachka, M Markov, E Dimova and Z Lilyan, *The new aspects in the Public Procurement Act* (Sofia: IK Trud i Pravo, 2006)

MZ Hillebrandt, D Curtin, A Meijer, *'Transparency in the EU Council of Ministers: An Institutional Analysis'* <http://www.clientearth.org/reports/aarhus-centre-resources-library/scholarly-articles/Transparency%20in%20EU%20Council,%20Curtin.pdf>, accessed 2 October 2016

P Trepte, Public procurement in the EU (Oxford: Oxford University Press, 2007)

R Avramov, *The communal capitalism – among the Bulgarian economical past* (vol. III, Sofia: Centre for Liberal Strategies, 2007)

R Balfour and C Stratulat, *The enlargement of the European Union* (2014) Discussion Paper <http://www.epc.eu/documents/uploads/pub_3176_enlargement_of_the_eu.pdf> accessed 24 October 2016

R Oliver, What is transparency? (New York: McGraw-Hill, 2004)

S Arrowsmith, 'Towards a multilateral agreement on transparency in government procurement' (1998) 47 *International and Comparative Law Quarterly*

S Arrowsmith, 'Transparency in Government Procurement: The Objectives of Regulation and the Boundaries of the WTO' 37 (2003) *Journal of World Trade*

S Arrowsmith, *The law of public and utilities procurement* (London: Sweet & Maxwell, 2005, 2014)

S Schooner, 'Desiderata: Objectives for a System of Government Contract Law' (2002) 11 *Public Procurement Law Review*

T Kotsonis, 'The Extent of the Transparency Obligation Imposed on a Contracting Authority Awarding a Contract Whose Value Falls Below the Relevant Value Threshold: Case C-195/04, *Commission v Finland*, 26.4.2007' (2007) 5 *Public Procurement Law Review*

Chapter 3
Corruption – Definition and Characteristics

'Corruption and fraud are sometimes a matter of mentality.'
(Alessandro Buticce, OLAF, in an interview for the Bulgarian TV channel 'BNT')

3.1 The Reasons for This Chapter

Hardly a day passes without corruption being discussed as a hot topic in the media or even casually, over coffee. Corruption is commonly described as the 'curse of humanity' and national governments and international organisations unite in their efforts towards combating this phenomenon. This work is also orientated towards the options available for combating corruption but which also provide a different angle to analyse the problem. It is focused more specifically on the manifestation of corruption in public procurement and the aspirations for transparency to act as the main instrument in this fight.

This chapter will thus examine the origin of corruption, its elements and its various forms of manifestation, as well as its most common consequences. It also discusses the main reasons for the abundance of corruption in an example Member State (Bulgaria), elucidating the reasons for and the national specificities of corruption, as well as the perception of corruption in the field of procurement, based on recent empirical research.[1]

The chapter will uncover the specific features of corruption as a common phenomenon deliberately and, further, as a phenomenon which has its own distinguishing characteristics approached from the perspective of a particular country. I consider it particularly important to have enumerated these differences in detail before a 'bad example' such as Bulgaria is researched and compared with Member States with lower levels of corruption. This is because when the reasons behind a negative phenomenon are clearly understood, then the measures needed to address it are easier to

---

[1] eg K Pashev, A Dyulgerov and G Kaschiev, Corruption in Public Procurement – Risks and Reform Policies (Sofia: Center for the Study of Democracy, 2006); S Stoychev, Corruption Violations in Public Procurement in Bulgaria (Sofia: Transparency International Bulgaria, 2007); K Pashev, Controlling corruption in public procurement: Indicators for assessing policy impact (Sofia: Management Monitoring Association, 2009).

© Springer International Publishing AG 2017
I. Georgieva, *Using Transparency Against Corruption in Public Procurement*,
Studies in European Economic Law and Regulation 11,
DOI 10.1007/978-3-319-51304-1_3

identify. Moreover, from the wider perspective of the EU and the New Procurement Directives, the effectiveness of the anticorruption tools in the legislation could have been greater if the rules had relied not only on good practices (such as those of Germany, and Austria to some extent, as analysed in this work), but had accounted for the specificity of the individual Member States and the sheer impossibility of imposing methods proven as effective from some Member States across the whole EU. However, this conclusion will crystallise from the analysis performed in later chapters and the benchmarking part of the book.

3.2   Corruption – Common Definitions

As opposed to the transparency principle, the definition of which is still subject to debate, as observed in Chap. 2, a straightforward general definition of corruption has been almost unanimously accepted in the literature – the 'abuse of power'. Nonetheless, despite this common definition, the various authors researching the phenomenon tend to expand on its characteristics and it has become widely recognised in society in all of its manifestations. Some authors however, argue that a unified definition of corruption has not yet been reached[2] due to its multifaceted structure and the clandestine nature of its related activities, but this opinion refers rather to the different forms and elements of corruption than the term in its entirety itself.

While the abuse of power can take many forms, the most frequent and easily recognisable form of corruption involves any kind of bribery. However, any activity abusing legally delegated power for personal interest and benefit, no matter whether it takes the form of simple 'gift giving', fraudulent actions, provision of misleading information or unacceptable lobbying is also defined as corruption.

TI supplements the general definition by describing corruption as the 'abuse of entrusted power for private gain', and distinguishes between 'according to rule' (eg a bribe paid for a service, required to be implemented by law, where the purpose of the bribe may well be to procure the service more speedily) and 'against the rule corruption' (eg a bribe paid to obtain services which are explicitly prohibited by law).[3]

Authors like Klitgaard et al. (1996), Lambsdorff (2007) and Ackermann (2006) have also left their trace in theory by providing their own definitions of corruption, which have over time become textbook examples:

> [C]orruption means the misuse of office for personal gain. The office is a position of trust, where one receives authority in order to act on behalf of an institution, be it a private, public, or non-profit. Corruption means charging an illicit price for a service or using the power of office to further illicit aims.[4]

---

[2] eg M Farrales, What is Corruption?: A History of Corruption Studies and the Great Definitions Debate (2005) SSRN <http://ssrn.com/abstract=1739962> accessed 21 April 2016.

[3] Transparency International (Website FAQs) <http://archive.transparency.org/news_room/faq/corruption_faq> accessed 21 April 2016.

[4] R Klitgaard, R MacLean-Abaroa and HL Parris, 'A practical approach to dealing with municipal malfeasance' (1996) UNDP/UNCHS/World Bank-UMP Working paper No 7 <www.bezkorupce.cz/documents/studie/klitgaard-parris-strategie-pro-mesta.pdf> accessed 21 April 2016, 1.

> Corruption, the misuse of public power for private benefit.[5]
> Corruption occurs where private wealth and public power overlap. It represents the illicit use of willingness to pay as a decision making criterion.[6]

The distinctive view of Klitgaard et al. (1996) on corruption proposes a different definition in their attempt to explain corruption using a mathematical formula, arguing that 'corruption is a crime of calculation, not passion'. The formula runs as follows: C=M+D-A, where '[c]orruption equals monopoly *plus* discretion *minus* accountability'.[7] This approach is rather different from the theoretical definitions mentioned above, but the concept is almost the same – monopoly (or power) and discretion (in other words the freedom to exercise personal judgement) without the necessary sense of accountability (liability, moral interdiction) will lead to corrupt actions. Following from this mathematical approach, Klitgaard (1998) also defended the proposition that combating corruption must reciprocally be more precise, calculated and focused on systematic actions. He proposed a more radical approach towards corruption by 'administering a shock to disturb a corrupt equilibrium'.[8]

At any rate, the definitions tend to be very close in meaning and cover the main characteristics of the phenomenon, which can be summarised as follows: *(i) corruption is an action (or inaction) of an official in violation of the rules of his or her public position, (ii) it is commenced consciously and (iii) it is intended to bring personal benefit to the official, third parties or organisations involved, where (iv) the benefits are usually not (otherwise) accessible for the beneficiary.*[9]

3.2.1 Forms of Corruption

There is a wealth of literature resulting from research, studies and notes analysing corruption and trying to categorise it. Although the definitions of corruption employed in most theories are similar, as commented above, the form and level of corruption often differs according to nationalities, cultures, historical heritage and different level of development.

Nevertheless, the most widely-known and prevalent forms of corruption appear to be the following, in descending order of frequency of occurrence[10]:

---

[5] JG Lambsdorff, The Institutional Economics of Corruption and Reform: Theory Evidence and Policy (Cambridge: Cambridge University Press, 2007) 1.

[6] S Rose-Ackerman, International handbook on the economics of corruption (Cheltenham: Elgar, 2006) xvii.

[7] See above (n 4); R Klitgaard, International Cooperation against Corruption (Finance & Development, 1998) 3–6; and R Klitgaard, R MacLean-Abaroa and H Parris, Corrupt cities (Oakland, Calif.: ICS Press, 2000) 26.

[8] R Klitgaard, International Cooperation against Corruption (Finance & Development, 1998) 3–6.

[9] Except in the case of 'according to rule corruption', as explained by TI.

[10] In 2004 the United Nations Office on Drugs and Crime (UNODC) presented the 2nd edition of its Anti-corruption toolkit (<www.unodc.org/pdf/crime/corruption/toolkit/AC_Toolkit_Edition2.

(a) *Bribery* – This is the most common form of corruption. It is the act of paying for service, special treatment and/or influencing a decision. The purpose of bribery is to gain personal benefit by receiving money, information, position or the award of a desired project etc. Bribery can be related to or cause the other forms of corruption listed below. The UNODC[11] distinguishes several specific types of bribery, such as the influence-peddling of privileges; offering or receiving improper gifts; bribery to avoid liability for taxes or other costs; bribery in support of fraud; bribery in support of unfair competition (which could be linked to the most common form of corruption in the public procurement sector) etc.;

(b) *Embezzlement, theft and fraud* – these involve individuals obtaining money, privileges or possessions to which they have access, but to which they are not entitled;

(c) *Extortion* – this form of corruption uses the threat of violence or exposure of information to assure the cooperation of one or more individuals;

(d) *Abuse of discretion* – this is commonly seen in state or other public institutions, which have the opportunity to dispose of or purchase goods or services. UNODC[12] provides the example of an official responsible for government contracting who exercises his discretion to purchase goods from a company in which he holds personal interest. A variation of this form of corruption in the public procurement sector can be seen where a representative of the contracting authority chooses eg as supplier, a company in which he or she has an interest or other connection and consequently benefits from the profit gained by the supplier as a result of the award of the contract; this frequently takes the form of the next type of corruption;

(e) *Favouritism, nepotism and clientelism* – this form of corruption is commonly encountered in countries which were previously behind the Iron Curtain,[13] such as Bulgaria. The abuse of power favours someone related to the official concerned (eg a family member, or a member of the same political party, or a fellow-member of a particular group of people);

(f) *Conduct creating or exploiting conflicting interests* – the name of this form is self-explanatory, whereas, as UNODC also observes,[14] most of the other forms of corruption can be linked with the conflict of interest form (such as embezzlement and favouritism);

---

pdf> accessed 21 April 2016). It is one of the most comprehensive elaborations of the different categories of corruption. The UNODC categories have been used in the summary above.

[11] Ibid.

[12] Ibid.

[13] The political, military, and ideological barriers erected by the Soviet Union after the Second World War to seal off itself and its dependent Eastern and Central European allies from open contact with the West and other non-communist areas.

[14] See above (n 10).

(g) *Improper political contributions* – this form involves improper attempts to influence the activities of a political party or its members, usually by 'donations' either to the political party itself or to a body linked to it.

(h) *Bid rigging (i.e. concerted practice)* – this form is associated with the award of public procurements and infringement of competition rules in the sector; it relates to different forms of 'arranging' the outcome of a public procurement procedure between the bidders, with or without the consent of the contracting authority;

(i) *Kickbacks* – a form of bribery which has also its place in procurement award; the contracting authority considers accepting a bribe which will be accounted for in the tendering process;

(j) *Conflict of interests* – the contracting authority (or a member or employee of it) is personally interested in the outcome of the procurement procedure.

Most of these forms of corruption can be for personal gain (individual corruption) or to ensure the adoption or application of a certain policy (institutional corruption).

Of great significance for the manifestation of the different forms of corruption is the level of social and economic development of the country concerned, as well as the historical background of that country. To a large extent, these factors, along with the existing mindset and social mentality, play a role in the prevalence of certain corrupt practices and in the field in which they will be manifested, as will be explained further in this book. In this sense, an excellent addition to the definitions and characteristics of corruption is the opinion that '[c]orrupt is not only the individual accepting (receiving) undue benefits. Corrupt is also the individual abusing public trust'.[15] Precisely for this reason, the historical preconditions for the existence of corruption and the attitudes of society towards this phenomenon are reviewed in this work.

3.2.2   Origins

Corruption, both in its entirety and in its infinitely varied forms of manifestation is not in the focus of this work, but its origins and main historical and social milestones are important for the comprehensiveness and understanding of the conclusions of the research made. With this in mind, the following discussion will briefly outline the roots of corruption and its development in the course of time and across the world as well as its forms in public procurement, which will be the subject of detailed discussion in the subsequent chapters.

The historical roots of corruption as a world phenomenon go back to ancient times: the customary presentation of gifts for someone's benignancy is well-known in all countries. However, even in primeval days the moral principles of society

---

[15] G Boyadjiev, E Tsenkov and K Dobrev, Corruption in 100 answers (Sofia: Civil Connection Foundation, 2000) 1.

drew a distinction between a simple gift given out of gratitude and a gift provided with the expectation of something in return. Later, the complicated state apparatus in the various nations began to require an increase in bureaucracy and, as a consequence, other forms of corruption than straightforward bribery began to appear.

Historical evidence about corruption and the fight against it can be found as early as the twenty-fourth century BC.[16] One of the first documents discussing corruption is the Indian treatise *Arthaśāstra* from the sixth century BC. One of the two authors[17] of *Arthaśāstra* – Kautilya – describes around forty forms of embezzlement of government funds.

In more modern times, wars and the resulting hardship and privation constitute one of the main catalysts for corruption; therefore it is mainly after the two World Wars and the massive-scale corruption which set in at that time that more serious analyses of the topic were carried out, and some attempts were made by the fragile democratic societies to deal with the problem.

After the First World War, ideas started to take shape towards creation of a global system against the acts of corruption. Investigations into the causes and consequences of corruption commenced and politicians began to search for the best weapon to combat this scourge.[18]

Academic interest in corruption escalated after the Second World War and especially in the fifties,[19] reaching a peak with the onset of the Cold War and the later dissolution of the Soviet Union – a time where widely quoted and well-known authors such as Johann Graf Lambsdorff, Rose Ackermann, Robert Klitgaard and many others were active.

Today, as the existence and increasing extent of corruption continues as a source of concern, whether at local, national or even international level, curbing corruption is a priority for many international organisations. Even though a catch-all instrument against corruption has yet to be found, the scrutiny of corruption lays bare its different manifestations, its causes and its negative consequences in various spheres of life.

---

[16] One of the first rulers to dedicate a great deal of attention to fighting corruption was the ruler of the city of Lagash, Mesopotamia – Urukagina (c. 2380–2360 BC). The Code of Urukagina is known for its anticorruption provisions and stipulated penalties. However, historical evidence indicates that his policy met with limited success.

[17] Kautilya and Vishnugupta.

[18] This was one of the main goals of the 'Progressive Era' in the United States, during which the idea crystallised that exposure of the machinery of government and its heads can serve as a weapon to combat corruption. In Europe, the idea of stronger government policies and the role of the elite class in constitutional governments (influenced by the Japanese intellectual leader Yoshino 1878–1933) as a reaction against corruption attracted followers in the wake of the First World War.

[19] Authors and seminal works from this period include: E Banfield, The Moral Basis of Backward Society (New York: New York Free Press, 1958); E Banfield, Corruption as a Feature of Governmental Organisation (1975) 18(3) Journal of Law and Economics 587–605; SH Alatas, The Sociology of Corruption: The Nature, Function, Causes and Prevention of Corruption (1968) 1(2) Journal of Southeast Asian Studies 142–143; M McMullan, A Theory of Corruption (1961) 9(2) Sociological Review ix; J Nye, Corruption and Political Development: A Cost-Benefit Analysis (1967) 61(2) American Political Science Review 417–427.

3.2.3   Causes and Consequences

Based on the definition of corruption and its historical development, and considering its main and ultimate goal – personal benefit – the causes of corruption are relatively easy to determine. Usually, lack of governmental transparency is identified as the first precondition for corruption to flourish, combined with underpaid officialdom. Other noted causes of corruption include limited freedom of speech and freedom of the press, weak judicial control and concentration of power in the hands of unaccountable persons.

The different factors which can cause corruption also depend on the sphere of life considered, such as the governmental, economic, political or social environments. Corruption manages to find its niche in all of these spheres and its systematic development could lead to catastrophic consequences. Perhaps the most negative consequences for a society suffering from systematic and increasing corruption are the *resulting hindrances for economic development* as well as the *growing climate of distrust in society*.

3.2.4   International Organisations Against Corruption

Numerous well-known organisations view combating corruption as one of their priorities, including:

(i) *international organisations* such as the WTO, the World Bank, the International Monetary Fund and the United Nations;

(ii) *regional organisations*, such as the European Union, the Council of Europe and the European Bank for Reconstruction and Development;

(iii) *trade union initiatives* such as the Trade Union Advisory Committee to the Organisation for Economic Cooperation and Development (TUAC to OECD);

(iv) *private sector initiatives* of the International Chamber of Commerce and the Business and Industry Committee to the OECD (BIAC to OECD)[20]; and

(v) *non-governmental organisation* such as Transparency International (TI).

Some of the findings of the present work are based on research carried out by these organisations, although not all of their initiatives are related particularly to corruption in the field of public procurement. Chapter 2 has already made a brief note of the work of the WTO, the OECD and TI: these three organisations investigate the correlation between corruption and transparency in detail and have been particularly active in analysing corruption in government procurement.

---

[20] See the OECD Working Group on Bribery methodology.

3.3   Corruption in Figures

TI has published the CPI corruption index annually since 1995, which allows for international comparisons of corruption based on the subjective perceptions of businessmen, experts, risk analysts and citizens.[21]

This index, which TI created, is currently deemed to be one of the most reliable sources of information on the corruption status round the world.[22] As described by TI itself, '[it] is a composite index, a poll of polls, drawing on corruption-related date from expert and business surveys carried out by a variety of independent and reputable institutions.'[23]

CPI ranks around 170[24] countries in terms of corruption, using at least three reliable, high quality data sources, published no earlier than within in previous 2 years. These are usually polls and surveys which rank different countries and territories.

As mentioned, the CPI[25] presents the generally accepted and recognisable statistical data on the level of corruption globally. However, the *modus operandi* of the CPI is open to criticism for lack of objectivity and reliability. Because corruption inherently manifests itself behind the scenes and exists as furtively as possible, it is obvious that there can be no valid method that could clearly reflect the amount of corruption in a given country. For this reason it must be admitted that CPI uses somewhat hypothetical and subjective formulas based on the perception, estimation and attitudes of the examined sample population. This is quite limited in terms of its methodology, and the following points demonstrate its shortcomings[26]:

(a) The assessment of the development and spread of corruption are based entirely on subjective factors;

---

[21] 'It is the deep conviction of the authors of the corruption index that in an area as complex and contradictory as corruption there may exist a single source or survey method, to provide the ideal framework model with a sufficiently wide coverage of countries and fully convincing methodology for comparative study. That is why the corruption index is designed based on the generalised index method. That is, it is composed of reliable studies that use different methodologies and framework models and is statistically the most convincing means of recording subjective perceptions of corruption', Center for the Study of Democracy 'Corruption and Anticorruption' (Sofia: Center for the Study of Democracy, 2003) <http://www.sliven.bg/doc/Announ/01.pdf> accessed 21 April 2016, 238.

[22] Other frequently used sources are also the EU Commission's Special Eurobarometer Surveys, the Business Environment and Enterprise Performance Survey of the EBRD and the World Bank, the Nations in Transit survey of Freedom House etc.

[23] Transparency International, 'Frequently Asked Questions' (Transparency International Corruption Perception Index 2009) <www.transparency.ch/de/PDF_files/CPI/CPI2009_FAQ.pdf> accessed 21 April 2016.

[24] 168 countries for 2015.

[25] As an international barometer of corruption, along with the Global Corruption Barometer.

[26] Despite the fact that the initial CPI was later supplemented by the Global Corruption Barometer based on their own sociological polls, reflecting not only the perceptions of the respondents, but also their experience of involvement in corrupt acts.

(b) The CPI does not use its own studies of the prevalence of corruption but rather relies on independent studies and expert assessments;
(c) The index predominantly takes into account cases of bribery and extortion in the business field, without reflecting a number of other significant forms of corrupt practices[27];
(d) The CPI has been criticised for its one-sidedness as it only reflects the corruption of those 'taking', but not of those 'giving';
(e) The CPI is unable to measure trends in the prevalence of corruption, although it is often interpreted that way. In this sense it can hardly be regarded as a measure of the success of ongoing anticorruption policies and reforms[28];
(f) The CPI does not reflect the national, economic and political characteristics of the surveyed countries in any way. Post-socialist and Balkan countries are traditionally considered corrupt in this sense. Therefore, even if corruption at all levels of government has actually declined considerably, the CPI will not reflect this positive change for a long time, as it relies solely on the subjective perceptions of respondents, who often do not reflect the true situation;
(g) TI uses sources from the previous 2 years for its annual CPI. These sources might mirror social perceptions which in turn were formed earlier in the past. That is why any significant changes in the CPI are only likely to emerge over longer periods.

These shortcomings should not be considered fatal; so far, the CPI is one of the few attempts to measure the immeasurable. If there is a perception of corruption in a country, there must surely be some unresolved issues at the national level. However, such indices should be considered very carefully, since people's perceptions are a factor which is influenced much more slowly than the actual changes (either an increase or decrease in corruption). Obviously therefore, when analysing the annual results of this index we must be conscious that the truth likely falls between two extremes.

3.4 Corruption in Government Procurement – A Global Review

The economic significance of public procurement in Europe is considerable. Despite not all areas of public expenditure being covered by public procurement rules, the market reached EUR 447 billion (19% of EU GDP) in 2010[29] and slightly decreased,

---

[27] In this sense it is completely superfluous to assessing corruption schemes in public procurement.

[28] In this connection see also: F Galtung, Measuring the Immeasurable: Boundaries and Functions of (Macro) Corruption Indices in C Sampford, Measuring corruption (Aldershot: Ashgate, 2006).

[29] Based on total estimated value of tenders published in the Tenders Electronic Daily (TED), according to Council (EU), 'Annual Public Procurement Implementation Review 2013' SWD(2014) 262 final, 1 August 2014, 5.

due to the financial crisis worldwide, to EUR 425 billion in 2011.[30] According to a study[31] conducted in 2013:

> [T]he direct public loss encountered in corrupt/grey cases amounts to 18% of the budgets involved, while this figure is 6% in clean cases. Hence, the overall public loss due to corruption is estimated at 13% (rounding errors), thus explaining over 2/3 (69%) of the direct public losses of corrupt/grey projects.[32]

Understanding government procurement as a public sector activity which operates with the state budget and redistributes public funds to the private sector (in most cases) in return for the supply of goods and services readily brings to mind the 'thin line' between procurement and corruption. The tempting opportunity for entrepreneurs and traders to gain benefit from the distribution of public funds has been one of the most commonly encountered reasons for 'abuse of power' for many decades. In Grødeland's (2005) words:

> Given the large sums of money involved in public procurement, it is not surprising that a number of individuals and groups have vested interests in promoting certain outcomes with regard to public tenders.[33]

In addition, the whole process of participating in one procurement procedure and the preparation of a cost-efficient offer is a time-consuming and expensive process and therefore many candidates decide to improve their chances by engaging in corrupt practices such as bribery. Moreover, most of the candidates take the view that 'everyone else is involved in such kind of business'.[34]

The forms of corruption in procurement are as various as the imaginations of the participants – from bribery through fraud to abuse of discretion. The different manifestations of corruption depend on the type of procurement (construction, supply etc), the type of procedure (open, restricted, competitive dialogue etc), the type of contract to be concluded (fixed price or variable, framework contract etc) and of course the personal interests involved. Common forms of corruption in the public procurement award process remain 'bid rigging', 'kickbacks' and 'conflicts of interest' (where the contracting authority is personally related to the winning bidder).

Corruption can occur at any phase of the procurement process; however, the most common cases of corruption are connected with the candidate qualification/evaluation phase. Because contracting authorities are often (depending on the domestic legal framework) free to decide the methodology of evaluation of candi-

---

[30] Ibid.

[31] W Wensink and J Maarten de Vet, Identifying and Reducing Corruption in Public Procurement in the EU – Development of a methodology to estimate the direct costs of corruption and other elements for an EU-evaluation mechanism in the area of anti-corruption (prepared for the European Commission by PwC and Ecorys, with support of Utrecht University, 2013).

[32] Ibid, 174.

[33] A Grødeland, Bulgaria, Czech Republic, Romania and Slovenia: The Use of Contracts and Informal Networks in Public Procurement in Fighting Corruption and Promoting Integrity in Public Procurement (Paris: OECD Publishing, 2000) ch 7, 60.

[34] See T Søreide, Corruption in Public Procurement: Causes, Consequences and Cures (Bergen, Norway: Chr. Michelsen Institute, Development Studies and Human Rights, 2002) 4.

dates, the respective instance of corruption may very well remain undetected. The contracting authority is always interested, in its capacity as bribe-taker, to motivate the evaluation of candidates in such a way that the 'impartially chosen' winner would appear, beyond all doubt, to be the candidate who has presented the most economically advantageous tender. Where the procurement award criteria is the lowest price, corrupt practices regarding candidate qualification are naturally somewhat more sophisticated.[35]

The specific hypothesis of corruption in procurement procedures and at the various phases will be studied in detail in the next chapters of this work. This chapter discusses the most common and likely types of corruption and the phases at which it occurs, as presented in the table below. For these purposes the procurement process is divided into four main phases (not considering specific differences between different procedures)[36]:

1. *Choice of Object Phase* – when the contracting authority decides that it needs to purchase goods, procure construction work or have certain services performed. In this phase the contracting authority determines the basic parameters of the procurement, such as technical specifications, presumed price and the relevant period; it also calculates the budget for the procurement. This phase concludes with the selection of a particular procedure and the decision to commence the procurement procedure.
2. *Announcement Phase* – in which the contracting authority and the experts (if required) prepare the required documentation for the launch of the procurement procedure (such as the official announcement of the procedure, the application forms, the technical specifications and other parameters of the procurement).
3. *Procedure Conduct Phase* – this is the core phase of the whole procedure, involving the contracting authority and all the participants/approved candidates. In this phase potential bidders have a limited period to present their offers/applications; the contracting authority examines their offers and may make a preliminary selection of candidates; the contracting authority ranks the candidates and announces a winner. This phase is considered most susceptible to corruption, as bidders can seek to bribe the contracting authority prior to or during the evaluation of the tenders.
4. *Contract Implementation Phase* – this involves the conclusion of the contract between the contracting authority and the successful bidder, as well as the performance of all contractual obligations.[37] Corruption here is also frequent, as it is

---

[35] In this respect it would be interesting to track practice following the transposition of the New Procurement Directives and (at least theoretically) the elimination of the lowest price criteria. This point is discussed in relation to corrupt intent during the award process in the following chapters of this book.

[36] In this context see also OECD, 'Bribery in Public Procurement: Methods, Actors and Counter-Measures' (OECD online publication 2007) <www.oecd.org/daf/anti-bribery/anti-briberyconvention/44956834.pdf> accessed on 21 April 2016, 19–22.

[37] This outcome is initially uncertain, as the contracting authority may decide to award the contract to none of the bidders. Such an outcome rarely involves corrupt practices and is therefore not discussed further.

mainly the procurement award which is the focus of regulation, while control over implementation often takes a backseat. This trend is expected to change as a result of the much more strictly defined cases in which lawful amendment of a concluded procurement contract is possible under the New Procurement Directives. Whether this will achieve a satisfactory result in most Member States remains to be seen.

Table 3.1[38] contains the most frequent elements of corrupt policies with regards to the award process phases listed above.

Table 3.1 Manifestation of corruption in the procurement process

Procurement process phase	Manifestation of corruption
Choice of object	The contracting authority is corruptly requested by the interested party to open a procurement procedure which does not correspond to the contracting authority's justifiable need for particular services and/or goods;
	The contracting authority is corrupted by the interested party to the effect that the contracting authority's correct appraisal of the type of the procedure to be conducted is altered etc.
Announcement	The contracting authority is corrupted by the interested party so that the parameters of the procedure chosen suit the interested party's candidate;
	The contracting authority is corrupted so that the assessment criteria and/or the methodology of the formula used for determination of the winner of the procedure are presented vaguely and ambiguously;
	The contracting authority is corrupted so that the procurement requirements are phrased in such a way that some of the possible bidders are automatically excluded from participation etc.
Procedure conduct	The contracting authority is corrupted by the interested party to provide confidential information about the tenders submitted by other participants in the procedure;
	The contracting authority is corrupted to misrepresent the evaluation of the candidates;
	The contracting authority is corrupted to prevent it from examining the use of subcontractors by a particular bidder;
	The contracting authority is corrupted to accept and assess additionally provided and manipulated information/documentation not contained in the offer etc.
Contract implementation	The contracting authority is corrupted to accept substantial changes in the preliminary draft of the procurement contract which fundamentally alter the parameters of the procurement from those initially announced.

---

[38] An inexhaustive list provided for the comprehensiveness of this section, as this topic will be the object of analysis of the next few chapters.

As for those involved in corrupt schemes in public procurement, it must be noted that in addition to the purely 'briber-bribed' scheme, the specifics and complexity of the award process involve many persons up to the final decision of the contracting body (eg experts, committee members, consortium members). The participation of numerous different actors in a corrupt scheme renders its detection all the more difficult. Moreover, public spending whets the appetites of political parties and 'the powers that be' in government. For this reason, in some countries (including Bulgaria, as shown in this book), where there is a lack of sufficiently independent bodies to exercise control over the award process, the burden falls (to a big extent) on legislation in the field. This leads to rules which are created and monitored by decision-makers, which leaves corruption loopholes in the regulation of the award process and further, to the absence of effective control.

3.5   Members States with Higher Levels of Corruption – The Example of Bulgaria

As explained above, in the search for the specificities of the phenomenon this part of the chapter will pay more detailed attention to the origin of corruption in Bulgaria, and the historical and economic factors which have brought corruption to today's magnitude in this Member State.

3.5.1   Historical Explanation of the Predisposition to Corruption

Bearing in mind that the Bulgarian state is one of the oldest in Europe,[39] historical sources provide evidence of corruption and the offering of 'gifts' – and of the fierce struggle of the Bulgarian khans against this problem, under the influence of the Byzantine Empire – dating from as early as the ninth century CE. Historical records indicate that combating corruption was one of the priorities of the rulers of that time, along with measures against alcohol abuse and theft.[40]

Later on, the Bulgarians (similar to other nations part of the Ottoman Empire) used elementary bribery on a daily basis in order to survive the oppressive conditions and the rocketing taxes which subjugated populations were obliged to pay their rulers. A historical fact worth noting in this context is that the Ottoman Penal Code of 1857, written in precisely those times (partially adopted in Bulgarian legal

---

[39] Established in 681 CE.

[40] In this context see, for example I Bojilov and V Gyuzelov, History of Bulgaria in Three Volumes (Sofia: Anubis Publishing, 1999) vol 1, ch 6.

practice as well), contained very detailed provisions defining bribery and how it was to be sanctioned.[41]

In the nineteenth century, after ceasing to be part of the Ottoman Empire and during the period that Bulgaria began to rebuild itself as a nation, bribery, as well as other forms of corruption continued to be common and widespread behaviour. A start was made towards fighting corruption with the adoption of legislation such as the Law on Ministerial Liability (1880), which stipulated that a minister could be sued in the event of allegations that he/she places personal gain before state interests. Later, the Bulgarian Penal Code of 1896 criminalised bribery: the receiving party was liable for imprisonment of two to ten years.[42]

Elenkov (1998)[43] reviewed the development of various measures against corruption in Bulgarian penal legislation, and analysed in detail the special laws which were enacted to combat the phenomenon. Accordingly, prior to the end of the Second World War the following laws were enacted: the Law on Prosecution of Illegally Enriched State Officials (1894); the Law on the Mercenary Abuse of Office (1934), and the Law on Appointment of Family Members in State, Municipal and Autonomous Institutions (1935). Numerous decrees were also adopted, and many anticorruption measures implemented.

After the Second World War and the subsequent distribution between Stalin and Churchill of spheres of influence over European countries,[44] Bulgaria fell under the Russian sphere and accordingly, a communist regime was imposed on the country for a particularly extended period – from 1944 to the early 1990s. During this period, private property ownership was prohibited (real estate and material possessions could be acquired only under strict control of the state and in predetermined quantities), and the pursuit of material wellbeing was generally condemned (at least in theory) as 'capitalistic' and 'destructive'.

Slowly, but surely, the human desire to possess more (be it goods, information or opportunities) or to simply reach out to and taste the 'worldly goods' of the Western world prevailed over the communist ideal. In order to satisfy those neglected needs, people once again opened the door to corruption at all levels of social and political life. As Krastev (2002)[45] described it:

---

[41] I Elenkov, Corruption in Contemporary Bulgaria: Analytical Overview , 1998, ch V, 2, which contains section III, entitled 'On Bribery' from the Ottoman Penal Code of 1857. 'A bribe is everything which is taken and given under any name in order to reach a goal: Gifts, small or big, given under any name or pretext, are regarded as a bribe…'; 'Where officials, appointed to offer state revenue for sale, are shown to take money from someone, or to sell state revenue at a lower price in order to fulfil personal interest although other buyers were also available, such officials shall be punished as embezzlers of state property'.

[42] Ibid.

[43] Ibid.

[44] ie the so called informal 'percentage agreement' made during the Moscow Conference in October 1944, right after the end of the Second World War.

[45] I Krastev, 'How to Control Corruption in Southeastern Europe: The Case of Bulgaria in Southeast European and Black Sea Studies Sofia' (2002) 2(1) Southeast European and Black Sea Studies 119–125.

> Under communist rule dominated by an economy of shortages, corruption manifested itself
> in the form of bartering. In most cases, it took the form of exchange of influence and ser-
> vices – straightforward bribery was the exception rather than the rule. The monetisation of
> corruption as a business transaction between buyers and sellers has made it more visible
> and disruptive for the majority of the population.

This form of 'bartering corruption' became habitual in Bulgarian society (as well as in the other countries behind the Iron Curtain, such as the Czechoslovak Republic, Poland, Hungary, Romania, Albania etc) and, moreover, remained unpunishable and even tolerated for the entire period until the end of the Cold War in 1991. Consequently, the transitional period after *Perestroika*[46] confronted Bulgaria with one of the most challenging issues – *how to change the mentality of a society which considers corruption as a normal and indispensable part of life*. At the state admin-istration level, the idea that civil servants would expect to receive an additional incentive (in the shape of cash or a gift) and that this incentive would ensure the preferential treatment of the bribe-offering party, remained an integral part of the national mentality for a very long time.

The transitional period saw an immediate increase in corruption, since centralised control over the phenomenon exercised by the former totalitarian elite was lost; this was a time when governments began to enter the market of corruption independently. As Linarelli (1998) notes, '[t]he weakness of central government allows various gov-ernment agencies to impose independent bribes, when entry into the market of cor-ruption is free or relatively inexpensive, high levels of corruption result.[47]

Some commentators[48] have argued that corruption in post-communist Bulgaria is basically different than the form practised during the communist administration. In other words, the 'bartering corruption' became 'straightforward'[49] in the transitional period. Although it may be the case that corruption has changed to an extent, it is rather the *direction* than the *character* of corruption which has shifted. Since the simple needs of society for a better life have today (more or less) been satisfied, the downfall of the Iron Curtain opened up new opportunities and new horizons for bribery. The privatisation process or the accumulation of funds under operational programmes, including through public procurement procedures, are sufficient proof that corruption can most certainly remain undetected and not be exactly 'straight-forward', but still active at all institutional levels.[50]

---

[46] The policy of governmental and economic reform instituted by M. Gorbachev in the Soviet Union during the mid-1980s.

[47] See J Linarelli, 'Corruption in developing countries and countries in transition legal and eco-nomic perspectives' in S Arrowsmith and A Davies (eds) Public Procurement: Global Revolution (Alphen aan den Rijn: Kluwer Law International, 1998) 125–128.

[48] B Ellison, 'Public Administration Reform in Eastern Europe: A Research Note and a Look at Bulgaria' (2007) 39(2) Administration & Society 221–232.

[49] As described by Krastev (2002) – See above n 44.

[50] Completing the picture, Pashev (2006) notes as follows: 'In the early 1990's, when democracy and the rule of law were quite fragile, political corruption was mainly in the form of pumping resources out of the state-owned enterprises and their preparation for cheap privatisation. The newly established private businesses stood at the input and output of state-owned enterprises with

After the privatisation process was basically completed, public procurement and concessions became a major sphere of large-scale corruption. Their place on the top of the pyramid
of corrupt practices is determined by the large financial resources distributed within the
public procurement system, and the related opportunities for personal enrichment.[51]

At legislative level these specific manifestations of corruption are reflected and
defined in the current Criminal Code (*Наказателен Закон*).[52] The offence which
covers to the largest extent the characteristics of corrupt behaviour is bribery.[53]
According to Bulgarian criminal law, a bribe can be passive or active. In terms of
the sanctions provided, passive bribery is a more serious public offence. In 2000
the legislator criminalised acts which were previously not punishable, such as the
promise or offer of a bribe to an official, as well as an official's request or acceptance of a promise of a bribe.[54] Thus regulation of corruption within the Criminal
Code now covers almost all forms of corruption. But '[r]egardless of the fact that
the criminal law framework regulating corruption appears satisfactory, the results
from the fight against the most severe forms of corruption are not particularly aus-
picious. [...] [T]his is mainly due to two factors outside substantive criminal law.
Firstly, offences related to corruption and especially bribery is difficult to prove
[...]. Secondly, the fight against the most significant forms of corruption is impeded
by purely psychological stumbling blocks. Alas, Bulgarian society has, as yet, not
developed a culture of intolerance towards corruption. [...] [I]t is regarded as
somewhat normal that one will have to pay in order to exercise one's legal rights.
This peculiar 'accustomisation' to corruption, which may gradually turn into stan-

---

the participation of the management of the latter. Against the backdrop of the underdeveloped
market economy and the price liberalisation, they got the opportunity to bleed state-owned enterprises out and the state budget thanks to the soft budget constraints prior to the introduction of the
currency board arrangements. Thus, the economic shock-therapy and financial liberalisation of the
early 1990's, together with the delayed structural reforms and the soft budget constraints, created
opportunities for channelling assets of the public sector to privileged private groups. After the
[political and financial] crisis in 1996–7 and the introduction of the currency board, those structures which were the main factor for the delay of the reform processes turned into major participants in the privatisation.'; K Pashev, A Dyulgerov and G Kaschiev, Corruption in public
procurement – risks and reform policies (Sofia: Center for the Study of Democracy, 2006) 12.

[51] Ibid, 13.

[52] Promulgated in SG 26/2.4.1968, effective as of 1 May 1968, as amended.

[53] Art 301 Criminal Code.

[54] ie Art 304 et seq Criminal Code. Other examples of the Criminal Code incriminating corrupt
behaviour in the wider sense are Art 282 Criminal Code 'An official who violates or fails to fulfil
his official duties, or exceeds his powers or rights for the purpose of acquiring a benefit for himself
or for another, or to cause damage to another'; Art. 283 Criminal Code 'An official who uses his
official position to acquire unlawful benefit for himself or for another'; Art 224 Criminal Code 'A
person who receives a gift or other material benefit in order to give, or because he has given, to a
foreign country, foreign organisation or company, or to a foreign citizen, information from which
considerable damage has ensued or may ensue for the economy' etc.

dard behaviour, artificially lowers the negative public perception of the phenomenon.'[55]

3.5.2   *Economic Factors for Corruption in Bulgaria*

Before focusing on the government procurement sector in Bulgaria it is also neces-sary to review corruption and its factors from an economic perspective, in order better to understand the causes of corruption in this sector and to discuss the optimal comprehensive measures against it. Ganev (1998)[56] reviews the relationship between economic factors and the state of corruption in Bulgaria in a very comprehensible and well-organised manner. His conclusions help outline the economic 'conditions precedent' for the increasing corruption in this Member State.

Ganev (1998) identifies three factors which determine the risk of corruption and the level of corruption:

(i)   The value of the resources placed under the public official's control;
(ii) The level of personal discretion of public officials in managing those resources; and
(iii) The degree of accountability for the actions and decisions of public officials.

Further, the factors determining the demand and supply for corruption correlates mainly to the anticipated consequences for the respective public official – eg the material losses which the public official in charge may suffer in case of disclosure of his/her corrupt behaviour, the amount of those losses, the moral principles of the officials etc. The demand for corruption, however, depends on much more specific conditions which Ganev (1998) divides into four types:

(i)   The number and nature of the permissions and/or licensing regime – the more complicated the regime, the greater the possibilities for corrupt practices, since any permission regime is usually viewed by traders as an obstacle to their busi-ness activities;
(ii) The tax system – entrepreneurs are ready to offer bribes in order to decrease their tax liabilities[57];
(iii) The total value of state-supplied goods – traders are willing to bribe in order to 'buy low and sell high'; and
(iv) State expenditure on goods and services – this factor is directly connected to the public procurement regime in the country and therefore is of a particular interest for the present work. This factor attracts increasing corruption, as the

---

[55] L. Gruev and B Velchev, Criminal Law Issues in Combating Corruption (Sofa: Coalition 2000, 2000) 14–15.

[56] G Ganev, 'Corruption and economic development in Bulgaria' in Transparency International, Corruption in contemporary Bulgaria: Analytical overview (Sofia: Transparency International, 1998) 56.

[57] Ibid, 56 .

state authorities have to decide how and to whom to distribute enormous sums from public funds. Needless to say, entrepreneurs are anxious to win procurement contracts and to sell their services and/or productivity in large quantities. 'Corruption always occurs when an 'outside' resource is placed under somebody's control.'[58]

The macroeconomic effects of corruption in Bulgaria and the state's ability to react, based on the above observations, can be conveniently illustrated in a graphic (Graph 3.1).

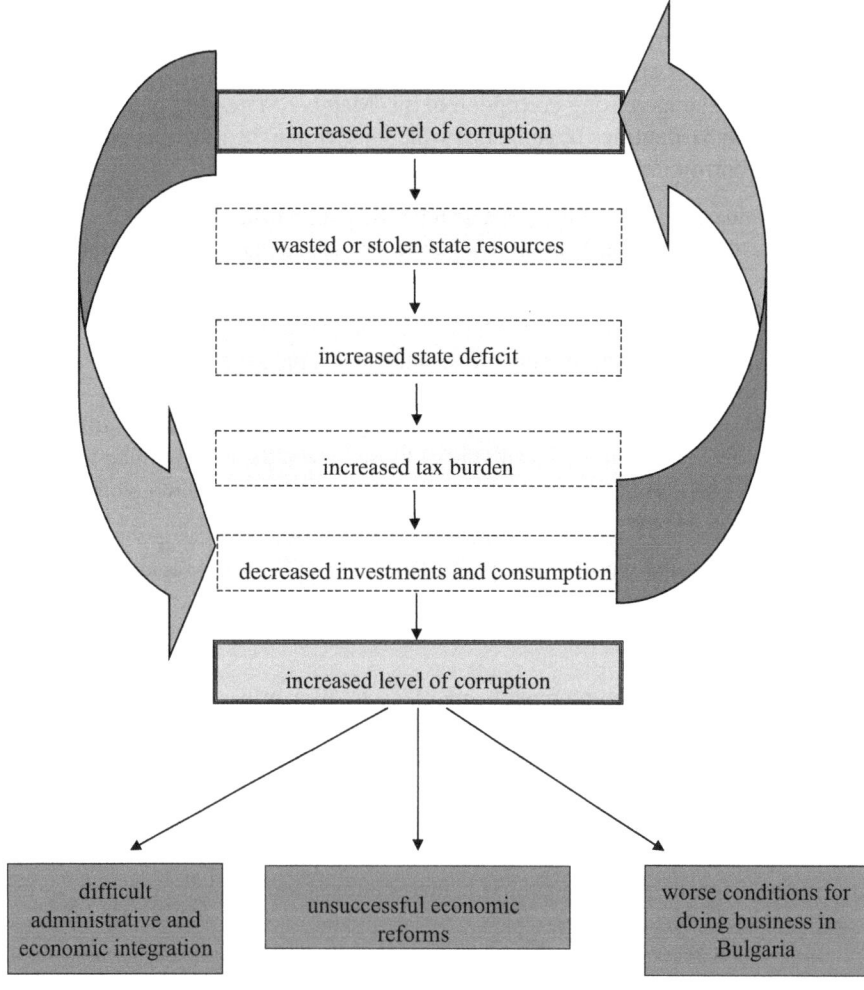

Graph 3.1 Macroeconomic effects of corruption

---

[58] Ibid, 57.

As a general conclusion, all of the effects of corruption sketched out above reflect the quality of the economic environment in Bulgaria. The entire institutional framework is distorted, where one of the expressions of this distortion is that mistrust has become a conceptual staple of economic behaviour in Bulgaria, as is the willingness to breach norms.

Another, equally comprehensive 'dissection' of the features of corruption in Bulgaria has not emerged in the last decade. However, nothing has changed, neither at a macroeconomic nor at a sociocultural level sufficiently to mark any substantial departure from Ganev's (1998) main observations. In light of the above, the latest EU country report sounds somehow sadly familiar: 'The fourth and fifth benchmarks for Bulgaria [...] concern the need for effective measures against corruption, including high-level corruption as well as corruption more generally in public institutions. Bulgaria consistently ranks among the EU Member States with the highest perceived level of corruption, and corruption is considered to be one of the most important barriers to doing business in Bulgaria'.[59]

3.5.3   Corruption in Bulgaria in Figures

TI's CPI and the Corruption Monitoring System (CMS), developed by the Center for the Study of Democracy[60] present verified statistical data on the level of corruption in the country for almost the last two decades. These two independent institutions regularly examine corruption in Bulgaria hence their achievements and conclusions merit further analysis.

The present section, however, will only address the statistical aspect of their activity in order to provide a visual representation of corruption levels in Bulgaria: (a) as compared to global trends, and (b) as assessed at local level.

CPI

Bearing the shortcomings of the CPI, already discussed in this chapter, in mind, below are presented the recent figures for Bulgaria.

Bulgaria was included in the CPI for the first time in 1998 and was awarded an index value of 2.9. Since then, the annual CPI values in Bulgaria have gradually come to be favoured by the media and civil society as a key indicator and an objective measure of the level of corruption in the country.

The CPI for the period from 1998 to 2008 establishes Bulgaria as a country with a moderate level of corruption. The index indicates improvement for the period

---

[59] Commission (EU), 'Report from the Commission to the European Parliament and the Council on Progress in Bulgaria under the Co-operation and Verification mechanism' SWD (2016) 15 final, 7.

[60] As a domestic complex of indexes measuring the level of corruption in Bulgaria.

from 1999 to 2002 (from 3.3 to 4) and relatively stable scores from 2002 to 2007 (figures vary for those years from 3.9 to 4.1). Against this background, a significant drop was registered in 2008,[61] and that low score of 3.6 was almost exactly reproduced in 2009 with a small improvement to 3.9.[62]

The CPI scores for Bulgaria in 2012 and 2013 and 2015 is 41.[63] At this level, Bulgaria draws closer to Greece and Romania at 69th position.

The graphic below illustrates the movement in CPI over the last decade[64] (Graph 3.2).

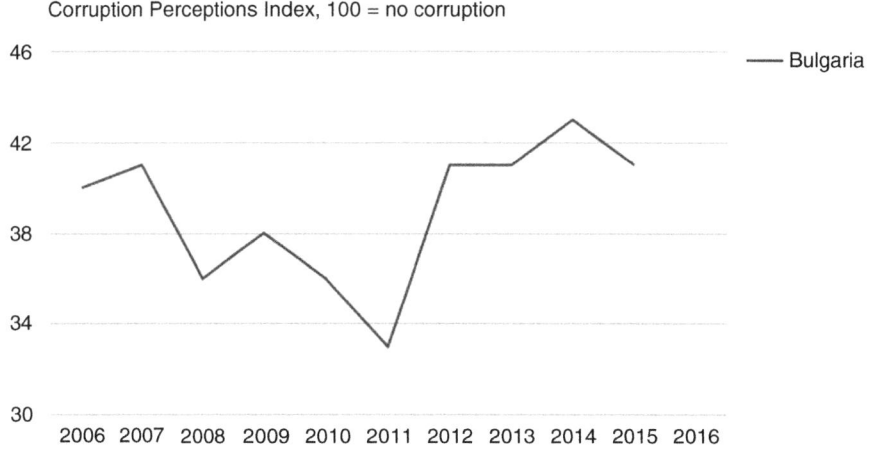

Corruption Perceptions Index, 100 = no corruption

Source: TheGlobalEconomy.com, World Bank

Graph 3.2 CPI for Bulgaria (2006–2016)

---

[61] A particular example of the evaluation of Bulgaria as a country with increasing corruption in 2008 was the 'shattering' report from OLAF of July 2008, which mysteriously leaked to the media and was made publicly available. In this report OLAF described Bulgaria as a country which tolerated fraud, money laundering, and forgery etc. In particular it exposed the criminal activities of one organisation in Bulgaria, which was under investigation for SAPARD projects fraudulently funded with EUR 7.5 mln in cash. The report also noted that Bulgaria had injured the EU's financial interests to a cost of over EUR 32 mln due to fraudulent and corrupt actions concerning SAPARD projects.

[62] The assessment scale used until (and incl. 2011) was of 0 (highly corrupt) to 10 (very clean).

[63] The now applicable assessment system (from 2012 on) uses a scale of 0 (highly corrupt) to 100 (very clean).

[64] Source: TheGlobalEconomy.com, 'Global economy, world economy' (2015) <www.theglobaleconomy.com> accessed 21 April 2016; and Transparency International.

CMS

The CMS is the first of its kind in the post-socialist countries and has been success-fully applied in Bulgaria ever since the 1990s, having been subsequently included in the United Nations Anti-Corruption Toolkit[65] and assessed by the UN as the best national corruption monitoring system.

The CMS provides data on the prevalence and dynamics of corruption in the public and the business sector. The study group includes representative samples of different social strata, public servants and business executives, press, radio and tele-vision media monitoring etc. The CMS records the actual level and the trends in the spread of administrative corruption in a country, as well as the related public atti-tudes, opinions and expectations. It uses nationally and internationally tested indi-cators to assess the level of corruption and the public attitudes towards it.

The CMS is a system comprising four different categories of indicators which vary in their ultimate research goal:

(a) The first set of indicators explores the *attitudes towards corruption* – the extent to which Bulgarians perceive the corrupt behaviour of MPs and public sector employees through the prism of their own value system. It explores the suscep-tibility of the population to corruption and in particular the susceptibility of public sector employees to corrupt behaviour;

(b) The second group of indicators examines *corrupt behaviour itself* – described as 'corruption pressure', both on citizens and on public employees. These explore the extent of the actual use of corrupt schemes by analysing the specific manifestations of corruption (from the most mundane offering of gifts to an employee to the more serious forms of abuse of power);

(c) The third set of indicators reflects the *assessment of the size of corruption* according to the population during the monitoring period, the degree of mani-festation of corruption and the actual result of corrupt behaviour;

(d) The last group of indicators analyse the *corruption expectations* of the public for effective limiting of corruption in the country.[66]

By applying this methodology, the CMS enormously expands the scope of its analysis, using various sources of information and different methods of assessment, specifically designed for the country and the attitudes of the Bulgarian population to the spread of corruption. Finally, this helps achieve comparability between the information collected and processed for Bulgaria on the one hand and the informa-tion about other European countries on the other. The CMS reports provide data from international comparative studies, reflecting different aspects of corruption.

---

[65] In 2011 CSD joined the UNCAC Coalition, also known as The Coalition of Civil Society Friends of the UN Convention against Corruption.

[66] The methodology adopted by the CMS is detailed in Center for the Study of Democracy 'Corruption and Anticorruption' (Sofia: Center for the Study of Democracy, 2003) <http://www.sliven.bg/doc/Announ/01.pdf> accessed 21 April 2016, 229–237.

A major difference between the CMS and the CPI is precisely that in addition to public attitudes and perceptions, the CSD's system also registers the actual distribution and manifestation of corruption in Bulgaria, thus allowing for a much more thorough analysis of corrupt practices in the country and therefore contributing to the search for different and effective methods of prevention. The subjective assessments offered by the CPI may sometimes distort the actual situation in the country within the period covered, while the CMS completes the picture and provides significantly more detailed and personalised data enabling assessment of the negative and positive trends in the levels of corruption in the country. That is why, it should be noted, that with respect to Bulgaria, the CMS set of indicators is far more objective in reflecting corruption levels and trends.[67]

The CMS index shows a significant and constant decrease in corrupt transactions (from 1.0 to 0.3) as well as in corruption pressure (from nearly 2.1 to 0.8) for the period from 1998 to 2004. However, after 2004, the CMS registered a rising trend in the corruption rate in the Bulgarian population. In this respect, the CMS accorded Bulgaria a 0.7 score for involvement in corruption transactions and 1.7 for corruption pressure in 2008. These results show that Bulgaria witnessed a slowdown in its anticorruption efforts in the years just before and right after its accession to the European Union.

Since 2009 a certain improvement compared to the previous periods has been observed in the index concerning corruption pressure and involvement in corrupt transactions, as part of the complex CMS. A general trend of declining numbers of people involved in corrupt transactions in the 1999–2013 period became apparent. For 2012 and 2013 this trend was reversed, and the number of participants in corrupt transactions increased.

> Subjective assessments by citizens indicate that corruption has been growing in recent years. Corruption practices are perceived to get more widespread, with the index going up from 6.1 in 2010 to 6.7 in October 2013. Even stronger is the increase in the perception of the practical efficiency of corruption (the probability of resolving problems by means of corruption). That index changed from 5.9 in 2010 to 6.9 in 2013.[68]

According to the latest report of the Center for the Study of Democracy published in 2014, the CMS has registered the highest levels of participation of the Bulgarian population in corrupt transactions for the last 15 years.[69] Over this particular year approximately 158,000 corrupt transactions have been carried out on a

---

[67] As of mid-2015 the Center for the Study of Democracy launched a new and additional index system for mapping of anticorruption enforcement instruments – the Monitoring Anti-corruption Policy Implementation (MACPI) tool which is 'intended to evaluate the anti-corruption preparedness of public organisations by identifying areas of corruption vulnerability' and actually supplements the achievements of CMS, as explained in Center for the Study of Democracy, 'Mapping Anti-Corruption Enforcement Instruments', Policy Brief 51 (Sofia: Center for the Study of Democracy, 2015) 1.

[68] Center for the Study of Democracy 'Corruption and Anticorruption (2012–2013)', Policy Brief 43 (Sofia: Center for the Study of Democracy, 2013) 5.

[69] In its Annual Corruption Assessment Report 'Anti-Corruption Policies against State Capture', the Center for the Study of Democracy provides an overview of the state of corruption and anticor-

monthly basis. What is even more striking, against this generally negative picture, is the fact that the percentage of those requesting bribes is falling at the expense of those offering bribes without a request being needed. The report draws particular attention to the public procurement sector as one with an increasing and generally high risk of corruption.

The figures for 2015 are slightly better – according to the CMS the perception of corruption has decreased from 29.3% of people participating in corrupt activities in 2014 to 18.6% for 2015; also from 39.4% of people exposed to corruption pressure in 2014 to 27.7% for 2015.[70]

3.5.4   Corruption in Government Procurement

Corruption can, beyond dispute, be detected in the Bulgarian public procurement system in all of its manifestations. Despite some a bit more optimistic assessments[71] of the level of corruption and the anticorruption measures launched in Bulgaria in the last decade, corruption in procurement has always remains at the forefront of all critical debate. Some of the particular issues which work towards creating such an inseverable link between corruption and procurement deserve attention here. The various manifestations of corruption in the different procurement procedures will then be considered. Based on the assessments of the quality of the legal regulation of procurement in Bulgaria, the literature[72] on the topic currently notes *inter alia* the following factors which facilitate corrupt practices in the public procurement sector: poor regulation of the various procedures; an insufficient level of transparency in the conduct of the procedures; predominantly *ex post* control over the conduct of procedures (partial *ex ante* control exists, but has not yet shown any definitely positive and constant results); amendments to contracts following conclusion of public procurement procedures; and a lack of publicity with respect to the procurement contracts concluded.

Most of these issues do indeed originate from the legal framework regulating public procurement and could possibly be remedied. However, the experience of the Bulgarian legislator unambiguously demonstrates that after almost thirty amendments and supplements to the PPA (before the entry into force of the New PPA in April 2016), the results are far from perfect. As Linarelli (1998) observes, and this closely fits the situation described:

---

ruption in Bulgaria for the period of 2013–2014. The report is produced within the framework of the Southeast Europe Leadership for Development and Integrity (SELDI).

[70] 'System for monitoring of anti-corruption politics' <http://www.csd.bg/fileSrc.php?id=22602 (2015)> accessed 21 April 2016 3

[71] eg JH Anderson and CW Grey, Anti-Corruption in transition 3: Who is succeeding… and Why? (The International Bank for Reconstruction and Development/The World Bank, 2006).

[72] Based on reports by Transparency International Bulgaria, the Center for Study of Democracy, the Bulgarian Public Financial Inspection Agency etc.

The elimination of corruption in public procurement in developing and transitioning countries depends on much more than good procurement rules. It will depend on long-lasting and credible reform of the executive, legislative and judicial organs of state that surround the procurement system and upon which a properly functioning procurement system depends for its viability. There are no easy solutions to combating corruption.[73]

Corruption in the procurement sector is further facilitated by the deliberate over-bureaucratisation[74] of public procurement procedures. The large number of bidding requirements and the administrative burden induces participants to seek political patronage in order to circumvent rules and requirements. With the transposition of the New Procurement Directives, and in view of the ambitious programmes which each subsequent government has pledged to undertake, one of the aspects on which reforms in the field are expected to focus will be precisely a reduction of the administrative burden, a lightening of the procedures and a gradual transition to e-procurement. It is still too early to draw any definite conclusions as to how exactly these plans are reflected in national legislation, but the New PPA offers no hope for any speedy simplification of the burdensome procedures which apply at present.

Finally, the global economic crisis has also impacted on Bulgaria, increasing competition between companies over public contracts and giving an additional impulse to both politicians and administration to obtain corruption fees. In this connection the political instability in Bulgaria and the frequent changes of polarised governments with either pro-Russian or pro-Western political and economic influence also play a part. The latter in particular has a disastrous effect on the legislative framework of public procurement, which is the inevitable subject of numerous modifications, many of which are dictated by purely political considerations.

Naturally, the losses incurred as a result of corrupt policies in the organisation, award and implementation of public procurement in a small country such as Bulgaria are enormous. Bearing in mind the national historical and social characteristics of corruption, as outlined above, it is perfectly justifiable to assume that the sums offered as bribes to win contracts are negligible in relation to the other benefits and privileges offered (including career advancement and political office) and also in relation to the direct economic damage and the loss of investment which are the natural consequence of increased corruption in the sector. This is precisely the angle one study took back in 2006,[75] which calculated the losses due to corruption as a percentage of national GDP and concluded that: 'if we abandon all conservative assumptions underlying the abovementioned optimistic estimate of the fiscal losses from corruption in the public procurement sector, they could reach 1 billion levs annually, ie some 20–25% of the size of the market or approximately 2.4% of GDP.'[76]

---

[73] See above (n 47).

[74] In this context see also above (n 15) 34–35.

[75] See above (n 1), 29–30.

[76] Though the study was published eight years ago and current figures will probably be slightly different, this in no way affects the conclusions drawn.

3.6   Concluding Observations

This chapter aims to present an overview of the origin and development of corruption worldwide and lastly focuses on Bulgaria as the 'benchmarking example' of this book, which is unable to fight corruption. The chapter outlines the main specifics of corruption at public procurement level.

The first part of the chapter allows us to trace the origin of this negative phenomenon and to highlight conclusions as to why it exists and what is typical of it. By summarising the various manifestations of corruption, those which are specific to public procurement are easily discerned. Obviously, certain infringements of the proper functioning of the procurement award process and the execution of procurement contracts describe the core problems of corruption in the sector and are recognisable at each stage of the procedure.

However, while corruption has its international dimensions, it also has its individual aspects with respect to each and every state. It is important to bear this in mind in the analysis of the three different legislations in the field of public procurement, in the assessment of the anticorruption policies so far pursued, and last but not least, in considering the best practices, thus to achieve maximum objectivity in the evaluation of possible positive developments in the procurement system of Member States with similar issues to Bulgaria.

That is why the historical 'walk' through the depths of corruption in Bulgaria presented in the second part of this chapter is essential to assess the causal relationships which have brought this Member State to this level of corruption. The features of this phenomenon in Bulgaria inevitably reflected the system of award of procurements as well as the legislative decisions aimed at tackling the problem. As will be seen in Chap. 5 of this book, which provides for a detailed analysis of the types of corruption infringements in the process of awarding and their relationship with the principle of transparency, there are types of violations which other countries have already overcome, but which are still relevant in Bulgaria.

Therefore, the conclusions drawn in the next chapters, in all cases relate to the points discussed so far and support the link between legal aspects and the socio-historical roots of corruption in the different Member States.

Bibliography

A Grødeland, *Bulgaria, Czech Republic, Romania and Slovenia: The Use of Contracts and Informal Networks in Public Procurement* in *Fighting Corruption and Promoting Integrity in Public Procurement* (Paris: OECD Publishing, 2000)

B Ellison, 'Public Administration Reform in Eastern Europe: A Research Note and a Look at Bulgaria' (2007) 39(2) Administration & Society

E Banfield, The Moral Basis of Backward Society (New York: New York Free Press, 1958)

E Banfield, *Corruption as a Feature of Governmental Organisation* (1975) 18(3) Journal of Law and Economics

F Galtung, *Measuring the Immeasurable: Boundaries and Functions of (Macro) Corruption Indices* in C Sampford, *Measuring corruption* (Aldershot: Ashgate, 2006)

G Boyadzhiev, E Tsenkov and K Dobrev, Corruption in 100 Answers (Sofia: Civil Connection Foundation, 2000)

G Ganev, 'Corruption and economic development in Bulgaria' in Transparency International, *Corruption in contemporary Bulgaria: Analytical overview* (Sofia: Transparency International, 1998)

I Bojilov and V Gyuzelov, History of Bulgaria in Three Volumes (Sofia: Anubis Publishing, 1999)

I Elenkov, Corruption in Contemporary Bulgaria: Analytical Overview, 1998

I Krastev, 'How to Control Corruption in Southeastern Europe: The Case of Bulgaria in Southeast European and Black Sea Studies Sofia' (2002) 2(1) Southeast European and Black Sea Studies

JG Lambsdorff, The Institutional Economics of Corruption and Reform: Theory Evidence and Policy (Cambridge: Cambridge University Press, 2007)

JH Anderson and CW Grey, *Anti-Corruption in transition 3: Who is succeeding… and Why?* (The International Bank for Reconstruction and Development/The World Bank, 2006)

J Linarelli, 'Corruption in developing countries and countries in transition legal and economic perspectives' in S Arrowsmith and A Davies (eds) *Public Procurement: Global Revolution* (Alphen aan den Rijn: Kluwer Law International, 1998)

J Nye, Corruption and Political Development: A Cost-Benefit Analysis (1967) 61(2) American Political Science Review

K Pashev, A Dyulgerov and G Kaschiev, Corruption in Public Procurement – Risks and Reform Policies (Sofia: Center for the Study of Democracy, 2006)

K Pashev, Controlling corruption in public procurement: Indicators for assessing policy impact (Sofia: Management Monitoring Association, 2009)

L Gruev and B Velchev, *Criminal Law Issues in Combating Corruption* (Sofa: Coalition 2000, 2000)

M Farrales, *What is Corruption?: A History of Corruption Studies and the Great Definitions Debate* (2005) SSRN <http://ssrn.com/abstract=1739962> accessed 21 April 2016

M McMullan, *A Theory of Corruption* (1961) 9(2) Sociological Review

R Klitgaard, R MacLean-Abaroa and HL Parris, 'A practical approach to dealing with municipal malfeasance' (1996) UNDP/UNCHS/World Bank-UMP Working paper No 7 <www.bez-korupce.cz/documents/studie/klitgaard-parris-strategie-pro-mesta.pdf> accessed 21 April 2016

R Klitgaard, *International Cooperation against Corruption* (Finance & Development, 1998)

R Klitgaard, R MacLean-Abaroa and H Parris, *Corrupt cities* (Oakland, Calif.: ICS Press, 2000)

S Stoychev, Corruption Violations in Public Procurement in Bulgaria (Sofia: Transparency International Bulgaria, 2007)

SH Alatas, The Sociology of Corruption: The Nature, Function, Causes and Prevention of Corruption (1968) 1(2) Journal of Southeast Asian Studies

S Rose-Ackerman, International handbook on the economics of corruption (Cheltenham: Elgar, 2006)

T Søreide, *Corruption in Public Procurement: Causes, Consequences and Cures* (Bergen, Norway: Chr. Michelsen Institute, Development Studies and Human Rights, 2002)

W Wensink and J.Maarten de Vet, *Identifying and Reducing Corruption in Public Procurement in the EU – Development of a methodology to estimate the direct costs of corruption and other elements for an EU-evaluation mechanism in the area of anti-corruption* (prepared for the European Commission by PwC and Ecorys, with support of Utrecht University, 2013)

Chapter 4
The Public Procurement System in Bulgaria: Authorities, Participants, Control and Achievements

'[C]ommending himself with all his heart to his lady Dulcinea,
[...] he charged at Rocinante's fullest gallop
and fell upon the first mill that stood in front of him.'
(Miguel de Cervantes Saavedra
'The Ingenious Gentleman Don Quixote of La Mancha')

4.1 What Is Examined, and Why?

The participants in the procurement process, along with the control and supervision authorities in Bulgaria will be described, to render them recognisable and perceivable as possible contributors to corrupt practices and to distinguish their different levels of accountability. Of course, when attempting to differentiate between the 'actors' in corruption, it should be noted that '[c]orruption may be the act of a single person operating in his or her personal interest. Employees, representatives or associates, as well as intermediaries or agents, may engage in corruption practices without the knowledge or approval of the project owner or the company for which they carry out a task'.[1]

Further, the chapter focuses on the organisations and institutions which in recent years have been researching the manifestations of corruption in this sector in Bulgaria and have proposed a variety of remedial measures. Their chosen approach (whether by further expanding transparency rules or not) and the proposed schemes and projects aimed at preventing corruption in public procurement are presented in brief. An assessment of the various proposals is made based on current legislation, taking into account the level of modernisation of the procurement system in Bulgaria, its weaknesses and the EU Commission's expectations that measures to handle corruption in public expenditure need to be taken urgently.

The following chapter analyses the main types of infringements with corrupt intent observed in the public procurement process and the gaps and disadvantages in the legislations which contribute to the abundance of corruption in this area (where applicable). Therefore, and for the sake of simplicity in the subsequent benchmarking process, it is appropriate first to examine the Bulgarian system, look-

---

[1] N Ehlermann-Cache, *Bribery in public procurement*. (Paris: OECD, 2007) ch 4, 37.

© Springer International Publishing AG 2017
I. Georgieva, *Using Transparency Against Corruption in Public Procurement*,
Studies in European Economic Law and Regulation 11,
DOI 10.1007/978-3-319-51304-1_4

ing at the contracting authorities, the bidders and the institutions involved in the process. This approach will help outline those characteristics of the national legislation which differ from or supplement EU legislation, leaving aside the majority of the provisions which merely mirror the EU rules.

4.2   The Participants

4.2.1   Contracting Authorities

The applicable Bulgarian legislation does not provide a definition of the term 'contracting authority', but rather enumerates various possible authorities. The legal definition of 'contracting authority', as provided by Directive 2014/24/EC,[2] is as follows: the State, regional or local authorities, bodies governed by public law or associations formed by one or more such authorities or one or more such bodies governed by public law.[3]

The New PPA provides a relatively comprehensive list of Bulgarian contracting authorities. In accordance with the approach of the EU legislator, the main distinction can be drawn between contracting authorities in the standard (public) sector and contracting entities (which may or may not be authorities) in the utilities. The main obligation of contracting authorities is to conduct public procurement award procedures, where the grounds provided for in law exist. To facilitate the procurement process, contracting authorities may organise and conduct public procurement award procedures by authorising particular officials to act on their behalf (with appropriate anti-splitting rules), or two or more than two contracting authorities to conduct a joint procedure.

Standard (public sector) contracting authorities are typically public authorities which allocate mainly budget funds. These include the representatives and/or the managers of state authority bodies – such as the President or the manager of the Bulgarian National Bank – as well as other persons governing state institutions established by a statutory instrument, bodies governed by public law and all other bodies and/or combinations of bodies possible Directive 2014/24/EU.[4]

---

[2] Art 2(1) Directive 2014/24/EU.

[3] This definition does not substantively change the definition of 'contracting authority' under Art 1(9) item 1 Directive 2004/18/EC. It provides however for a new classification of central and subcentral contracting authorities.

[4] The most common sub-classification of central and regional standard contracting authority under Bulgarian legislation is that made by Krivachka in M Krivachka, M Markov, E Dimova and Z Lilyan, *The new aspects in the Public Procurement Act* (Sofia: IK Trud i Pravo, 2008), 54 et seq: (i) The central standard contracting authorities include the National Assembly, the NAO, the President, the Bulgarian Ombudsman, the Constitutional court, the CM, the whole ministerial apparatus, executive directors of state executive agencies, judges, and the Bulgarian National Bank; (ii) territorial standard contracting authorities are primarily municipalities and their mayors, as well as the municipal managers. However, with the New PPA legal entities could not be contracting authorities but only physical persons – representatives or managers of the respective institution, as explicitly enumerated in Art 5 New PPA.

With respect to the definition of 'body governed by public law' the PPA has suf-fered a poor transposition of the Procurement Directives and has artificially expanded the circle of contracting authorities, but now the New PPA is in line with the EU rules. Unfortunately, the definition of 'body governed by public law' remains unchanged at EU level within the New Procurement Directives. As Medeiros (2014) comments, despite the attempts at clarifying and structuring the definition of a 'body governed by public law' '[t]he truth, however, is that the final version of the Directive 2014/24/EU ended up dropping all these changes/amendments, register-ing a true return to the initial state. As such, the definition of what is a body gov-erned by public law does not suffer relevant changes'.[5]

Utility sector contracting authorities allocate funds received for the public services they provide, which are explicitly defined in law. In compliance with Directive 2014/25/EU, the New PPA distinguishes between (i) public undertakings and any combinations thereof, carrying out one or several utility activities; (ii) commercial entities and other persons who are not public undertakings, carrying out one or several utility activities on the basis of special or exclusive rights; and (iii) the heads of central purchasing bodies established to meet the needs of utility sector contracting authori-ties. The main difference between the first two types of utility sector authorities is that public companies perform utility activities without the need for any specific licensing or permission regime, as these activities are their state obligation. Private entities, on the other hand, may undertake utility activities only after they have been granted spe-cial or exclusive rights, as determined by the relevant national legislation. Utility activities are divided into groups according to the services provided, and all utility contracting authorities are specified in compliance with Directive 2014/25/EU.

The New PPA also presents the figure of the '*contracting authority for a particular case*'[6] – when public funds are financed directly by more than 50% of any of the fol-lowing activities: buildings with an estimated value less than or equal to BGN 5 million (approx. EUR 2,556,460); and services related to construction under item 1 when the estimated value is greater than or equal to BGN 408,762 (approx. EUR 208,997). In these cases the person awarded the contract is considered to be a contracting authority regardless whether he/she is the financing body or the financed one. Therefore, in these particular cases the more strict procurement rules would apply for entities which are not contracting authorities and which are normally purely commercially oriented.

Further, back in 2012 the PPA[7] provide for the establishment of a *central pur-chasing body* (CPB) through which procedures can be conducted and public pro-curement contracts or framework agreements be concluded to meet the executive's needs. The purpose of this body was to achieve efficient spending of budget funds and the highest possible quality in return for the best possible price. The intention was to give the Council of Ministers the opportunity to create another contracting authority responsible for the effective distribution of funds and also to meet the

---

[5] L. Tavares, R Medeiros and D Coelho *The new Directive 2014/24/EU on Public Procurement* (Lisbon: OPET, 2014) ch 2 (The New Directive 2014/24/EU on Public Procurement: A First Overview), 34.

[6] Art 6 New PPA.

[7] As amended by SG 93/2011, effective as of 26 February 2012.

requirements of EU law to ensure more transparent and less corrupt procedures. The first (and only) CPB was created by the Minister of Finance. Contracting authorities are able to avoid the complicated procurement procedures and to contract with the CPB instead (for deliveries and services only). However, the remit of this body remains rather vague and it is used only by the Ministry of Finance and only for sundry expenses.[8] In practice, the original idea of using the CPB to award contracts and to facilitate transparency has ended up in a quite trivial body, the need for which is rather questionable.

The advantage of this type of award bodies is all the more obvious given that the New Procurement Directives have increased the functions and scope of activity of these bodies,[9] which is a clear encouragement as to their introduction and use. In addition to the interim figure of the CPB providing centralised purchasing activities and, possibly, ancillary purchasing activities for contracting authorities, the new rules define a 'procurement service provider'.[10] Aligned to this EU trend, the New PPA has expanded the legal options for regulating the functions of such purchasing bodies,[11] but it is still too early to speculate whether these provisions will once again remain a purely palliative reconstruction of award rules or will have an actual practical and anti-corruption effect (eg as is proven to exist according to the practice of other Member States, as discussed below).

4.2.2   Bidders

With respect to the determination of candidates and participants in public procurements, the Bulgarian legislator has followed the requirements of the New Procurement Directives fairly closely. Accordingly, those of their actions or omissions which define their relationship with contracting authorities and are conducive to corruption, are addressed later in this work. For this reason, and solely for the sake of completeness of this chapter, it is sufficient to note briefly their most basic characteristics: (i) any Bulgarian or foreign natural or legal entity, as well as (ii) any combination thereof, and (iii) any other entity entitled to carry out works, supplies or services under the laws of the country in which it is established may be a candidate or participant in a public procurement procedure.[12] Where the candidate or participant envisages participation of subcontractors in the contract performance, the requirements and/or exclusion grounds apply, in general, also to such subcontractors.

---

[8] eg different types of office supplies and fuel, building maintenance and purchasing of plane tickets; Art 3, para 1 of *Decree No 112 of the Council of Ministers*, dated 4 June 2010.

[9] Art 2(14), (15) & (16) and Art 37 Directive 2014/24/EU.

[10] ie a public or private body offering ancillary purchasing activities on the market.

[11] Art 95 et seq of the New PPA. A new CPB has just been established, organised to work for the Ministry of Healthcare.

[12] Art 10(1) New PPA.

4.3 Authorities Involved in the Public Procurement Process. Controlling and Appellate Authorities

The authorities involved in the process of assignment of public procurements differ not only in responsibilities and functions, but also in their hierarchical position – from the highest level of state government (eg the Council of Ministers) through controlling authorities (eg the Public Procurement Agency, National Audit Office and Public Financial Inspection Agency) and down to appellate authorities (eg Commission for Protection of Competition, Supreme Administrative court).

4.3.1 Council of Ministers

The Council of Ministers of Bulgaria (*Министерски Съвет*, CM), although not directly involved in the public procurement process, has several significant functions in procurement:

(a) The CM issues all secondary legislation in accordance with the New PPA, including the Regulations for the implementation of the New PPA;

(b) CPBs are created by an Act of the CM.

(c) The CM may designate areas where public procurement must be divided into lots according to specialised SME sectors and the capabilities of SMEs.

(d) The CM determines which procurements are reserved in accordance with the aims of enhanced social engagement in the new procurement package, as transposed in national legislation.

4.3.2 Controlling Authorities

The use of different criteria leads to the definition of different types of control over the public procurement awards (as described below). Despite the differences, almost all of the functions of controlling authorities are related to legality control, ie compliance with the regulatory requirements of the national legislation. Efficiency control, ie the monitoring and sanctioning of the effectiveness, efficiency and cost-effectiveness of procurement (including any corruption actions undertaken) is narrowly limited and regulated fragmentarily in the procurement legislation. This is one of the characteristics of the legal framework in public procurement which is criticised for creating conditions in which various corrupt schemes can avoid censure, regardless the regime's apparent compliance with legal requirements and maximum transparency in making awards. Accordingly, the suggested anti-corruption models of most of the organisations working on curbing corruption in public procurement in Bulgaria seek the development of 'a system of risk assessment, and the transfer of the weight from the currently dominant legality control to the control of efficiency and effectiveness'.[13]

Depending on the phase of the public procurement award process under control, control can be divided into *ex ante*, ongoing and *ex post* control.

Ex ante control is exercised at the pre-award phase and is concentrated in a single body – the Executive Director of the Public Procurement Agency. Before the New PPA, control was directed (i) towards public procurement procedures fully or partially funded by EU resources, valued above the thresholds defined in the New PPA; (ii) towards public procurement procedures for works of value equal or higher than the European thresholds; and (iii) towards decisions to initiate negotiated procedures without prior publication of procurement notice, which are at or above national thresholds (except where such procedures are conducted by contracting authorities in the utilities sector). Under the New PPA, (i) and (ii) are no longer applicable as there are three new options for *ex ante* control, which are rather curious and their applicability in practice is particularly interesting[14]: First, *ex ante* control can now be exercised 'randomly' over selected procedures. Second, control 'over some exemptions from the scope of the law' is also envisaged (which covers control over in-house procurements (ie the *Teckal*[15] exemptions). Finally, the New PPA also provides for the possibility of preliminary control of envisaged amendments in already concluded procurement contracts, but only over some of the permitted exceptions and only above the EU thresholds. This extension to the scope of the *ex ante* control is made in response to the constant EU criticism that the control in the award process should be strengthened and able to restrict corruption incentives.[16] However, only future practice will reveal whether this legislative solution was right and effective; and some concerns have already been voiced over the new types of control, only at the level of theory, and discussed below in greater detail.

Ongoing control can *de jure* be exercised at any stage of the public procurement award process – from the moment a procedure is launched until completion of the contract – by any contracting authority. Its purpose is to ascertain in good time, any possible inaccuracies, omissions or irregularities in the conduct of specific procedures; it is therefore considered to be the most comprehensive type of control, covering both the legality of the procedures and also the effectiveness of implementation. Ongoing control can identify infringements of such gravity as may force the contracting authority to terminate the procedure.[17] It is conducted in adherence to the principles of publicity and transparency in the various phases of the award process

---

[13] Corruption in public procurement: risks and counteractions. Development of public-private partnership, *Centre for the Study of Democracy*, Csd.bg (2015) <www.csd.bg/artShow.php?id=8621> accessed 23 April 2016.

[14] Art 121 et seq New PPA.

[15] Case C-107/98 *Teckal Srl v Comune di Viano and Azienda Gas-Acqua Consorziale (AGAC) di Reggio Emilia* [1999] ECR I 8121.

[16] See eg Council (EU), 'Recommendation for a Council Recommendation on Bulgaria's 2013 national reform programme and delivering a Council opinion on Bulgaria's convergence programme for 2012–2016' (Document) COM (2013) 352.

[17] Pursuant to Art 110(1) New PPA, it 5.

and in compliance with the internal regulations adopted by each specific contracting authority. The functions of internal control[18] are set out by the applicable procurement legislation,[19] the Financial Management and Control in the Public Sector Act (*Закон за финансовото управление и контрол в публичния сектор*)[20] and the Internal Audit in the Public Sector Act (*Закон за вътрешния одит в публичния сектор*).[21] Some authors[22] maintain that internal control objectively has the greatest potential to limit corruption opportunities, due to the fact that these controlling activities also include elements of risk management. However, they also consider that: '[t]he problem with internal control is that, comparatively speaking, it suffers from the lowest level of independence in comparison to external audit and state inspections and examinations'.[23]

Ex post control concerns the examination of those public procurement awards procedures which resulted in a contract or a contractor selection decision and which were not disputed. The purpose of *ex post* control is to determine (i) whether and to what extent the contracting authority acted in accordance with legal requirements, (ii) whether it made any omissions or infringements of the relevant rules, and (iii) whether its conduct resulted in infringement of the basic principles of public procurement awards – publicity and transparency, free and fair competition, and equal treatment of all candidates. *Ex post* control is entrusted to two bodies which must always be independent of the contracting authority. These are the Bulgarian National Audit Office and the Public Financial Inspection Agency, whose functions are discussed below. Although these two bodies have different functions and different lines of responsibility, they both focus their control powers solely on one of the participants in the public procurement award process – the contracting authority.

The types of controls and their relationship to corruption detection and transparency are examined below in the light of the functions of the respective responsible institutions.

The Public Procurement Agency

The Public Procurement Agency (*Агенция по обществени поръчки*, PPAgency) was the first separate administrative structure with relatively clearly defined powers in the public procurement system in Bulgaria. The law establishing the Agency responded to a specific condition for the country's accession to the European Union.

---

[18] Which should together cover *ex ante*, ongoing and *ex post* control.

[19] Until 2011 the procurement legislation did not contain any provisions to allow the contracting authority to control the review, evaluation and ranking of offers by the procurement selection committee.

[20] Promulgated SG 21/10.3.2006, as amended.

[21] Promulgated SG 27/31.3.2006, as amended.

[22] K Pashev and K Marinov, *Reducing corruption risks and implementation of good practices by the management of public procurements*. (Sofia: Center for the Study of Democracy, 2009) 20.

[23] Ibid.

The implementation of a sustainable policy in the public procurement field and the fulfilment of the commitments for harmonisation of legislation required the establishment of a separate administrative body to be responsible for these goals.

The PPAgency assists in the implementation of state policy in the public procurement field. It is a legal entity entirely financed by state funds, it does not generate its own revenue and all of its services are provided free of charge. The administration is managed and represented by an Executive Director.

The responsibilities and functions of the PPAgency are aimed at ensuring the legality of public procurement awards, the application of the horizontal policies of the EU, efficient use of public resources, including those from European funds, and adherence to the principles of publicity, transparency and fair competition. The PPAgency is responsible for the preparation of various draft regulations and develops methodologies which assist participants and candidates in the procedures. The main functions of the Executive Director of the PPAgency are set out in the New PPA[24] and are spelled out in detail in the relevant secondary legislation. Generally, the functions of the PPAgency's Executive Director can be classified as follows.[25]

(a) *methodological functions* – the Executive Director of the PPAgency issues methodological guidance which aims to consolidate practices in the application of the procurement legislation and the relevant secondary legislation; draws up draft statutory instruments and standard forms for the publication of information in the Public Procurement Register to the PPAgency; and gives opinions on international treaties in the public procurement realm etc.

(b) *cooperative functions* – the Executive Director of the PPAgency pursues cooperation with other authorities, branch organisations as well as with organisations in other countries in the public procurement field; it encourages good practices in the award of public procurements, including those related to the application of environmental, social and innovative requirements etc.

(c) *informative functions* – the Executive Director of the PPAgency provides summarised information from the Public Procurement Register through its website and produces annual statistical reports and notifications of the enforceable rulings of the Commission for Protection of Competition for the EU Commission; it notifies the EU Commission of any difficulties, in law or in fact, encountered in connection with participation of Bulgarian entities in public procurement award procedures for services in third countries etc.

(d) *assistance* – the Executive Director of the PPAgency maintains the Public Procurement Register, a list of contracting authorities and (with the assistance of the professional associations and organisations in the relevant sector) a list of persons whom contracting authorities may recruit as external experts in the

---

[24] Art 229 New PPA.

[25] Part of the information collected by the Executive Director in implementation of his/her functions is publicly accessible on the official website of the PPAgency – Aop.bg, (2015) <http://www.aop.bg> accessed 23 April 2016.

preparation and conduct of public procurement award procedures; it assists in the implementation of electronic public procurement award processes etc.

(e) *control and sanctioning functions* – The Executive Director of the PPAgency supervises the competent authorities so as to exercise control over compliance with the procurement legislation; it lodges appeals to the Commission on Protection of Competition against decisions of contracting authorities, as identified by the EU Commission prior to contract conclusion; it organises *ex ante* control over public procurement awards etc.

The functions of the Executive Director of the PPAgency relate mainly to the development of legislation, providing support to public procurement participants and promoting good practice, exercising *ex ante* control on the enforcement of legislation, maintaining the Public Procurement Register and information monitoring. The one function on which the Executive Director should concentrate most of his/her efforts in order to contribute to the limitation of violations and corruption in the public procurement field is in fact the *ex ante* control of procedures. This would also be the main challenge in its functions for the period after transposition of the new procurement package and the implementation of the regulations set out in the New PPA.

At the EU level, the Council Recommendation on Bulgaria's 2013 national reform programme, expressing the Council's opinion on Bulgaria's convergence programme for 2012–2016[26] stated in Recital 15 of the Preamble:

Effective implementation of EU funds remains critical to necessary public investment. The 2011 reform of public procurement legislation was a significant step towards improving the monitoring, prevention and punishment of irregularities. While new rules covering *inter alia* EU co-funded projects have entered into force,[27] giving broader powers to the Public Procurement Agency would further enhance the effectiveness of *ex ante* control.

It is precisely with a view to these and similar EU recommendations that the PPA was amended several times to increase the Executive Director's possibilities for *ex ante* control, with the New PPA now introducing three new controlling options.[28]

---

[26] Above (n 16).

[27] In 2012.

[28] In addition to this *ex ante* control conducted by the PPAgency, control over the spending of European funds (*ex ante* and *ex post*) is carried out by the Managing Authorities of each Operational Programme (for Bulgaria these are: 'Transport', 'Environment', 'Regional Development', 'Competitiveness', 'Technical Assistance', 'Human Resources Development' and 'Administrative Capacity') as well as the audits performed by the Audit of EU Funds Executive Agency. The Managing Authorities also exercise *ex post* control over all procedures implemented by beneficiaries. In addition, the Managing Authorities are assisted and controlled by the Audit of EU Funds Executive Agency in its capacity as responsible body for specific audit activities for EU funds and programmes in accordance with international agreements for the provision of funds from the EU and the respective EU regulations on the management and control of contributions by the Structural Funds, the Cohesion Fund and the EU pre-accession funds. The Audit of EU Funds Executive Agency is appointed to act as an Audit authority and Compliance Assessment Authority for the management and control systems of all operational programmes co-funded by the European Regional Development Fund, the European Social Fund and the Cohesion Fund. Given that these additional control activities are performed by those two independent bodies on the basis of direct

As already summarised, the Executive Director of the PPAgency is empowered to conduct *ex ante* control on the decisions of contracting authorities to initiate negotiated procedures without prior publication of a procurement notice or to choose direct awarding, as this function was inherited (although amended) from the PPA. It is worth mentioning that contrary to the overall ambition that control would be expanded, monitoring of negotiated procedures without prior publication is actually restricted. The thresholds above which such procedures will be controlled are significantly higher than they were in the PPA.[29] The anticorruption effect of such preliminary control over this type of procedure which is often used to circumvent the more severe rules for the implementation of open and restricted procedures, is now lowered and a much smaller number of such facilitated procedures will actually be controlled.

The new options for control, although as yet unexamined in practice, have also raised some doubts and questions about their preventive effect:

1. The random *ex ante* control[30] would cover 5% of the published procurement procedures and would be chosen according to methodology and criteria which are currently quite unclear and already sound burdensome.[31]

Such randomness in which procedures are controlled could have a disciplining effect on the contracting authorities to be more precise in the preparation of the documentation for their procedures and to escape discriminatory and/or restrictive competition requirements. However, it is of utmost importance that the methodology for choosing which procedures to control be rigorous, particularly as regards to the random selection. Otherwise, this step could easily be turned into another tool in the hands of the offenders, where 'random selection' becomes in reality an 'actual alert' for a particular contracting authority.

---

implementation of EU rules their activity is of no particular interest for this work as it is not the product of national legislation. It is worth noting, however, that the control exercised by these authorities is again solely control over the legality of contracting authority's acts, while the efficiency of public spending remains outside their scope. It is therefore quite possible in practice to encounter (and, according to individuals working in the field, quite common) public procurements which are controlled of all the possible control bodies pursuant to national and European legislation, where formal technical errors in the conduct of the procedures are detected and penalised under financial rules, but corruption schemes nevertheless remain 'elusive'.

[29] According to the PPA the thresholds for control over negotiated procedures without prior publication of procurement notice were BGN 264,000 (approx. EUR 134,981) for construction works and BGN 66,000 (approx. EUR 33,745) for goods and services. Now, under the New PPA (Art 232) the threshold for goods and services is closer to the previous one for construction works, and the new construction works threshold is BGN 5,000,000 (approx. EUR 2,556,459).

[30] Art 232 et seq New PPA. In full force and effect after 1 September 2016.

[31] According to Art 121 et seq Regulation for Implementation of the New PPA (SG 28/08.04.2016, in force as of 15 April 2016) the controls would be performed in two stages in which different types of documents would be examined. This type of control would delay the start of a procedure by at least 10–15 days more.

We assume that the procedures to be inspected will be determined on the basis of specially designed objective mechanism based on clear and sound criteria, enabling each of orders to fall into the control sample according to its object, subject and value.[32]

2. The supervisory functions of the Executive Director of the PPAgency include further *ex ante* control over the in-house awarding by standard contracting authorities above certain thresholds, which so far is met with approval because this type of award actually needs serious control in order to avoid circumvention of the law and the handing out of contracts to affiliated undertakings. Its application in practice, however, is what is yet to be demonstrated as the right way to supervise the contracting authorities using the *Teckal* exemptions.
3. *Ex ante* control now also covers the legal grounds for amendments of already concluded procurement contracts.

Unfortunately, the latter includes only cases where the contracting authority is using the condition of 'unforeseen circumstances' to amend the procurement contract and the preliminary review includes only contracts above the EU thresholds. Indeed, this is the reason for amending already signed contracts, which is most commonly used to circumvent the burdensome procurement rules and not rarely with corrupt intent. However, the expectations of the new legislation were to strengthen the control over the implementation of contracts entirely and not just in one case. Certainly it is better to have something than nothing.

It is too early to assess the applicability of these monitoring functions but it is more than clear that if the control over the actions of the contracting authority and the selected contractor after the contract has been concluded, is exercised properly (even despite the fact that it covers only particular procurements) this in any case could reduce the number of cases of uninvestigated and easy substitution of basic contractual parameters by corrupt means. Of course, one could only hope that this would remain only wishful thinking.

National Audit Office and Public Financial Inspection Agency

The National Audit Office[33] (*Сметна палата*, NAO), along with the Public Financial Inspection Agency[34] (*Агенция за държавна финансова инспекция*, PFIA), are the main bodies to which the procurement regulation entrusts the implementation of *ex post* control in the public procurement field.

Control by the NAO concerns contracting authorities falling within the scope of the National Audit Office Act (*Закон за сметната палата*, ANAO)[35] (in general,

---

[32] V Panchev, *Procurements under control. Past, present and future of the preliminary control exercised by the Public Procurement Agency under current legislation and draft new PPA* (2016) 1 ZOP+ 15.

[33] An independent organisation accountable to the National Assembly (ie the Parliament).

[34] An executive authority accountable to the Minister of Finance.

[35] Promulgated SG 12/12.2.2015, as amended. Art 6 ANAO '(1) The National Audit Office shall audit: 1. the state budget; 2. the budget of the state social security scheme; 3. the budget of the National Health Insurance Fund; 4. the budgets of municipalities; 5. other budgets adopted by the

these are standard contracting authorities). Such control covers procedures which have already ended in a contract or termination decision, completed contracts and, as of July 2014 – the implementation of procurement contracts (although control over performance quality is explicitly excluded) and thus is, in most cases, *ex post*.[36] However, the scope of control by the NAO includes the effectiveness and cost-efficiency of procurements,[37] which is a huge advantage over the narrower control exercised by the PFIA. In fact, the NAO audit is the only type (compared to all other types of external institutional control) which goes beyond issues of legality (ie compliance with legal rules). Pashev (2009) notes, moreover, that: 'the control functions of the NAO cover such crucial pieces of anticorruption legislation as the Prevention and Detection of Conflicts of Interests Act, the Party Finances Act and the Disclosure

National Assembly. (2) The National Audit Office shall audit also: 1. the budgets of spenders of budget appropriations under the budgets referred to in paragraph (1) and the management of their property; 2. the budgets of budget organisations under Art 13(3) & (4) of the Public Finances Act; 3. budgetary resources granted to persons engaged in business; 4. accounts for funds from the European Union and other international programs and contracts under Art 8(2) & (4) of the Law on Public Finance, including the management thereof by the relevant authorities and final beneficiaries; 5. The budget expenditures of the Bulgarian National Bank and their management; 6. The formulation of any annual surplus of income of expenditures of the Bulgarian National Bank that is payable to the state budget, and any other dealings of the Bank with the state budget; 7. The generation and management of government debt, government-secured debt, municipal debt and the use of debt instruments; 8. privatisation and concession of state and municipal property and of public resources and public assets provided to individuals outside the public sector; 9. The performance under international agreements, treaties, conventions or other international instruments, where so provided for in the respective international instrument or assigned by an empowered authority; 10. Other public resources and activities, where so assigned by law. (3) The National Audit Office shall audit: 1. state-owned enterprises falling within the scope of Art 62(3) of the Commercial Act; 2. commercial undertakings with more than 50 per cent state and/or municipal interest in capital; 3. legal entities that have obligations guaranteed by the state, or obligations guaranteed with state and/or municipal property. (4) The National Audit Office audits the management and disposition of public assets and liabilities regardless of the reason for this management and disposition and the status of those who carry it out. (5) The National Audit Office produces reports with opinions on the implementation of the state budget, the budget of the state social security, the budget of the National Health Fund and the budgetary costs of the Bulgarian National Bank which it then submits to the National Assembly. 6) The National Audit Office may also audit the foreign funds accounts of budget organisations'.

[36] By way of exception, ongoing control is regulated by Art 44 ANAO 'Where, in the course of the audit, it has been found that certain actions result in opportunities for legal irregularities in collecting or spending budgetary or other public funds, and for damaging the property of the auditee, the head of the respective department or the regional division director shall, upon a proposal by the head of the audit team, notify the relevant competent authority so that measures can be taken to discontinue such actions'.

[37] §1, item 4 (supplementary provisions) ANAO - 'Performance audit' shall refer to an inspection of activities involved in the planning, implementation and control at all management levels of the auditee to ensure their effectiveness, efficiency and economy, where (a) 'effectiveness' is the achievement of the objectives of the auditee when comparing the actual and expected results of its operations; (b) 'efficiency' is the achievement of maximum results from available resources in the activities of the auditee; (c) 'economy' is the acquisition, at the lowest possible cost, of the resources required for the activity of the audited entity in compliance with the quality requirements to such resources'.

of Assets of High-Rank State Officials Act. These are important safeguards against abuse of contract-awarding power, which aim at weakening the sources of corruption in the political system'.[38]

The PFIA exercises *ex post* control over the actions of contracting authorities which fall within the scope of the Public Financial Inspection Act (*Закон за държавната финансова инспекция*, APFIA).[39] Its control functions cover not only standard contracting authorities but also those in the utilities sector. The control exercised by PFIA is limited to the legality of the public procurement. Nevertheless, it is more targeted from the standpoint of detection of corruption in public procurement due because it is based *inter alia* on alerts from state authorities, individuals and legal entities, as discussed below.

A significant difference between the two types of *ex post* control performed by NAO and PFIA is that the NAO's control in all cases covers a particular period (the 'audited period'), while the PFIA inspects specific procedures, contracts or costs incurred for the particular type of public procurement, expressly specified in the financial inspection order. This means that the control exercised by the PFIA has a better chance of detecting infringements in public procurement procedures in time.

PFIA control activities may be initiated (i) on receipt of requests, complaints or alerts for violations of the budget, financial, economic or accounting activities of the organisations and entities audited by PFIA and submitted by state authorities, natural persons and legal entities; (ii) on request by the PPAgency or the NAO; (iii) with respect to the monitoring of the use of state aid and the spending of target subsidies provided under the State Budget Act for the respective year, and according to the decrees issued by the Council of Ministers; (iv) on request by the Council of Ministers or the Minister of Finance; and (v) on assignment by the Prosecutor's Office and upon alerts for irregularities, affecting the financial interests of the EU, established by the Ministry of Interior.[40] In addition to the above options, financial inspection of the award and implementation activities in public procurement can also be carried out, from time to time, on the basis of an approved annual plan which is mandatory for the Agency.[41]

Unlike the PFIA, which may, in addition to planned inspections, perform inspections when alerted, the NAO may only audit organisations on the basis of the annual

---

[38] K Pashev, *Reducing Corruption Risks and Practices in Public Procurement: Evidence from Bulgaria*, Paper presented at the First Global Dialogue on Ethical and Effective Governance (Amsterdam, 2009), 21.

[39] Promulgated SG 33/21.4.2006, as amended. Art 4 APFIA 'Public financial inspections shall be performed in: 1. budget organisations; 2 state enterprises […], as well as municipal enterprises; 3. commercial companies with blocking quota of state or municipal share in the capital; 4. commercial companies, in whose capital the blocking quota belongs to an entity on item 2 or 3; 5. legal entities, having liabilities guaranteed with state or municipal property; 6. legal entities under the Non-Profit Entities Act and the non-personified partnerships under the Obligations and Contracts Act, where the state or municipalities participate directly or indirectly in their property; 7. state aid beneficiaries, entities financed with funds from the central government budget or municipal budgets, under international agreements or under European Union programmes, as well as the entities funded by state-owned enterprises […] – as regards the spending of such funds'. Control over other contracting authorities which do not fall under Art 4 is implemented through inspections.

[40] Through the 'Protection of the financial interests of the European Union' directorate.

[41] Art 5(1) and (2) APFIA.

programme adopted for its audit activities. The National Assembly may also assign to the NAO to carry out up to five extra audits per year, in addition to those included in the annual programme.[42] Bearing in mind that the NAO is the only control body in public procurement which is relatively independent and not under the umbrella of the executive power and is also the only body monitoring the appropriateness of procedures, the lack of options for alerting this body at the request of individual natural persons and organisations is a serious drawback to its ability to fight organised corruption in the award.

The two *ex post* control bodies in the public procurement field can be further distinguished on the basis of the type of control they apply to contracting authorities. Under the ANAO, the only form of control applied to entities inspected by the NAO is an *external audit*. Control conducted by the NAO authorities not infrequently results in the detection of inaccuracies, weaknesses and even infringements of regulatory requirements in the public procurement field.

PFIA auditors verify compliance with the procurement rules by means of *financial inspections* of the contracting authorities covered by APFIA (the standard contracting authorities). On the other hand, compliance with the legislation on the part of entities which are not subject to financial inspection (the utilities) is controlled by the PFIA by means of *examinations*.[43] Depending on the inspection results, the Director of PFIA or officials authorised by him, as the case may be, are entitled to: (i) offer written instructions for the suspension of violations and for elimination of the harmful consequences thereof; (ii) make proposals to the competent authorities to cease actions leading to the commission of an offence or the causing of damage; (iii) make proposals to the competent authorities for the annulment of illegal acts; (iv) propose to the competent authorities that the property be searched and/or disciplinary action be taken, as appropriate; (v) propose to the Minister of Finance that the transfer of subsidies allocated for that year be suspended, or that the accounts of the budgetary organisations be blocked until the infringements are eliminated.[44] The results of a PFIA audit which finds infringements in award procedures are also sent to the PPAgency: if there is evidence of crime, the inspection materials are sent to the Prosecutor's office again. As with the consequences of PFIA-detected violations, this institution may, as discussed above, act as a regulatory authority with the power to impose fines and other sanctions.

---

[42] Art 7(1) ANAO.

[43] A different form of control (from financial inspections) stipulated by the Public Financial Inspection Act. In carrying out examinations the PFIA bodies are entitled to free access to the inspected entity. They can check any documentation related to a public procurement award and to activities requiring the award of public contracts. PFIA bodies have the powers to search premises, vehicles and other places where the inspected entity's records are kept, and to seize documents, computer data and the storage media thereof as evidence. Assistance from the Ministry of Interior may be requested to conduct these actions. The individuals in the inspected entities are obliged to assist the PFIA authorities and provide the necessary documents, information and reports. Failure to do so is punishable by fines.

[44] Art 18 APFIA.

The current position of the NAO, however, verges on the absurd. Precisely due to the fact that this is the only control body in Bulgaria in a position to act as a significant actor in the fight against corruption and detecting of material infringements, its structure, functions and organisation have suffered repeated and radical changes at legislative level, with two of these changes occurring in less than a year. The NAO has thus been reduced to an object of political games and revanchism for each new government and is currently almost unable to function because it is paralysed by the constant ambiguity about its rights and authority. Between May 2014 and January 2015 alone, the NAO was successively stripped of its administrative penal functions and then had them restored, was transformed into a collectively governed commission and then conversely was assigned a chairman and members, and it was tasked with auditing small municipalities and then divested of these powers if the value of the inspection falls below BGN 10 million (approx. EUR 5,113,148).

Ultimately, the NAO may sanction inspected entities when violations are detected.[45] Whether or not this function, as well as any of the other key responsibilities of the NAO in detecting public spending under corruption pressure will, once again, be pared down following the next change in government is unclear. The analysis of legislative amendments regulating the NAO, however, clearly indicates that the ambition of each new government is to restrict the independence of this body, created *a priori* as an independent corrective force, or at the very least, to limit its activity severely to ensure that the NAO will not act as intended and will not detect corruption deals to the inconvenience of the powers that be.

The analysis of the similarities and differences between the two bodies performing *ex post* control on the award process and (as of very recently) on public procurement implementation reveals that PFIA has greater responsibilities, but is limited to the implementation of legality control only (monitoring mainly accordance with procedural rules in the conduct of the procedures). On the other hand, the NAO is also entitled to analyse the efficiency and effectiveness of the awards and it would be more proper if it were the more independent body of the two. The NAO, however, does not act on alerts. Both institutions currently act on the basis of planned inspections (PFIA may act on alerts made by natural persons and/or organisations as well) and both act as administrative regulatory authorities with the power to impose sanctions. From this perspective, and bearing in mind the economic level of Bulgaria and the limited resources allocated to individual institutions, it can be concluded that it would be much more effective if only a single authority existed, dedicated to *ex post* control over public procurement. Efforts should be concentrated around the NAO, upholding its independence and ensuring a sufficient number of employees with the necessary qualifications instead of experts whose legality control activities in the PFIA and the NAO unfortunately often overlap. An independent audit office, combining responsibility for both legality and efficiency, able to sanction perpetrators and to act on alerts, could become one of the main pillars in the fight against corruption in the sector and could significantly limit efforts to restrict competition and manipulate public spending for personal gain. Unfortunately, European legislation (even the New Procurement Directives) provide significant freedom to the national legislator to choose how and through which institution to carry out *ex post*

---

[45] Art 59 ANAO.

control over contract award and implementation. The national legislator has thus clearly embraced the 'the more, the better' principle, which in this particular case appears quite inefficient and inadequate to counter corruption. In this context, it should be also noted that both institutions not only superimpose in their functions but maintain and promote different practices and different recommendations which causes consternation among the contracting authorities as they often do not know which practice and what opinion to consider relevant and to apply. The New PPA therefore envisages a permanent methodological council with the participation of the NAO, the PPAgency and the PFIA to be created for the purposes of unifying practices in the implementation of control activities under the law.[46] The council will adopt guidelines for the implementation of *ex ante* and *ex post* control as well as the internal control of the contracting authorities. Hopefully this measure will somehow unify the practice of these institutions so that they start working in the interests of adequately monitoring the procurement process at national level.

Nevertheless, the control functions of these two authorities, external to the contracting authorities, are of particular interest, regardless their failings. Given the fact that *ex post* control cannot prevent or resolve any shortcomings in the behaviour of the contracting authority, but can only establish and sanction it, the role of the two other types of control over public procurements – *ex ante* and ongoing, the introduction and implementation of which depends largely on the will of the contracting authorities – ought gradually to be strengthened. However, the work and reports of the NAO and PFIA over the years[47] have led to the identification of the most common offences committed by contracting authorities. For this reason, their conclusions, along with those of various other national and international non-governmental organisations, are used in the following chapter of this book to provide a comprehensive classification and examples of infringements of procurement procedures, involving corrupt behaviour.

4.3.3 Appellate Authorities

The appellate instances dealing with procurement are the Commission for Protection of Competition (at first instance) and the Supreme Administrative Court (at second instance, but the only judicial instance). Their functions, as well as the controversial role of the Commission for Protection of Competition in this process, are detailed below.

---

[46] A similar body existed until recently, although it was not legally established. Its work did not yield the expected results however, and now the hope is that with the regulation in the New PPA, its functions will be strengthened.

[47] Not including the NAO's activity in the past two years, since, as has been already discussed, the said body has been rather sluggish to take action of late due to its being subjected to constant organisational and functional changes.

Commission for Protection of Competition

As originally created, the Commission for Protection of Competition (*Комисия за защита на конкуренцията*, CPC) is the national regulator in the competition sector. It is an independent, specialised government authority empowered to apply competition legislation in Bulgaria, the main purpose of which is to ensure the protection and expansion of competition and free commercial enterprise. In 2006 the CPC was elected as the competent administrative authority to decide on claims against the acts of contracting authorities (as a first instance of appeal).[48] The control that the CPC currently exercises is control of the legality of the actions and/or inactions of the contracting authorities. Efficiency control cannot be carried out by the CPC because of its specific proceeding's nature, which differs in terms of appeal under the general administrative rules. Nevertheless, the scope of control over contracting authorities by CPC is maximised – almost all decisions of contracting authorities up to the conclusion of a public contract (or, as the case may be, a framework agreement) may be appealed.[49] It should be borne in mind that the actions/inactions of the selection committee itself are outside the scope of appeal before the CPC. The selection committee is considered a subsidiary body to the contracting authority; its acts do not constitute individual administrative acts and are therefore not subject to separate appeal.[50]

Under the present legislation, decisions of the contracting authorities on the following matters are open to appeal: generally any decision taken by the contracting

---

[48] Despite the close connection between competition and procurement, the decision of the legislator to grant jurisdiction to a non-judicial authority was criticised as unconstitutional for a long time (According to the Bulgarian Constitution 'extraordinary courts are prohibited', meaning that any court other than the Supreme Court of Cassation, the Supreme Administrative Court, the appellate, county, military and district courts, and any other specialised courts established by law, is prohibited). Under the general administrative rules in Bulgaria, administrative acts issued by administrative bodies can be appealed before a court or before a higher ranking administrative body. The CPC is not a higher ranking administrative body than contracting authorities. However, it would appear that after almost a decade of established experience, the CPC is considered by legislators to have appropriate expertise with public procurement issues and, despite several attempts to transfer appeals to administrative courts, this special authority continues its activities. The transposition of the New Procurement Directive presented another opportunity to discuss the transfer of the first instance appellate jurisdiction to the administrative courts. However, such a move would have distributed appeals among various district courts, with perhaps the somewhat unfortunate result that appeals could be expected to become more burdensome in terms of decision making deadlines. The situation with the appellate institutions thus remains quite similar under the New PPA.

[49] The only procurement procedures which can be appealed before the general administrative courts and not before the CPC are those connected with the defence and security of the state under Art 296 TFEU. Relatively detailed analysis of the decisions of the contracting authority excluded from the scope of the CPC is made by T Nikolova in the article 'Highlights in the process of appealing the decisions, actions and omissions of the contracting authority under the new Public Procurement Act' (2016) 3 ZOP+ 44–53.

[50] In this sense - Definition No 273 of 2007 of the SAC, as well as A Kovacheva, *Public Procurements Award* (Sofia: Fenea Publishers, 2008) 138. However, acts of contracting authorities based on selection committee protocols can be appealed.

authorities in respect to (i) public procurements, including the conclusion of a framework agreement, dynamic purchasing system or qualification system; (ii) the conclusion of a framework agreement; (iii) the establishment of a dynamic purchasing system or qualification system; and (iv) design contests. The decisions of the contracting authorities rejecting the subcontractors chosen by a candidate in procurements related to defence and security are also appealable. Last but not least, all the actions and/or inactions of the contracting authority which hinder the access or participation of the parties in the procedure are subject to an appeal. These decisions may be appealed to the CPC as to their legality, including the existence of discriminatory economic, financial, technical or qualification requirements in the notification, or any other parts of the documentation prepared by the contracting authority. Following completion of the investigation and research into the complaint, the CPC schedules an open meeting to consider the matter. After clarifying the dispute from a legal and factual perspective, the CPC decides in closed session; this marks the end of the administrative proceedings before the CPC.

The CPC generally has the following legal options in its decisions. *First*, it may decide to take no further action. This means that the CPC finds the complaint unfounded because the defects in the tender process alleged by the applicant are not proved. Another situation in which no further action may be taken is when the contracting authority has concluded the procurement contract and a temporary measure 'suspending the execution of the contract' was not imposed[51] either due to the CPC's refusal to grant it, or due to cancellation of this temporary measure by the court. *Secondly*, the CPC may find the complaint justified and conclude that illegal actions (or inactions) have been committed, or that illegal decisions have been made during the award procedure. In this case the decisions are regarded as taken in violation of substantive or procedural norms. The CPC may impose sanctions or annul the act, inaction or decision concerned, and can return the procedure to the stage of the last lawful decision or action undertaken, thus requiring the procedure to be re-run in a lawful manner from that stage onwards. There is also the opportunity for the CPC to provide instructions on the future course of the public procurement: these are binding upon the contracting authority. *The third option* for the CPC is the decision of the contracting authority to be declared void.

Supreme Administrative Court

The party whose legal interests are affected by the operative part of the decision of the CPC may lodge an appeal within 14 days of notification of the parties, to a three-member panel of the Supreme Administrative Court (*Върховен Административен Съд*, SAC). This is the second, but first judicial, instance of appeal under the New

---

[51] According to Art 203(1) New PPA, there is no automatic suspensive effect of the appeal. This is possible only if the appeal is directed 'against the decision on the selection of contractor'. In all other cases an interim 'measure of suspension' may be requested, to be decided on by the CPC, with the decision of the CPC being appealable to the Supreme Administrative Court.

PPA. The complaint is filed through the CPC and copied to all parties concerned. The consideration of the legality of the CPC's decision takes place in open court. The decision of the three-member panel is final and not open to further appeal. The SAC can confirm or annul the CPC's decision in whole or in part.[52]

Despite the fact that a contracting authority's decisions can be appealed by a wide variety of interested parties – stakeholders or candidates[53] – before the CPC (and at a later stage before the SAC) on the basis of 'the presence of discriminatory economic, technical or qualification requirements in the procurement notice, the procurement documentation and any other document related to the procedure',[54] given that only the legality of the statements issued by contracting authorities is examined, no significant corruption prevention effect can be expected to arise from the activities of these two instances. Some of the criteria used by contracting authorities have indeed been branded discriminatory over the years,[55] but others are constantly being invented to take their place, the detection of which requires expert analysis which, though possible under the procurement legislation, is very rarely carried out at appeal level. The two institutions simply lack the financial means to employ such experts: certain very specific criteria concealing purely corrupt motives for contract conclusion with a desired candidate thus remain undetected.

As part of the research conducted in this book, several interviews were conducted with SAC judges who chose to remain anonymous. Some of the interviewees, when commenting on the most common violations in public procurement awards, said that they did not feel that the award procedures suffered from frequent corruption. Their standpoint confirms the view that legality control over decisions issued by contracting authorities up to the contract conclusion stage is and could not be an effective corruption detection and anticorruption mechanism in the award process. Appellate authorities can declare that certain procedures are completely lawful and demonstrate sufficient transparency of documentation and of the award process, even when these same procedures are in reality 'tailor-made' for a specific candidate, with the corrupt scheme revealing itself only after contract conclusion.

---

[52] A less common hypothesis is for the SAC to repeal the CPC decision. SAC Decision No 13193 of 10 October 2013 is to that effect (due to unsubstantiated legal conclusions reached by the CPC), as well as Decision No 1760 of 2 April 2011 (due to lack of grounds for the legal conclusions and discrepancy with the evidence provided under the case); No 13781 of 17 November 2010 (lack of substantiation) etc.

[53] Art 198(1) New PPA.

[54] Art 196(3) New PPA.

[55] CPC Decision 531/2007 and CPC Decision 1136/2007 declare the criterion 'number of subscribers of the mobile operator at the date of tender submission' as discriminatory; CPC Decision 983/2007 defines the criterion 'number of roaming agreements concluded' as discriminatory in some cases; CPC Decision 39/2007 declares the requirement that each participant indicate a list of major construction contracts performed in the country and EU states over the preceding 5 years as discriminatory etc. See also above Kovacheva (2008) (n 50) 29–41.

4.4   Why Not Less Burdensome But More Effective?

It is apparent from the above that the relationship between the separate authorities and their functions is extremely complex, partly because of the background EU legislation, but partly because of the choices made by the national legislator. The review of the types of control and appellate authorities is further relevant for this work, insofar as Directive 2007/66/EC (the Remedies Directive)[56] imposes on Member States the general obligation to provide effective remedies for violation of the public procurement rules. The conclusion is that most of the institutions discussed (the PPAgency, the PFIA, the CPC and the SAC) essentially exercise *control over the legality of contracting authority actions.* All procedural rules are exclusively and strictly observed in line with the basic principles of public procurement, and reports on any inaccuracies found are presented annually. In recent years, there has been significant progress towards achieving greater transparency in the actions of the contracting authorities and individual bodies. The annual reports of controlling institutions demonstrate the higher degree of accountability for the actions of participants in the procedures. However, this in no way creates insurmountable obstacles for candidates and contracting authorities in their quest to create increasingly ingenious and resourceful routes to corruption and ensuring that a predetermined candidate comes out on top. This will be discussed further in the following chapters.

In addition, the structure of control and appellate authorities is too burdensome and multi-instanced (as seen on Graph 4.1 below). Some of the institutions have vague powers to interfere in or to improve the procurement process. Further, *ex ante* control is concentrated mainly within the powers of the Executive Director of the PPAgency and reduced in scope (the new possibilities for control are still far from being clear and consistent and only practice will reveal their result). Ongoing control is internally implemented, not independent enough and prevents corruption at the lower and middle level of administration only. *Ex post* control is distributed too fragmentarily among the different authorities, without achieving serious results in exposing corruption and infringements. The PFIA has greater responsibilities, but is limited to the implementation of legality control only (mainly monitoring compliance with procedural rules in the conduct of procedures). The NAO is entitled to analyse the efficiency and effectiveness of the awards but has no powers to act on alerts. It was observed above that this body has so far been (virtually) inoperative due to constant restructuring and changes in its functions. Finally, the appellate authorities – the CPC and the SAC – also focus solely on compliance with the letter of law. In other words, as Pashev and Marinov (2009) conclude 'the responsibility for fighting corruption remains mostly a national obligation',[57] which is certainly insufficient at present.

---

[56] Directive 2007/66/EC of the European Parliament and of the Council amending Council Directives 89/665/EEC and 92/13/EEC with regard to improving the effectiveness of review procedures concerning the award of public contracts [2007] OJ L335/31, as amended.

[57] See above (n 22) 114.

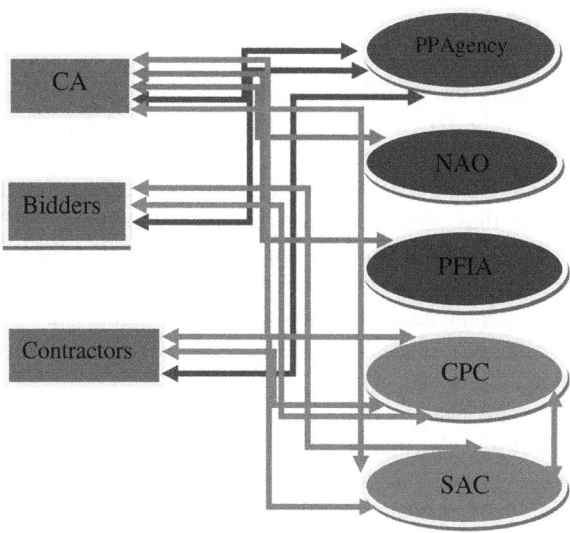

Graph 4.1 Participants in procurement procedures and control and appeal authorities

4.5 Some Warriors in the Uneven War Against Corruption in Bulgarian Public Procurement

While discussing corruption in the implementation of public procurement procedures and offering a comparative analysis of the best practices in some Member States,[58] it is appropriate to evaluate *what has been accomplished so far* in this area in Bulgaria, as a country chosen to exemplify Member States who are unable to limit corruption in the procurement process, despite the transparency of its conduct.

Precisely for this reason, and also with the purpose of highlighting the conclusions which this work will draw, the final section of this chapter will focus briefly on the organisations and institutions which in recent years have been researching corruption in this sector in Bulgaria and which have proposed a variety of measures to combat it. Their recommended course of action and the proposed schemes and projects aimed at preventing corruption in public procurement are summarised here. An assessment of the various proposals is made based on current legislation, taking into account the level of modernisation of the procurement system, its weaknesses and the EU's expectations that measures to tackle corruption in public expenditure be taken urgently.

---

[58] See Chaps. 5 and 6 of the book.

4.5.1 Who Are They?

In the years following the transition from communism and especially in the pre-accession period to the EU, corruption at all levels and spheres of activity was quickly identified as a major problem for the development and establishment of Bulgaria as an economically stable and democratic country upholding the Rule of Law. Bulgaria was thus one of the first signatories of the OECD Anti-Bribery Convention, UNCAC and the Civil and Criminal Law Conventions against Corruption. Bulgaria is also a member of GRECO. However, as this in itself did not help, numerous governmental and non-governmental organisations and institutions emerged which claimed to investigate corrupt practices and to offer various solutions to prevent and sanction it.

The state apparatus also created various committees and agencies tasked with exposing corruption and alerting the prosecutor's office, but, given their dependence on political structures and the executive power, they have not achieved any satisfactory results.[59] On the other hand, the Bulgarian public and media tend to react critically to any initiative in this area. Each new preventive measure is quickly stigmatised as ineffective, overly expensive to the taxpayer, politically driven, and/or funded by countries of varying economic influence.

In light of the above it should be stressed that the present work examines those methods and analyses put forward by these organisations, which, in the present author's view, have had some beneficial impact on curbing corruption or have at least (i) laid the groundwork for an effective system to limit tender manipulation or (ii) have made proposals for measures which could prove effective.

There are three active organisations in Bulgaria which have made major contributions to the development of projects and models designed to prevent corruption, to studying its specific manifestations in the different stages of the public procurement process and its implementation, as well as to the sharing of certain models which have already proved their efficacy in other countries. These organisations have very different approaches and focuses for their activities and therefore their 'end products' offer radically different viewpoints as to how corruption in public procurement should be treated:

(a) *The Center for the Study of Democracy* – a non-profit organisation that continuously invests in the collection and analysis of information on current anticorruption practices at various levels of government (including in the area of public procurement), exploring the 'national traits' of corruption and establishing a

---

[59] ie (i) the Commission for Prevention and Countering of Corruption – chaired by the Minister for the Interior. It coordinates and monitors the drafting and implementation of anticorruption strategic documents; (ii) the State Agency for National Security – an agency acting under the umbrella of the Council of Ministers and focusing on protecting national security – one of the aspects of its activities is the detection of 'large-scale' corruption; and (iii) the Commission for Prevention and Ascertainment of Conflict of Interest – an independent body focusing on the detection of conflict of interest in the public sector. It has predominantly supportive functions as regards the detection of corruption in public procurement etc.

complete set of indicators to measure the level of corruption in a country, although these are not the only means of measuring subjective perceptions of corruption in a society.

(b) *Transparency International in Bulgaria* – the national branch of TI also invests a lot of effort locally to analyse corruption in Bulgaria and in particular the weaknesses of public procurement procedures compared to the provisions of the law and how those provisions are currently implemented. Apart from applying the Corruption Perception Index, in late 2013 the national representative organisation announced that it would attempt to implement an Integrity Pact in public procurement, following the example of many other European and non-European countries where this initiative of Transparency International has yielded positive results (e.g. Germany, as reviewed in Chap. 6 of this book). A special report was produced on the Bulgarian model of the Integrity Pact and the results of its pilot implementation, its impact and applicability, which is discussed below.

(c) *The Center for Prevention and Countering Corruption and Organised Crime and the BORKOR project* – the Center for Prevention and Countering Corruption and Organised Crime was established in response to constant criticism by the EU and its insistence that a centralised body should be established to develop a successful and effective model for fighting corruption in close cooperation with the government of Bulgaria. The BORKOR project was widely criticised both by civil society (for being too expensive for the taxpayers) and in the EU Commission's 2014 report on Bulgaria,[60] as being ineffective. However, this state budget funded body has its own strategy and has offered a corruption prevention model with a particular focus in the area of public procurement.

4.5.2   Center for the Study of Democracy

The Center for the Study of Democracy (*Център за Изследване на Демокрацията*, CSD) is a non-profit organisation with a broad scope of activities. The CSD engages in various social initiatives, international cooperation and exchanges of information, research and sociological studies, economic analyses, training and consultancy etc. In recent years it has become an active participant in the formation and implementation of a number of Public Policies. The CSD deals specifically with the development and monitoring of anticorruption policies and practices.[61]

One of the CSD's major achievements is the implementation of a national corruption index, the CMS, as discussed in detail in Chap. 3. It was the first of its kind and has been successfully applied in Bulgaria since the 1990s. In addition to estab-

---

[60] Commission (EU), 'Report on Progress in Bulgaria under the Co-operation and Verification Mechanism' COM(2014)36 final, 22 January 2014.

[61] The CSD is the Bulgarian partner for many European institutions, networks and initiatives such as the European Union Fundamental Rights Agency, the World Bank Global Distance Learning Network and the International Institute for Management Development in Switzerland's World Competitiveness Yearbook.

lishing this national corruption monitoring system, CSD has pursued a number of other ambitious goals in the field of fighting corruption, some of which have achieved positive results.

One of the CSD's fields of study is naturally the manifestations of corruption in public procurement. In a series of analytical reports, learning materials and methodologies developed over the past 20 years, the CSD outlines very clearly the bottlenecks in the implementation of the procurement legislation, the corruption models used by contracting authorities and tenderers in the implementation and award of public procurement contracts and the main recommendations, in legislative terms, aimed at more timely prevention of corruption in public procurement procedures.[62] Sadly, some of the recommendations made by the CSD for changes in legislation and for combating corrupt practices in one of its earliest works – its 2002 Corruption Assessment Report[63] – continue to sound relevant today, and despite the more than 30 amendments made to the former legislation since then, as well as the presentation of the now applicable New PPA, these recommendations have not been fully addressed yet:

[I]t is further necessary:

-   to institutionalise responsibility for the overall implementation and monitoring of public procurement in an independent Public Procurement Agency[64];
-   the National Audit Office and the State Internal Financial Control Agency[65] should be authorised to perform preliminary control over public procurement, ie before contracting[66];
-   […] evaluation committees' technical skills should be improved while their member's administrative and criminal liability should be defined more clearly.[67]

These recommendations, made back in 2002, are fundamental to the organisation of successful measures to combat corruption and to reduce the rate of violations and omissions in the implementation and awarding of public procurement contracts, regardless their nature. As the analysis in this chapter revealed, the strengthening

---

[62] The CSD issues Policy Briefs annually on the levels of corruption and their impact in different public sectors, as well as annual reports on the level of corruption in the country and its manifestations, with a special focus on public procurement. It is from these studies that the above conclusions can be drawn. The recent CSD analyses are entitled 'Corruption and Anti-corruption in Bulgaria (2013–2014)' Policy Brief No. 46/2014, and 'Anti-corruption Policies against State Capture. 10th annual report providing an overview of the state of corruption and anticorruption in Bulgaria 2013–2014'. That report was prepared as part of the Southeast Europe Leadership for Development and Integrity (SELDI) initiative.

[63] 'Corruption Assessment Report 2002' (Sofia: Coalition 2000/Center for the Study of Democracy, 2002).

[64] Under the New PPA, the PPAgency already exists, as noted in this chapter, but it has definitely not undertaken overall implementation and control of public procurement procedures – a fact which has been further noted in EU reports.

[65] Now the Public Financial Inspection Agency.

[66] Only partially possible nowadays.

[67] 'Corruption Assessment Report 2002' (Sofia: Coalition 2000/Center for the Study of Democracy, 2002) 92.

and proper organisation of control over public procurements is a key factor in the attempts to limit corruption. The above observations, updated to reflect the current political and economic environment have also been confirmed by the CSD to be valid for the last few years.

> The lack of control over public spending in 2013 and 2014 coupled with long leadership vacuum at key revenue agencies and the de-facto blocking of anti-corruption law enforcement has resulted in the rise of public procurement and administrative corruption.[68]

The CSD continues to carry out serious analytical work each year.[69] Despite the fact that the CSD (unlike the two institutions discussed below) does not claim to provide working mechanisms for prevention of corruption in public procurement, the analytical and science-based categorisation of the main problems and outlining of the urgent legislative measures that need to be taken constitute an undeniably sound basis for the development of anticorruption policies tailored to the individual characteristics of the national system of public spending. Unfortunately, however, there is a tendency in Bulgaria to not always take into account the achievements of the theoretical mind, and '[s]ignificant legislative changes are made without any appropriate justification of the need for such changes and without any prior expert and public consultation'.[70]

4.5.3   Transparency International in Bulgaria

The National representative organisation of TI in Bulgaria (*Прозрачност без Граници България*, TIBG) was founded in 1998. Ever since then, for nearly 20 years, it has established itself in the country as one of the organisations undertaking broad-ranging activities directly aimed at the creation and implementation of projects to combat corruption at national and regional level.

Like the CSD, TIBG conducts research initiatives related to the problems of corruption by mobilising the efforts of researchers, public figures and experts in the relevant fields, collecting, presenting and disseminating the necessary analytical information among governmental institutions and civil society organisations, developing civic initiatives and projects aimed at reducing corruption etc. Further, one of the major functions that TIBG is associated with is the publication of the annual Corruption Perception Index (CPI), the mechanism and functions of which were reviewed in Chap. 3.

Of the recent works of the TIBG deserving the greatest attention is the Bulgarian version of the 'Integrity Pact' developed in the public procurement field, which presents TIBG's idea of an effective anticorruption model in public expenditure.

---

[68] 'Corruption and Anticorruption in Bulgaria (2013–2014)' (Sofia: Center for the Study of Democracy, 2014) Policy Brief No 46/2014, 19–20.

[69] One of the recent works of the CSD, analysing once again the issue of corruption in public procurement is – A Stoyanov, R Stefanov and B Velcheva, 'Bulgarian Anti-Corruption Reforms: A Lost Decade?' (2014) European Research Centre for Anti-Corruption and State-Building and Center for the Study of Democracy Working Paper No 42.

[70] Above (n 68) 8.

TIBG's project was launched in 2009 under the title '*Increasing Integrity through Advocacy: Counteracting Corruption in Public Contracting*' and was based on the Integrity Pact created by Transparency International and used worldwide.[71] The Integrity Pact is a tool developed in the 1990s by Transparency International as a solution to the development and use of corrupt and untransparent practices and inefficient management of public resources. 'This is a model applied in over 15 countries worldwide, including EU Member States, which are characterised by varying degrees of socio-economic development and have different management cultures'.[72]

The Integrity Pact in Public Procurement in Bulgaria (the Pact) is a voluntary contract between a contracting authority, the participants in a public procurement procedure and an independent monitor which enables external monitoring of all the actions of the participants and all documentation, to be conducted by such an independent monitor throughout all the phases of implementation of the public procurement procedure, including contract execution. The Pact establishes specific monitoring rules and binding commitments for the participants, requiring the latter to provide information and allow direct monitoring at all stages. In addition, the Pact provides guarantees for the imposition of effective penalties on tenderers and/ or penalties on individual staff members whose conduct fails to meet ethical standards. On the other hand, the Pact also creates incentives to encourage participants to fulfil their commitments of openness and transparency in the implementation of the public procurement contract.[73]

Public procurement procedures carried out in compliance with the Pact's monitoring terms and conditions are deemed both to help limit the possibilities of using corrupt schemes and to create conditions for more effective management of public funds and expand the access of businesses to public procurement contracts.

The pilot implementation of the Pact in Bulgaria, developed by TIBG, involves four Bulgarian ministries.[74] The results of this pilot with respect to several public procurement procedures (in the period February 2012 to December 2013) and the basic principles and benefits of the Pact were presented in the analysis '*Indicators of transparency and integrity in public procurement*'.[75]

---

[71] The TIBG has endeavoured to adapt the Integrity Pact version proposed for Bulgaria to the Bulgarian reality, to comply with the legal framework and the functions of administrative structures (see below (n 73) 9). Quite how much it has succeeded in 'tuning' the Integrity Pact to the needs effectively combating corrupt policies in procurement is, in my opinion, somewhat disputable, as explained further herein.

[72] Transparency.bg. <www.transparency.bg.> accessed 23 April 2016.

[73] 'Integrity Pact – Conceptual Framework' <http://integrity.transparency.bg/media/cms_page_media/1/IP_CONCEPT_BG_1.pdf>; and 'Integrity Pact – Bulgarian Model' <http://integrity.transparency.bg/media/cms_page_media/1/IP_BULGARIAN_MODEL_BG_1.pdf> accessed 23 April 2016.

[74] (i) The Ministry of Regional Development and Public Works, (ii) The Ministry of Labour and Social Policy, (iii) The Ministry of Health, and iv) The Ministry of Transport and Communications.

[75] V Kashukeev-Nusheva, K Hristova-Valtcheva, K Slavov, L. Roumenova, P Slavov and A Gulubov (eds), *Indicators of transparency and integrity in public procurement* (Sofia: Transparency International Bulgaria, 2013).

This analysis clarifies how the specific characteristics of the Pact model correct the use of corrupt schemes in public procurement. According to TIBG, the three highest risk points in public procurement are: (a) the decision announcing the procurement and the method for its implementation; (b) the public contract parameters and (c) the implementation of the awarded procurement.[76] The Pact has developed various sets of mechanisms for each of these areas, aimed *inter alia* at strict compliance with all applicable rules, objective personnel selection and monitoring.

In addition, TIBG has provided the results of the pilot implementation of the Pact as part of the above analysis, which permits a number of observations to made on the Pact and the results of the pilot implementation:

1. *Voluntary act*

This may be signed between the public institutions and the tenderers in a public procurement procedure. What does it mean in practice? It means that not only is the choice of whether to use the Pact left to the discretion of the contracting authority (and possibly the tenderers), but also the choice of which public procurement procedure to apply the Pact to. This, in turn means that monitoring of a contracting authority's overall activity can be omitted. Put cynically, if the contracting authority and a tenderer or candidate intend to use corrupt practices for some contracts, then the Pact can simply not be signed (or will not be proposed for signature) for those contracts. What is more, the contracting authority may use the Pact for those specific contracts where it has decided that it has no interest in manipulating the procedure to select a favoured candidate, (who on his turn will make use of the incentive effect of the Pact and thus getting listed in the White List, as described below).

2. *The figure of the independent monitor*

According to TIBG's analysis, an independent monitor is:

> [A]n organisation, publicly renowned and long active in combating corruption, which has proven itself independent, objective and impartial, which has experts with exceptional professional and moral qualities who would not hesitate from taking measures to prevent or counteract offenses and socially unacceptable business practices. The independent monitor is selected by the contracting authority and by joining the Pact, all participants unconditionally and irrevocably undertake to assist it in carrying out its duties and to comply with its recommendations and decisions.[77]

The intended independent monitor is TIBG, which fits completely with the above description. The independent monitor would certainly have a disciplining and restraining influence on the participants in public procurement, who will not only have an incentive to prevent corruption or any irregularities in the implementation of public procurement procedures but will also have the opportunity to use the monitor at a later stage as a mediator in resolving disputes and problems in the implementation of the contract once the procurement contract has been signed. However, given this formulation, the contracting authority is free to select another indepen-

---

[76] Ibid, 10–11.
[77] Ibid, 12.

dent monitor (whose only required characteristics are those specified above). It is not clear from the text of the analysis and the model Pact Agreement (apparently signed in this form in the pilot implementation of the model) precisely how the contracting authority should select this 'independent monitor', what professional requirements it would have to meet, what the selection criteria should be,[78] and how its relationship with the contracting authority should be settled so that the monitor can express its intention to participate in the public procurement procedure. There is no indication, for example, whether there should be a register of 'respected' and 'impartial' organisations, or whether it should be the contracting authority which assesses the qualities of the monitor; does the monitor participate on a *pro bono* or paid basis; how is the absence of relatedness to be proved between the contracting authority and the monitor on the one hand, and between the contracting authority and the tenderers on the other etc. Therefore, there is no mechanism in place to prevent applicants or tenderers related to the monitor from participating in a public procurement.[79] Only Article 28 of the Pact states: 'Along with the text of the Pact information regarding the independent monitor is provided, on the basis of which conclusions as to the professional qualifications, reputation and impartiality of the independent monitor was reached'.[80]

3. *The Pact White List*

To focus on encouraging participants towards fair and transparent conduct and implementation of public procurement in accordance with the monitoring and rules of the Pact, and in an effort to adapt the Pact to the specific characteristics of the Bulgarian economic reality and legislation, TIBG designed a White List to be maintained and updated by the individual contracting authorities, to champion for and promote those participants who clearly emphasise their anticorruption commitments and behaviour. This is of note in analysing and comparing the different Pacts implemented worldwide by TI as anticorruption models in public procurement.

Sanctions for failure to fulfil the commitments undertaken under the Pact and for 'unacceptable behaviour'[81] are minimised and shifted to the background as

---

[78] In the case of a competitive dialogue, for example, where the complexity of the public procurement and its more complicated nature make it impossible for the contracting authority to specifically determine its object, the pre-selection of an independent monitor with good professional qualification would be even more difficult.

[79] The monitor is apparently present at a much earlier stage in the implementation of the procedure – as early as the preparation and announcement of the criteria.

[80] Integrity Pact – Bulgarian Model <http://integrity.transparency.bg/media/cms_page_media/1/IP_BULGARIAN_MODEL_BG_1.pdf> accessed 23 April 2016.

[81] Art 24(1) Pact: 'Unacceptable behaviour shall be: (a) Any behaviour that may adversely affect the judgement and motivation of the contracting authority, its employees, the tenderer or third parties, including such behaviour, that is permitted by law, but is inconsistent with the best practices, the morals, the goals and the spirit of this Pact; (b) The provision to a tenderer, the contracting authority or a third party of information which has become known in the course of implementation of this Pact or the public procurement award or implementation procedure by a tenderer, the contracting authority, their employees, contractors or subcontractors'.

incentives are foregrounded. Such an incentive model, yet, is not a good way forward: its educational function with regard to anticorruption measures in public procurement is unclear. Moreover, the White List serves to 'advertise' the proper behaviour of the relevant participants in public procurement, which is intended to give contractors some confidence for subsequent participation in other procedures. The participants' positive reputations are built solely on the cases in which the Pact was applied (at the discretion of the contracting authority and the participants). As noted above, it is quite possible for the same organisations to have been involved in corrupt schemes in other public procurement procedures in which the Pact is not used. This prepares the ground for favouring certain public organisations and representatives of individual businesses.

4. *The time factor*

Time should also be taken into account when considering the Pact's merits. The deadlines for open procedures are relatively long (although severely shortened with the new procurement rules), but not for negotiated procedures (with or without call for proposals) or electronic tenders, and it might be difficult for the analysis and evaluation of the documentation by the independent monitor to fit statutory deadlines. This problem is also evident in the reported results of the pilot implementation of the Pact:

> The lengthy period for agreeing the commitments under the Integrity Pacts resulted in monitoring actually starting after drafting the tender documents for the relevant public procurement procedures. This predetermined the method which was applied to review the drafted documentation – subsequent monitoring of already completed documentation. Access to contracting authority decisions and tender documentation was not provided until after the start of the procedures.[82]

The Pilot implementation of the Pact demonstrates that at a certain stage of the award and implementation process (might be, due to lack of time) the tenderers themselves ignore the independent monitor, communicating with each other without notifying the monitor, or not taking advantage of all monitoring and assistance options available in the Pact at the document preparation stage. Their stance towards popularisation of the White List is also too lukewarm and lacking in enthusiasm.

5. *Questions remaining open*

Matters such as e.g. the implementation of the Pact with subcontractors and/or third parties and the use of framework agreements remain unsolved.

An initial conclusion from the analysis of the corruption prevention model proposed by TIBG is that the model is no 'panacea' for the profound corruption problems in the implementation of public procurement procedures in Bulgaria. However, this anticorruption initiative definitely creates conditions for the implementation of more effective control at the three main phases of public procurement (Announcement Phase, Procedure Conduct Phase and Contract Implementation Phase, as defined in Chap. 3 of this book) and has a disciplining effect on the parties to the Pact. Further adjustments in the Bulgarian model are definitely required for

---

[82] See above (n 80), 30.

the initiative to be successful and its popularisation to be effective. To this end, the individual approach in the creation of the Bulgarian Pact should be strengthened so that it can address the specific needs of Bulgaria to a much greater extent. Though this model is not a novelty in Scandinavian countries (the countries with the lowest level of corruption, according to the CPI) and older EU Member States and its merits are clear and bring positive results, for Bulgaria this type of prevention sounds a bit exotic, at least for the time being. Many elements of the rules of the Pact which are 'implied' or rely on statutory provisions in the relevant legislation therefore need to be further elaborated in much more details for the purposes of the Bulgarian public procurement system. This of course is not impossible, but it does require additional research and work in the field. Last but not least, strengthening the punitive element in the implementation of the Pact in Bulgaria will not have a disincentive effect on participants in public procurement, but will, on the contrary, have an even stronger disciplining effect. 'Other sanctions could include the forfeiture of the bid or performance bonds, liability for damages and debarment regarding future contract opportunities for a period of time reflecting the seriousness of the violation'.[83] This can be seen particularly well in addressing the Integrity Pact, as applied in Germany, in Chap. 6 of this book.

4.5.4   The BORKOR Project – An Attempt to Transfer German Experience in Bulgaria

In November 2009 the Bulgarian government adopted the 'National Strategy for Preventing and Combating Corruption and Organised Crime'. A national project called BORKOR (БОРКОР)[84] was established in this context.

The Center for Prevention and Countering Corruption and Organised Crime (Център за превенция и противодействие на корупцията и организираната престъпност, CPCCOC) was set up for the purposes of the BORKOR project.[85] The CPCCOC is a state budget funded body. Its objective is to develop comprehensive, effective and long-lasting preventive measures against corruption and organised crime.

The BORKOR project is a 'complex cybernetic model of centralised planning and development of effective measures and systems of measures against corruption'.[86] The concept behind BORKOR is a combination of technical and analytical methods aimed at the establishment of a highly productive system for the identification of weaknesses ('gateways to corruption')[87] which cause or encourage

---

[83] *Integrity in Public Procurement* (Paris: OECD Publishing, 2007) 87.

[84] An acronym formed from the Bulgarian words '*Борба*' (Fight) and '*Корупция*' (Corruption).

[85] Council of Ministers Decree of 29 July 2010.

[86] Borkor.government.bg. <http://borkor.government.bg/bg/page/5> accessed 23 April 2016.

[87] This is the term that CPCCOC uses for those weaknesses in the procedures which open the doors for corrupt behaviour.

corruption.[88] The model is based on the provisions of the project implementation standard adopted by the German Federal Government (the 'V-Modell XT'). This established standard is adapted, according to CPCCOC, to the local conditions in Bulgaria.[89]

One of the first areas on which the CPCCOC focused its attention through the BORKOR project was precisely the award and implementation of public procurement contracts in Bulgaria as an area representing a concentrated risk of corrupt schemes.[90] The 'Solution Model in the Area of Public Procurement' (the Solution Model) is essentially web-based, with six electronic platforms operating within its framework. It uses the methodological standard adopted under the BORKOR project. The Solution Model is fully consistent with the recommendations of the expert group on electronic procurement eTeg[91] (part of the EU Commission's strategy to introduce fully electronic procurement across the EU).[92] It incorporates four main aspects:

The technical part of the model consists of the development of six electronic platforms that interact with each other and support the procurement procedure from the first to the last stage and closely linked to the proposals in the New Procurement Directives.[93] Since the Solution Model was also forwarded to Parliament, some of

---

[88] An anticorruption formula has also been developed specifically for the purposes of the CPCCOC, which helps analyse the relationship between the factors that affect the behaviour of offenders.

[89] The author of the concept is the German expert Rolf Schlotterer, an adviser to the Bulgarian government (March 2009–October 2013).

[90] On 21 February 2012, the Advisory Board of CPCCOC charged the head of CPCCOC with the development of a *Solution model in the area of public procurement*.

[91] <http://ec.europa.eu/internal_market/publicprocurement/docs/eprocurement/conferences/121214_etendering-expert-group-draft-report-part1_en.pdf>; and <http://ec.europa.eu/internal_market/publicprocurement/docs/eprocurement/conferences/121214_etendering-expert-group-draft-report-part2_en.pdf> accessed 23 April 2016.

[92] <http://eur-lex.europa.eu/LexUriServ/LexUriServ.do?uri=COM:2012:0179:FIN:EN:PDF> accessed 23 April 2016.

[93] (i) e-Register – an electronic register, which is the central platform for all stakeholders in the award process; it contains information and documents for the procedure and predominantly supports the necessary legal and administrative steps to be undertaken prior to contract conclusion; (ii) e-Bidding – active online bidding software applications; (iii) e-Catalogue – an online platform supporting public procurement procedures that cover standardised products or products that can be visually presented (machinery, equipment, furniture etc); (iv) e-Auction – a classic form of announcing and awarding through online applications. Suitable for all three types of procurement contracts (works, services and supplies), where the procedure is more complicated and complex and the E-Bidding and E-Catalogue platforms cannot be used; (v) e-Monitoring – a platform that collects data and performs centralised monitoring of all contracts, annexes, protocols etc., which are entered into between government bodies and legal entities (the ambition being that even contracts outside the scope of public procurement be included in the platform). Platform applications include monitoring, statistics, analysis, reporting and other applications; (vi) e-Audit – An online platform to conduct audits and analytical work for identification of violations of rules and laws. Access to this platform will be available to the state institutions responsible for auditing and reviewing the public procurement award process. In addition the platform contains a communication system that allows the receipt of alerts about suspected violations.

these platforms have already been included in legislation, but there is still no overview of what has been achieved so far. These were initially heavily criticised by the majority of the members of the expert group organised by the CPCCOC to discuss the Solution Model, as well as by members of the Parliamentary committee. Arguments were put forward to show how expensive and organisationally difficult the introduction of such almost completely electronic award process would be. The great need for precisely such platforms was poorly accounted for – platforms which can (a) significantly lighten and simplify the award process which would no longer be so very dependent on the cumbersome bureaucratic apparatus, and (b) limit the human factor effect to a minimum and hence the spread of corrupt practices.

At a later stage, however, the legislator took note of the trends underlying the New Procurement Directives as it became clear that the Solution Model could not simply be a copy-paste version of a similar working model in Germany, but that as the EU[94] had expressly chosen a path towards electronic procurement, this model is regarded as a logical response to corruption in the sector. The e-Catalogue was explicitly created to facilitate contracting authorities in the award of standard procurements and its existence has already been codified in European legislation.[95]

Data collection for detection of corruption is the second aspect of the Solution Model. All information and documentation relating to procedures for the award of public contracts is collected and reviewed, even information and documentation which falls outside the scope of the legal framework. Therefore, according to the CPCCOC's proposal, the weaknesses in the system and the patterns of corruption are revealed in full. Perhaps in response to this proposal or in view of the trends set by the New Procurement Directives, in this case the Bulgarian legislator hastened to provide for even more 'publicity and transparency' in procedures by introducing the requirement for the entirety of the procurement documentation to be compiled in the 'buyer's profile'. This legislative decision was ill-advised and burdensome, although a good idea in principle. The drawbacks of this decision have already been reviewed in the previous chapters of this work, arriving at the unequivocal conclusion that this is not the right way to detect corrupt intent.

Active involvement of supervisory bodies is the aspect of the Solution Model which aims to achieve better coordination between all the supervisory bodies involved in *ex ante*, ongoing or *ex post* control of the individual stages of the procurement process. The CPCCOC established that regardless of the significant number of violations detected in and complaints made of corruption in public procurement procedures, the number of cases which actually reach the courtroom is negligible, and effective sentences are almost non-existent. Therefore, the CPCCOC

---

[94] ie the New Procurements Directives, although the issue of wider application of e-procurement was discussed in different acts preceding these Directives, eg in the course of gathering responses for: EU Commission Directorate General Internal Market and Services, 'Green Paper on the modernisation of EU public procurement policy towards a more efficient European Procurement Market' COM(2011) 15 final, 1 January 2011; EU Commission, Single Market Act II (Communication to the European Parliament, the Council, the European Economic and Social Committee and the Committee of the Regions) COM(2012) 573 final, 3 October 2012 etc.

[95] Art 36(1)–(6) Directive 2014/24/EU.

considers it necessary to require active involvement of the control authorities in the Solution Model. As already discussed, this is one of the key elements which could serve as a weapon against corruption in the country. Existing control bodies, along with the introduction of electronic platforms to facilitate access to information and to increase the distance in communication between the contracting authorities, the election committee and the tenderers, are the main ingredients for a successful campaign against corruption in the public spending process.

The last aspect outlined by the Solution Model is the creation of new *legal and organisational rules* to ensure its implementation, to help limit the opportunities for corrupt schemes and to maximise the efficient use of public funds at the legislative level.

It is precisely in connection with the implementation of these last four aspects of the Solution Model that the CPCCOC drafted a proposal for changes in the current legislation in the public procurement field and for the establishment of two separate institutions – this idea being once again entirely borrowed from the German legal system in the public procurement field: a) through 'pre-qualification' bodies and b) the establishment of the Central Public Procurement Services.

The two proposals comprise independent sets of measures which, according to the CPCCOC, are essential for the success of the Solution Model, as they are prerequisites for the implementation of the technical solution and address those weaknesses which were either not covered or only partially covered by the technical solution.

Pre-qualification[96]

All documents, registrations and certifications which are required as standard or which are usually received from all participants in the relevant sector[97] should be collected in a single register to facilitate significantly the contracting authorities in verifying the eligibility of candidates.[98] This will enable the identification and reg-

---

[96] This concept should actually be called 'pre-registration'. The German word used ('*Präqualifizierung*') has a different meaning in Bulgarian ('retraining') and therefore a more appropriate legal term was introduced; for the purposes of this work the term introduced and used by the CPCCOC in the Solution Model will be used.

[97] eg company registration in the Commercial Register, ISO certificates, proof of insolvency and construction certificates etc.

[98] To achieve the purposes of pre-qualification stage (following the model of German best practices), the idea was to establish two pre-qualification services based at the Ministry of Regional Development and Public Works: (a) a service for pre-qualification of companies and professionals in the field of public works contracts for, and (b) a service for pre-qualification of companies and professionals in the supplies, services and projects field. The internal structure and legal status of these pre-qualification services have also been defined. The CPCCOC expects that the unit providing these services will be established through far-reaching changes to national legislation: (i) adoption of a new procurement law for electronic procurement in accordance with the proposals of the CPCCOC; (ii) amendments to the legislation regulating the National Audit Office and the Public Financial Inspection; and (iii) amendments to the competition legislation.

istration of the professional skills, abilities and eligibility of each potential contractor and will allow for 'the widest separation between the administrative and the specific and qualitative components of a public procurement procedure'.[99] This concept is supposed to result in significant alleviation of the administrative burden and a subsequent focus on the specific qualities of the participants, thus expected to limit the existing 'gateways to corruption' in the award process. Another indisputable advantage is that the input of such formal data is envisaged to run separately and independently from the call for proposals, and that once entered (and updated where necessary), this data can be used repeatedly for different public procurement procedures.[100]

Central Public Procurement Services

Again borrowed from the German model, these are to be services with qualified and trained staff to assist with the preparation of the formal documentation required for a public procurement award procedure and to review the technical specifications prior to publication of the call. According to CPCCOC data, in Europe '[i]n 2011 already 5.73% of the announced public procurement procedures were conducted by the centralised services'[101] and this centralised approach has a proven organisational and anticorruption effect. The Solution Model envisages the establishment of at least five Central Public Procurement Services[102] with trained personnel to function as committee members, to advise and train contracting authorities and to draft and verify the quality of tender documentation.

By design, the Central Public Procurement Services are government entities which provide services and carry out their tasks independently of the contracting authority, and largely resemble the assigning functions of a CPB.[103] According to the initial Solution Model they are entrusted with functions which closely resemble the rights and obligations of a contracting authority and in some respects even take over the functions of those authorities.[104]

---

[99] R Schlotterer, 'First Report of CPCCOC on the draft Solution model in the area of public procurement' Summary version 1.52, (Sofia: CPCCOC, 2013) 13.

[100] According to the 'Towards a more efficient European Procurement Market' Green Paper (n 94), 14: 'The idea of a European-wide prequalification system finds some support from business but meets opposition from contracting authorities', but this refers to the administrative burden on contracting authorities and the extent to which such mode of operation will facilitate or further encumber them, rather than to the anti-corruption effect to be achieved by 'removing' formal documentation from the procedure itself.

[101] Schlotterer (n 99), 14.

[102] Ibid, 5.

[103] As envisaged in the Procurement Directives and advanced as a concept in the New Procurement Directives.

[104] For example, if the contract value reaches or exceeds the European procurement threshold, the Central Public Procurement Services will be responsible for announcing a public procurement tender. Accordingly, regardless of the thresholds, in all product and service procurement tenders the Central Public Procurement Services are responsible for matters such as: publishing the calls; reviewing and, where necessary, finalising tender documentation in consultation with the contract-

The establishment of such a centralised unit (with such extended functions and duties) suggests significant legislative changes, which include amendments to (or adoption of new) laws and regulations governing the activities of control authorities in public procurement.

The above description of CPCCOC's Solution Model and the BORKOR concept demonstrates the ambitiousness of the project, which offers both a purely technical improvement in public procurement (in line with the trend towards e-procurement) and an overall change in the current legislation. From this perspective, any constructive criticism of CPCCOC's project should try to avoid one-sidedness but instead requires analysis of the various aspects of anticorruption measures.[105]

The BORKOR project is actually a thorough piece of work, with quite a number of advantages.

Firstly, it is the first ever attempt in Bulgaria to create not only a single unit focused on fighting corruption (ie the CPCCOC), but also a comprehensive action programme and an IT model to be followed.

Secondly, the CPCCOC offers the only Solution Model so far which provides specific measures aimed at detecting corruption loopholes in public procurement in the country, as well as at their minimisation.

The technical part, as the first aspect of the Solution Model, deserves admiration since diminishing the human factor and auditing public procurement based on the BORKOR concept represents a serious anticorruption measure against the corruption schemes successfully developed so far.

The recording of corruption detection data and the active cooperation between supervisory authorities (as the second and third aspects of the Solution Model) also

---

ing authority; and the statistical recording and transmission of data relating to the tender to the relevant institutions responsible under the law. In addition, the Central Public Procurement Services should undertake matters such as: technical responsibility for the establishment and operation of electronic platforms in the field of public procurement; the preparation of tender documents and the conduct of public procurement procedures, including procurement and contracting; the preparation or implementation of high quality legal review of tender documentation, their publication and implementation or participation in the public procurement procedures up to contract award and conclusion; and assistance to the contracting authorities with legal and expert advice on the selection of the most suitable public procurement procedure.

[105] On the one hand, BORKOR proponents express rather bold predictions that: 'The BORKOR model is, at the moment, a key element of the fight against corruption and the prevention thereof in Bulgaria [...] The importance of the model for the neighbouring countries lies in its universal applicability. With slight modifications, it is possible to use the structure of the model in each country' (in L. Hensgen, *Fight against corruption in the Danube region: A study of regional best practices*, Max Planck Foundation for International Peace and the Rule of Law (Sankt Augustin: Konrad Adenauer Stiftung, 2013) 44). At the same time the *Report on Progress in Bulgaria under the Co-operation and Verification Mechanism*, (Brussels, 2014) 9, was sceptical as to what has been accomplished so far: 'The anti-corruption project BORKOR, which was promoted as a major instrument to identify and address corruption risks, still shows no concrete results, in spite of the resources which have been devoted to the project. In the area of public procurement, a complex and ever changing legislative framework has made it even more difficult to create a culture of objectivity and rigour. Some business voices are losing confidence that a tide of manipulation of tenders can be stemmed'.

deserve positive assessment. These two needs have repeatedly been identified both by the organisations which analyse the level of corruption in the country (as shown in this chapter) and the EU (in its monitoring reports).

The commentary on the terms of the legislative changes proposed and the establishment of 'pre-qualification' bodies and 'Central Public Procurement Services' is strongly polarised.

'Pre-qualification' is a good practice which has also had a positive impact in other European countries, as discussed in Chap. 6 here. Its implementation could significantly reduce the level of bureaucracy in an already sufficiently complicated public procurement system and will play a role in reducing corruption niches in the field. This is a worthy example of a constructive anticorruption solution that is not based solely on the principles of improving transparency and publicity in the award of public procurement contracts: pre-qualification virtually eliminates the possibility of unjust exclusion and/or refusal of admission of certain companies from participating in award procedures; the possibility of excluding a candidate on formal or technical grounds through unconventional qualification requirements is also removed and eliminated. However, viewed from the prism of the new European legislation, the need for such an institution at local level is not on the table for the moment. In case the e-Certis system turns out to be of sufficient help to contracting authorities and participants due to its similar functions,[106] this would replace the need for such an internal national pre-qualification system. Although in Germany the ambition now is that these two systems will work simultaneously, this is more appropriate for a country which has developed a national pre-qualification system long before the transposition of the New Procurement Directives, rather than for countries such as Bulgaria.

The assessments of the establishment of the Central Public Procurement Services are even more controversial. It is undisputable that centralised public procurement bodies have had a proven anticorruption effect due to their role as mediators between contracting authorities and tenderers and in supporting the needs of contracting authorities by largely eliminating the possibilities for 'covered arrangements'. This positive example is evident not only in Germany (as reviewed in detail in Chap. 6 here) but also in other countries where the levels of corruption have significantly dropped, such as in Hungary and Estonia for example. This premise is confirmed by the provisions of the New Procurement Directives, which expand on the provisions for the existence and functions of such centralised bodies. However, so far there has been no serious political will in Bulgaria to use such centralised bodies. The need for an increase in the number of such centralised bodies is obvious and the expansion of their functions would have an indisputably restrictive effect on corruption in the sector. Time and practice will tell whether the central and sub-central purchasing bodies envisaged in the New PPA[107] will once again remain a sham, as could well be said of the current situation, or if they will show their practical and anticorruption value.

The institution thus proposed by the Solution Model, however, is entrusted with too many and overly chaotic functions, which *de jure* render it obvious that the

---

[106] Based on Art 61 Directive 2014/24/EU.

[107] Art 95 et seq New PPA.

Central Public Procurement Services are in fact a type of CPB, although charged with further, atypical functions in addition to those delegated to the 'central purchasing body' in the New PPA.

Despite this criticism and the failings indentified in light of all the theoretical works developed so far, and of Bulgaria's attempts to deal with corruption, the measures proposed by the CPCCOC and the BORKOR project are really '[a] quite promising aspect in the development of intervention models that include multiple measures. [...] The development of a comprehensive approach is certainly more promising than targeted measures that are only limited to the analysis of weaknesses within the affected institution'.[108] Unfortunately, similarly to the NAO, the CPCCOC has also been reduced to a bargaining chip for the political classes and an object of all sorts of different appetites of the short-lived governments of recent years. The operation of the CPCCOC and indeed its very existence, have stalled due to the frequent changes in its management, the varying outlooks of politicians and the populist criticism claiming that the CPCCOC is a waste of resources. This institution may indeed thus turn out to be incredibly expensive for society, given that its projects were funded to a certain point, but thereafter its operation suffered serious decline. Therefore the scepticism of the EU and the public seems justified for the time being.

In 2015 the government began work on a new draft law to create a single national body to combat corruption, which would absorb the CPCCOC and several other institutions currently in force (such as the Commission for Conflict of Interest). According to the new Anti-corruption Strategy '[a]nalyses show that the existing system of bodies with often redundant or inefficiently distributed anti-corruption powers does not provide the necessary tangible and specific results in the fight against corruption. Each institution creates its own anti-corruption unit, but the results of its work are not visible. There is a general feeling that the problem is constantly being shifted between institutions, the approach to its solution is overly bureaucratic and actions in that direction fail to demonstrate the necessary determination and finality.'[109] Yet this new strategy does not comment in detail on the particular manifestations of corruption in public procurement, but merely states that measures should be taken to expand the preliminary and internal control in the field. It remains to be seen whether the latest purely political reshuffle and opening and closure of new institutions will once again occur or whether, finally, a truly effective and efficient body will be born, taking into account the positive guidelines laid down so far and leading the fight against corruption in the right direction.

---

[108] L. Hensgen, *Fight against corruption in the Danube region: A study of regional best practices*, Max Planck Foundation for International Peace and the Rule of Law (Sankt Augustin: Konrad Adenauer Stiftung, 2013) 50.

[109] 'Strategy for Prevention and Corruption in the Republic of Bulgaria 2015–2020' (2015) <www.government.bg/fce/001/0211/files/0804STRATEGY_anticorruption_april2015.pdf> accessed 23 April 2016, 5.

4.6   Where Does Bulgaria Stand Now?

The review of the participants in public procurement procedures in Bulgaria and the performance of the control and appellate authorities are fundamental to this book's conclusions, as they highlight the weaknesses in that Member State's award system and allow for more eloquent comparison with the systems of the other two countries examined in this work. Elements such as control efficiency, the functions of the institutions and the legal framework regulating the obligations of the contracting authorities are essential to determine adequate measures against corrupt activities in the sector, beyond the ensuring procedural transparency. In light of the findings in this chapter, as well as those in Chaps. 5 and 6, it is clear which anticorruption models and procurement regulations tackle corruption most satisfactorily. Apart from that, however, this chapter also helps distinguish the various political and legislative decisions forming the procurement systems of each of the reviewed Member States, making it clear that not every practice identified as good in developed Member States will work as well in Member States with problems like Bulgaria.

In addition, it is useful to assess the steps taken so far in a country which is making efforts to curb corruption in public procurement, but obviously not always in the right direction. The work of the organisations covered in this chapter again highlights the inability of transparency to limit corrupt procurement as the sole warrior against this phenomenon. Also, trying to make too sharp jump towards the practice in another country (ie Germany) is also not likely to meet with absolute success at the moment.

The CSD, TIBG and CPCCOC have definitely made a positive contribution to the monitoring and studying of the peculiarities of national corruption patterns in public procurement to date, the highlighting the problem areas in the procedure and the measures to be undertaken to minimise the negative effects of corruption.

Despite the very different direction of TIBG and CPCCOC, a parallel can nevertheless be drawn: (a) both projects started at about the same time and they both claim to offer an effective solution to reducing corruption in public procurement; (b) both projects use basically the best anticorruption practices from Germany (given the comparative nature of this work, these two projects, the analysis thereof, the public response to them and their results are of particular interest to the author); and (c) since both projects are in their initial stage and/or their development is currently suspended, it remains difficult to identify any actual positive and practical results. The approach of the two institutions, however, is completely antipodal, with the TIBG clearly championing increased trust between participants in the procedure and sufficient transparency, and the CPCCOC model offering measures which are far more radical and practical. In any case, both organisations' reports and work form an excellent basis for the development of an anticorruption mechanism which could 'save' public procurement from the constant waste of funds.

It is notable, however, that all of the prevention measures proposed so far, irrespective of whether they give priority to improving transparency or whether they are more constructive in nature, still fail to account for the individual characteristics of adverse national factors. Public administration in Bulgaria is not effective, it is deficient and poorly aligned to European standards: the level of technical and professional capability available in the individual contracting authorities is in most cases completely inadequate to address the proposed modern measures, and the legislative framework in the area of public procurement cannot be made fit for the purpose by further 'experiments' – a radical change of legislation is needed.

> In the attempts towards a comprehensive and all-embracing legal framework to regulate public procurement processes, the state not only fails to achieve a tangible improvement in the efficiency of investment of public funds, but also comes to the point of outright absurdities.[110]

In addition to the above, the proposed anticorruption measures must take into account the fact that the economic situation in Bulgaria does not allow for the allocation of substantial funds for the implementation of complex projects which would not deliver their first results until after the passage of several years, and that public attitudes are pessimistic and demand fast results and 'draconian measures'.

Bibliography

A Kovacheva, Public Procurement Award, (Sofia: Fenea Publishing, 2008)

A Stoyanov, R Stefanov and B Velcheva, 'Bulgarian Anti-Corruption Reforms: A Lost Decade?' (2014) European Research Centre for Anti-Corruption and State-Building and Center for the Study of Democracy Working Paper No 42

C Daskalov, 'Brain-Workshop' (2015) http://brain-workshop.org/index.php?option=com_content&view=article&id=231:2012-12-12-20-08-43&catid=29:politics&Itemid=37 and <http://borkor.government.bg/bg/pubs/3/124> accessed 23 April 2016

K Pashev and K Marinov, Reducing corruption risks and implementation of good practices by the management of public procurements. (Sofia: Center for the Study of Democracy, 2009)

K Pashev, Reducing Corruption Risks and Practices in Public Procurement: Evidence from Bulgaria, Paper presented at the First Global Dialogue on Ethical and Effective Governance (Amsterdam, 2009)

L Hensgen, Fight against corruption in the Danube region: A study of regional best practices, Max Planck Foundation for International Peace and the Rule of Law (Sankt Augustin: Konrad Adenauer Stiftung, 2013)

L Tavares, R Medeiros, and D Coelho The new Directive 2014/24/EU on Public Procurement. (Lisbon: OPET, 2014) ch 2 (The New Directive 2014/24/EU on Public Procurement: A First Overview)

M Krivachka, M Markov, E Dimova and Z Lilyan, The new aspects in the Public Procurement Act (Sofia: IK Trud i Pravo, 2008)

N Ehlermann-Cache, Bribery in public procurement. (Paris: OECD, 2007)

---

[110] C Daskalov, 'Brain-Workshop' (2015) <http://brain-workshop.org/index.php?option=com_content&view=article&id=231:2012-12-12-20-08-43&catid=29:politics&Itemid=37> and <http://borkor.government.bg/bg/pubs/3/124> accessed 23 April 2016.

R Schloterrer, 'First Report of CPCCOC on the draft Solution model in the area of public procurement' Summary version 1.52, (Sofia: CPCCOC, 2013)

T Nikolova 'Highlights in the process of appealing the decisions, actions and omissions of the contracting authority under the new Public Procurement Act' (2016) 3 ZOP+

V Kashukeev-Nusheva, K Hristova-Valtcheva, K Slavov, L Roumenova, P Slavov and A Gulubov (eds), *Indicators of transparency and integrity in public procurement* (Sofia: Transparency International Bulgaria, 2013)

V Panchev, *Procurements under control. Past, present and future of the preliminary control exercised by the Public Procurement Agency under current legislation and draft new PPA* (2016) 1 ZOP+

Chapter 5
Infringements in Procurement Procedures. Corruption Loopholes and Practices

'According to the 2013 flash Eurobarometer survey on corruption relevant to businesses, more than three out of ten (32%) companies in the Member States that participated in public procurement say corruption prevented them from winning a contract.'
(The First EU Anticorruption Report 2014)

5.1 Methodology

The methodology applied for the purposes of this chapter is as follows:

(i) description of the provisions of EU[1] (and national, where applicable)[2] law infringed;
(ii) description of the infringement itself;
(iii) violation of transparency rules, if any; and
(iv) analysis of the types of corruption loopholes opened by each particular infringement.

Each infringement is examined separately from the analysis of the specific corruption possibilities it opens, because a deviation from the rules does not necessarily mean an instance of corruption and *vice versa*:

---

[1] In cases where the new procurement package provides for different legislative solutions than before its entry into force the provisions of the Procurement Directives are also presented for the sake of easier comparison between rules.

[2] Certain provisions of the Bulgarian procurement legislation are extracted for illustrative purposes. Negative practice and legislative decisions are thus emphasised. Relevant provisions from the other benchmarked Member States are not provided to avoid duplicating the information provided and the discussions in the subsequent chapters.

© Springer International Publishing AG 2017
I. Georgieva, *Using Transparency Against Corruption in Public Procurement*,
Studies in European Economic Law and Regulation 11,
DOI 10.1007/978-3-319-51304-1_5

Even when an accusation of corruption surfaces, this provides no certainty that the case is actually corrupt. One must take into account false accusations, confusion of terminology [...] and other grounds before accepting something to be true.[3]

In any event, no attempt is made to provide a detailed description of specific actions per type of procedure, nor at a comprehensive review of existing legislative measures aimed at limiting infringements. The main parallel drawn is between the *numerous existing legal provisions regulating transparency of the procedure* in Member States, such as Bulgaria, that obviously cannot deal with corruption in the award process and present a bad example in terms of the legislative framework used, as reviewed in Chap. 2 of the book, and the *different types of infringements* described below and how they are affected, or, respectively, unaffected by the level of transparency provided.

Infringements are classified in the context of the four phases of the public procurement process as set out in Chap. 3 – ie Choice of Object, Announcement, Procedure Conduct and Contract Implementation.[4] Specific procedures are only examined where this is essential to make a particular point.

This chapter does not claim to catalogue all possible types of infringements comprehensively because, given the increasing resourcefulness of contracting authorities and of future contractors, this would be a hollow claim. Furthermore, 'ingenuity applies in full force for state administration which constantly identifies new 'loopholes' in legislation'.[5] The purpose of this chapter is to cover the most flagrant and still common infringements (along with comments on some of the infringements likely to arise under the new legal framework), especially those which remain without repercussions, and thus to outline the limited connection between what has been committed to and the actual demonstration of public, transparent conduct in public procurement.

In the public procurement field, 'it is the well-structured networks for targeted investments in politics that predominate rather than individual acts of random people from the lower tiers of authority taking advantage of lax oversight by their superiors.'[6] Despite this, and although the differentiation made by some authors between 'petty'[7] and 'grand'[8] corruption[9] is not without its problems, for the pur-

---

[3] W Wensink, J Maarten de Vet et al., *Identifying and Reducing Corruption in Public Procurement in the EU* (Brussels: PwC, Ecorys, with support from Utrecht University, 2013) 58.

[4] For a more detailed description of the method of classification, see Chap. 3.

[5] V Lazarov, representative of the National Association of Municipal Employees in Bulgaria, *Corruption in public procurement costs taxpayers an estimated 1.3 billion leva* (interviewed on 17 October 2008) <www.mediapool.bg/koruptsiyata-v-obshtestvenite-porachki-kostva-13-mlrd-leva-na-danakoplattsite-news144808.html> accessed 24 April 2016.

[6] K Pashev, A Dyulgerov, G Kaschiev, *Corruption in Public Procurement – Risks and Reform Policies*, (Sofia: Center for the Study of Democracy, 2006) 15.

[7] ie committed by low-ranking employees in return for minor rewards or services promised by a future contractor.

[8] ie committed by higher-ranking officials, often acting as contracting authorities themselves, and linked to considerable financial resources.

[9] In this sense see C Dahlström, 'Bureaucracy and the different cures for grand and petty corruption' (2012) University of Gothenburg, QoG Working Paper Series No 2011:20; S Stoychev,

poses of this chapter it is useful to adopt this provisional differentiation. The objective is to identify on the one hand, infringements aimed at significant financial abuse (generally involving substantial administrative capacity), and on the other hand, to point out instances of minor corruption, the repetitive occurrence and gradual accumulation of which also lead to a similar loss of resources.

5.2   Statistics

As is evident from the analysis carried out in the previous chapters, measuring corruption or forcing corruption into specific quantitative and qualitative dimensions is exceedingly difficult, especially in terms of its manifestations in the field of public procurement. The achievements of international and national organisations focused on combating corruption have already been noted; it has also been established that some of them do offer a methodology for quantifying the level of corruption (mainly subjectively), but their indices fail to account for corruption at higher levels of authority, which is precisely the type most often associated with public procurement.

In addition to using the information derived from the above sources and with a view to presenting a 'snapshot' of infringements and the corruption mechanisms employed in the field of public procurement, the most recently available statistical information is used.

The three figures below (Figs. 5.1–5.3) are an overview of the volume of public procurements *per annum* in Bulgaria, the contracts concluded and the number of contractors and contracting authorities. The figures shed light to some extent on the positive progression in terms of both the number of public procurements and the number of concluded contracts and help correctly assess the proportion of contracts affected by infringements in Bulgaria.

In terms of infringements as a percentage of the total number of procedures and/ or contracts there is, regrettably, no reliable statistical data neither for Bulgaria, nor for the other two Member States studied in this work – Germany and Austria. This significantly hinders the identification of realistic parameters to evaluate the size of the economic loss arising from misuse of public funds. Table 5.1 further below provides therefore a comparison of the most common infringements in the award process identified for the three Member States described in this book. The information is extracted from the special Eurobarometer flash on corruption in business for 2015 (Table 5.1).[10]

Corruption Violations in Public Procurement in Bulgaria (Sofia: Transparency International Bulgaria, 2007); and Transparency International <www.transparency.org/whoweare/organisation/ faqs_on_corruption/2/> accessed 24 April 2016 etc.

[10] Flash Eurobarometer 428 'Businesses' Attitudes towards Corruption in the EU/Report', Fieldwork: September–October 2015, published December 2015.

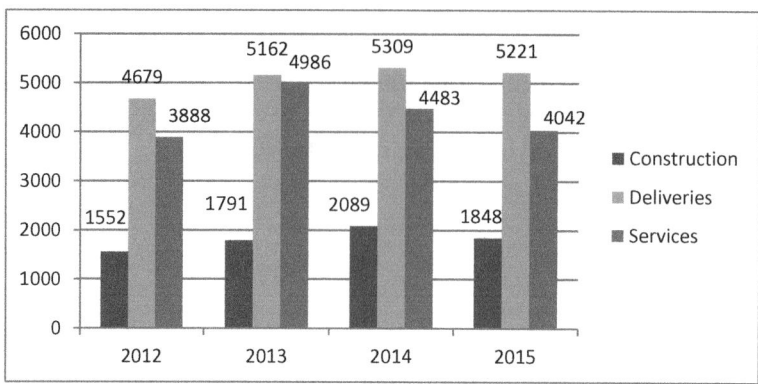

Fig. 5.1 Number of public procurement procedures in Bulgaria (2012–2015) (Figures taken from the bulletin of the PPAgency available at <http://rop3-app1.aop.bg:7778/portal/page?_pageid=93,1590259&_dad=portal&_schema=PORTAL> accessed 24 April 2016)

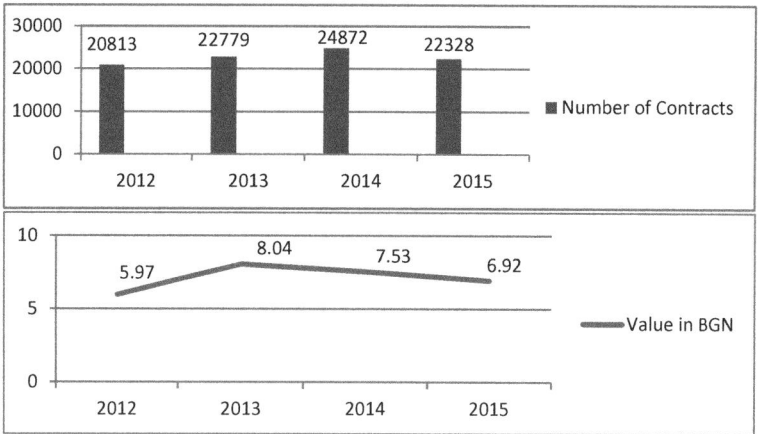

Fig. 5.2 Number of contracts concluded in Bulgaria (2012–2015) and their respective value (Figures taken from the bulletin of the PPAgency available at <http://rop3-app1.aop.bg:7778/portal/page?_pageid=93,1590259&_dad=portal&_schema=PORTAL> accessed 24 April 2016)

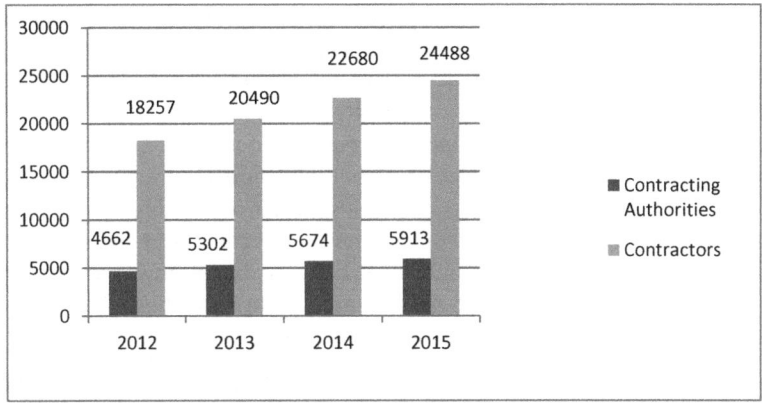

Fig. 5.3 Number of contracting authorities and contractors (2012–2015) (Figures taken from the bulletin of the PPAgency available at <http://rop3-app1.aop.bg:7778/portal/page?_pageid=93,1590259&_dad=portal&_schema=PORTAL> accessed 24 April 2016)

The PFIA provides in its annual reports statistical information on identified infringements, which is often used by the media and several public organisations to summarise their conclusions in the field of public procurements in Bulgaria. This information does not completely reflect the actual situation, especially for existing corruption mechanisms.[11] Nevertheless, the data contained in PFIA's report on public procurements for 2015[12] is a useful general guideline and reference point for further comments.

According to the PFIA report, 601 financial inspections were completed in 2014. A total of 2440 public procurement cases were reviewed under those audits, involving the disbursement of public procurement funds to a value of BGN 1,816,102,938 (approx. EUR 928,558,685). Of the total number of investigated procedures, infringements were detected in 924 cases, to a value of BGN 889,016,642 (approx. EUR 454,546,991), ie in 38% of all public procurements inspected. The infringements detected in the field of public procurements can, according to their nature, be classified as follows: breaches of law in the field of public procurement having a financial impact and resulting in violation of the principles of publicity and trans-

---

[11] (i) PFIA statistics fail to take into account the number of infringements detected by the PPAgency and the number of penal orders which are thereafter appealed and annulled by a court (which, in reality means that even if corruption is established by the PFIA, the penal orders are annulled by a court); (ii) these statistics cover an average of 2000–3000 cases per annum (due to, among other issues, lack of sufficient human and financial resources), only about a third of which fall within the scope of the annual PFIA plan, while the remaining cases refer to various previous years, ie the representative sample for a single year is too small to be compared to the total number of procedures and/or contracts as provided by the PPAgency; (iii) the larger portion of infringements covered by PFIA statistics relate to the patrons of municipalities (in their capacity as contracting authorities): these tend to be more easily detectable and demonstrable by means of available documentation and are usually classified as 'petty' corruption; and (iv) a significant proportion of detected infringements fall under the category of 'purely formal' and procedural infringements without financial effect.

[12] PFIA, 'Report on the activity of the Public Financial Inspection Agency for 2014' (2015).

parency, free and fair competition, and equality and non-discrimination, were identified in 416 procurements, ie 17% of all procurements investigated.

The above data may understandably give rise to numerous and various speculations but these can get in the way of objectiveness and comprehensiveness. In the particular case of analysing corruption in public procurements in the absence of complete statistical data and a clear system of indicators (restrictions, to which the majority of EU states are no strangers), such speculations are highly inappropriate, although there is no doubt of the worrying level of corruption in the sector. Pashev (2009) has rightly opined that the imbalance between the different groups of indicators and data sources could pose risks to monitoring activities. These risks will inevitably diminish the effectiveness of anticorruption policies:

> The first risk is to resort to monitoring of processes with a focus on input resources (input indicators) at the expense of monitoring of end results. The second risk is similar: a tendency to audit specific procedures […]. The third risk refers to the other extreme: focusing on public perceptions in order to evaluate corruption […].[13]

Despite the problems outlined above, data from the reports prepared by control bodies contribute significantly to the description of various infringements, their specific manifestations, prevalence and their classification, and therefore, where available, it is taken into account in this and in the subsequent chapters.

In addition, the table below (Table 5.1) ventures again into statistical data to illustrate the most common infringements in the procurement procedures in terms of what they represent as a proportion of all procurements for Bulgaria, Germany and Austria. The figures are self-explanatory (although based on the perceptions of the people interviewed) and will be considered in the course of the analysis below.

Table 5.1 Flash Eurobarometer 428 data for 2015[a]

Type of infringement – very widespread	Respondents in Bulgaria (%)	Respondents in Germany (%)	Respondents in Austria (%)
Abuse of negotiated procedure	26	5	5
Involvement of bidders in the design of specifications	28	20	18
Unclear selection or evaluation criteria	24	17	15
Conflicts of interests in the evaluation of the bids	32	13	8
Specifications tailor-made for particular companies	40	20	29
Abuse of emergency grounds to justify the use of non-competitive or fast-track procedures	17	12	11
Collusive bidding	17	21	23
Amendments of the contracts terms after conclusion of the contract	21	14	10

[a]Above (n 10)

---

[13] K Pashev, *Controlling corruption in public procurement: Indicators for assessing policy impact* (Sofia: Governance Monitoring Association, 2009) 17.

5.3 Types of Infringements and Incidents of Corruption

5.3.1 Choice of Object Phase[14]

Disbursement of Public Funds Without Regard to Legal Rules

Which legal provisions are breached? The main principles for conducting public procurements are completely ignored, both in terms of national[15] and EU law.[16]

What is the essence of the infringement? These are cases where the subject matter of the procedure, its value or the characteristics of the contracting authority have not been taken into account, and no procedure is thus conducted. In such cases the contracting authority directly proceeds to the conclusion of an agreement with the selected tenderer; disbursed expenses are not made public in any way and there is no control over the quality of procedural execution and the characteristics of the selected tenderer. This practice constitutes a gross violation of the law which naturally leads to lack of publicity and transparency and demonstrates obvious corrupt intent.

This practice is usually adopted by 'smaller' contracting authorities whose actions are guided by individual corrupt motives. Evidence and allegations usually point to authorities representing small municipalities, health and educational facilities, and regional institutions. Although they are obliged to act as contracting authorities, they conclude contracts with selected companies without organising a procedure of any kind. This type of infringement of public procurement law is considered as one of the most severe, as it not only infringes the publicity and transparency requirements but also restricts free and fair competition, equality and non-discrimination. Such infringements raise the question of whether public spending is effective and efficient and achieves value for money. The prevalence of this type of direct infringement involving the conclusion of public supply contracts in the absence of a proper tendering process continues to be relatively high in Bulgaria,[17] although it has long been identified both by control bodies and by sociologists and analysts. This infringement has not often been observed in Germany

---

[14] This includes cases of procedures negotiated without prior publication of contractual notice.

[15] Art 17 New PPA: 'Contracting authorities shall be required to implement the statutory procedure for procurement where the grounds provided for in the law exist'.

[16] The New Procurement Directives (and before, the Public Procurement Directives) set out the fundamental concept for regulation of this type of negotiation – 'for public contracts above a certain value, provisions should be drawn up coordinating national procurement procedures so as to ensure that those principles are given practical effect and public procurement is opened up to competition' (Recital 1, Preamble to Directive 2014/24/EU).

[17] According to the PFIA's data, a total of 330 cases were reported in Bulgaria for 2014, with contracts concluded within the preceding reporting periods amounting to a total value of BGN 347,216,268 (approx. EUR 177,528,859) without the use of any procedures for the award despite the presence of compelling legal grounds.

and Austria in the last decade. EU infringement procedures for non-observance of EU procurement rules against these Member States were most common back in 2001–2005.[18]

Naturally, this approach is rarely used to pursue 'grand' corruption precisely because of the high level of detectability. Nonetheless, although this type of infringement affects mainly small-scale contracting authorities, the cumulative effect is by no means negligible. In other words, almost one-fifth of the value of all infringements detected are the result of a deliberate failure to observe legal rules.[19]

> Even if we allow that the rate of detection within this market segment is much higher due to the direct nature of the infringement and the relative absence of political protection in contrast with large procurements, the relative share of direct infringements in the total volume of damages (including those that remain undetected) nevertheless appears significant. This is also an indication for the insufficient deterrent effect of sanctions as opposed to the benefits derived from acts of corruption.[20]

Are transparency rules breached? Yes, because the transaction is concluded without proper promulgation at the national and/or EU level, as required by law, in contravention of all other legal rules and guidance and in the absence of a healthy competitive environment.

What corruption loopholes are opened? The contracting authority concludes the transaction at its own discretion, with its favourite contractor, in violation of competition rules and proceeds to spend public funds which have not been duly evaluated and controlled as provided by law. In the absence of a procedure, the contracting authority pays for the relevant services, supplies or works on the basis of an ordinary commercial transaction, and driven by corrupt motives, deprives itself of the opportunity to assess the quality of implementation. Both the contracting authority and the contractor thus receive undue benefit by unlawfully allocating budget funds among themselves. Quite often in such infringements, the constituent elements of the offence include bribery and/or kickbacks in addition to abuse of power.

---

[18] See Commission (EU), 'Public procurement: Commission acts to enforce EU law in Germany, Greece, Spain, Italy, Austria, Portugal and Finland' (Press release 14 January 2005) <http://europa.eu/rapid/press-release_IP-05-44_en.htm> accessed 24 April 2016.

[19] Against this background, it is interesting to note that in Bulgaria the ANAO provides in Art 54(2) that the NAO will have discretion to determine the frequency of audits carried out on municipalities with a budget below BGN 10 million (approx. EUR 5 million) or whether to audit those municipalities on the basis of risk assessments. This would mean that the control of around 160 small municipalities is exercised on a highly subjective basis.

[20] Above (n 6) 30.

Splitting/Subdividing Public Procurements with the Purpose of Evading the Law

Which legal provisions are breached?

 (i) EU rules – Article 5(3) Directive 2014/24/EU, Article 16(3) Directive 2014/25/EU[21] (Article 9(3) Directive 2004/18/EC; Article 17(2) Directive 2004/17/EC)[22]
 (ii) National legislation – eg Article 7(3)[23] and Article 21(15) New PPA[24]

What is the essence of the infringement? The construction work, supplies or services required by a specific administration are subdivided by the contracting authority into sections so that each section falls below the tendering procedure thresholds (both national and European). The contracting authority then proceeds with either (a) direct negotiation or (b) a simplified award procedure by means of a public call for tenders.[25] Despite this split, the different sections are interconnected and comprise elements of one and the same procurement; the subdivision is performed solely in order to evade the public procurement rules, ie to allow for a simplified award process (or no process at all) rather than what would have been required in view of the total value of the procurement.

Not all cases of subdivision are deemed to be an infringement but only those cases in which deliberate behaviour (intent) of the contracting authority is evident and directed at circumventing the law.[26] In practice, proving intent in this type of infringement is very difficult for control bodies, hence a percentage of these violations remain undetected. Nevertheless, there are some very specific manifestations which indicate intent in the behaviour of the contracting authority.[27]

---

[21] Art 5(3) Directive 2014/24/EU and Art 16(3) Directive 2014/25/EU are identically worded: 'The choice of the method used to calculate the estimated value of a procurement shall not be made with the intention of excluding it from the scope of this Directive. A procurement shall not be subdivided with the effect of preventing it from falling within the scope of this Directive, unless justified by objective reasons'.

[22] Art 9(3) Directive 2004/18/EC: 'No works project or proposed purchase of a certain quantity of supplies and/or services may be subdivided to prevent its coming within the scope of this Directive'; Art 1(2) Directive 2004/17/EC: 'Contracting entities may not circumvent this Directive by splitting works projects or proposed purchases of a certain quantity of supplies and/or services or by using special methods for calculating the estimated value of contracts'.

[23] Authorisation for the conduct of procedures could not be used to split procurements and circumvent the law.

[24] Art 21(15) New PPA: 'Splitting of procurements on parts seeking the implementation of procedures for the award of lower values is not allowed'.

[25] Contracting authorities are not required to conduct the processes provided under the relevant legislation but can apply simplified terms or a public call for tenders taking into consideration the relevant thresholds.

[26] When a specific public procurement has been split but each of its parts are awarded by means of a procedure analogous to the one corresponding to the total value of the public procurement, no infringement will be deemed to have occurred as the prohibited result – circumvention of the law – has not been achieved.

[27] For example, the conclusion of numerous contracts with identical or similar subject-matter on the same date, and sometimes even with the same contractor.

In the case of Bulgaria, currently the New PPA provides for a rule which resembles the practice previously established by the NAO – it will not be considered splitting of an award when two or more procurements are awarded within a period of 12 months if: (i) the subject matter of the awards is construction or the design and execution of construction; or (ii) the awards have identical or similar subject matter, which were not known to the contracting authority at the time when a prior procurement process with the same subject matter was commenced.[28] Before the transposition of the New Procurement Directives both control authorities (as presented in Chap. 4) clashed in their practices with respect to interpretation of split procurement cases, which causes additional serious difficulties for contracting authorities and significantly increases the prevalence of infringements of this type, which in turn impedes the objective assessment of both the risk and the corrupt intent in such cases.[29] Given that the New PPA aims to unify the practices of these institutions, this clash is expected to be cured. However, the chosen course of action has already been criticised by some national institutions (eg BORKOR) because the new provision 'legitimises the possibility of improper separation of the order [and] could lead to the selection of a contractor without competitive tendering'.[30]

The splitting of public procurements currently continues to be one of the common types of infringement in Bulgaria, although some control authorities believe that the number of these violations is decreasing.[31] Practice reveals that the main route for achieving procurement splits are through (a) official authorisations and (b) division into lots.

(a) *Authorisation* in the field of public procurement is expressly permitted and is particularly suitable for contracting authorities with a complex organisational structure.

Contracting authorities, however, often fail to consider the fact that authorised entities do not act as independent contracting authorities and hence the value of contracts with an identical or similar subject awarded separately by such authorised entities needs to be consolidated. Although national legislations usually expressly prohibit the use of authorisation to split public procurements in order to circumvent the law, authorised entities apply an award approach depending on the needs of the separate unit under their direct control, and not on the total value of the procurement

---

[28] Art 21(16) New PPA.

[29] The practice adopted by the PFIA in this respect is radically different than the one of NAO, which is now adopted by the New PPA. In the opinion of PFIA's financial inspectors and in accordance with its policies, the contracting authority is obliged to consolidate incidental, newly arising needs with already contracted and planned activities, and the stricter award regime should also be applied to such newly arisen needs (despite neither being expected, nor capable of having been foreseen by the contracting authority).

[30] E Nikolova from BORKOR in an interview for the Bulgarian National Radio published in ZOP + issue 2/2016, 22.

[31] According to *Activity Report of the Audit Office of the Republic of Bulgaria for the period 11.6.2014–20.1.2015* (Sofia: NAO, 2015).

for the contracting authority as a whole. This inevitably results in circumvention of the law because a lighter regime than the one required is applied.[32]

(b) The other method for splitting public procurements is through *division into lots*.

It is wrongly assumed by some contracting authorities that an activity which can be regarded as a separate lot within the scope of a single public procurement, can be treated as an independent public procurement, and hence awarded in accordance with a procedure corresponding to its individual value. In fact, the contracting authorities are overlooking the fundamental characteristic of the lot, namely that it is an integral part of the project scope, which is systematically linked to its remaining parts. The estimated value of a project split into lots, which serves as basis for the determination of the relevant award regime, is calculated as the sum of the values of the individual lots. To prevent attempts by contracting authorities to circumvent the law by treating lots as individual contracts, the legislator has expressly specified that where the total sum exceeds the threshold for a mandatory procedure, then the rules applicable to the total value of the procurement must apply to each individual lot as well.

Considering the public procurement policies introduced by the New Procurement Directives, European trends are towards encouraging splitting procurements into lots with a view to supporting the entry of more small and medium enterprises (SME) to the field. Splitting will of course have to be substantiated and not result in circumvention of the rules. The logic from now on will be the reverse of what has hitherto been accepted for countries such as Bulgaria[33] – contracting authorities will have to justify their decision not to split a procurement into lots, while national legislation will possibly even oblige contracting authorities to split procurements. In particular in Bulgaria, the New PPA introduces a legislative approach which tries to achieve a 'happy medium' and proposes that the Council of Ministers designate areas where public procurement must be divided into lots according to specialised SME sectors and capabilities.[34] However, practice reveals that the determination of estimated values for procurements and the summing up of the various lots often results in errors, even unintentional ones. It is therefore difficult to say whether or not this new right/obligation of contracting authorities will result in even greater chaos in the award process and open up wider opportunities for 'adjusting' lots with corrupt intent in Member States such as Bulgaria. Further, potential conflicts of interest and/or relatedness between the individual contractors (eg SMEs, as desired

---

[32] A legal way for authorised officials to make public procurement awards without infringing the ban on splitting is for each authorised official to apply such an award regime as corresponds to the total value of the public procurement for the respective contracting authority as a whole. Accordingly, where ten authorised officials need to make awards for the supply of stationery and the total value of this activity for the entire contracting authority exceeds the thresholds set by law, then each authorised official must run a procurement procedure in order to satisfy the needs of the unit under its control. This is the only way not to circumvent the law.

[33] There are Member States where the obligation of the contracting authority to divide procurements into lots existed as a general legislative rule even before the transposition of the new procurement package (eg Germany).

[34] Art 46(3) New PPA.

by the EU legislator) will have to be monitored much more closely, since a frequently encountered corrupt practice is the winning of a contract by seemingly independent companies which turn out to be related parties or parties involved in concerted practices (bid rigging), as will be analysed further below.

Are transparency rules breached? (a) Yes, in cases where splitting is indeed carried out to circumvent the law. The relevant sections of the procurement are then awarded by means of direct negotiation in the absence of any publicity whatsoever; and (b) No, where the corrupt scheme is far more complicated and the idea is not to circumvent award rules but to exploit them to allocate lots to the desired candidates.[35] In the latter case, transparency rules are still observed in a strict sense and the corrupt scheme is not as easy to detect.

What corruption loopholes are opened? Splitting procurements opens up the possibility for different sections of the procurement to be awarded to freely selected tenderers which have entered into a corrupt relationship with the contracting authority (in most cases, on the basis of bribery). A relatively high detection rate is also typical of this type of infringement. In this light, the splitting of public procurements is predominantly used as a method of corruption by municipalities and also for relatively low value public procurements (ie 'petty' corruption). It is more common in countries suffering widespread corruption like Bulgaria, rather than in Member States with limited or not so flagrant types of corruption.[36] In addition, the unsubstantiated splitting of a procurement into lots, as a subcategory of this infringement (also deserving of comment in light of the New Procurement Directives), opens up avenues for corruption in terms of the coordination of anticompetitive activities not only for the contracting authority, but also between the different tenderers.

In addition, though it is not the aim of this work to adopt an excessively pessimistic stance, a theoretical analysis of the text of the New Procurement Directives suggests the initial conclusion that some corrupt practices would simply be replaced by others. If we expect that the practice of unlawful division into lots will be discouraged by the new rules,[37] some of the EU legislator's other proposals cannot be wholeheartedly welcomed. For example, the legislative decision under Directive 2014/24/EU to allow contracting authorities to award contracts for individual lots without applying procurement procedures (or by providing a procedure which

---

[35] An opportunity which will come to the foreground with the introduction of the New Procurement Directives, as noted above.

[36] Splitting of contracts is discussed further in Chap. 6 with respect to Germany and the measures undertaken by this country to limit the artificial splitting of procurements.

[37] In addition, the Bulgarian transposition of the rules for prioritising the division of procurements into lots is also not clear enough. Contracting authorities are indeed obliged to give some thought to the possibility of using lots. If they do not wish to do so, they have to motivate this refusal, also as per the EU legislation. Nevertheless, this decision is one of the few taken by the authorities which cannot be appealed. This would mean that the rights of companies denied lots in complex procedures cannot be defended further.

accords with the individual value of the respective lot),[38] provided that the estimated value net of VAT of the lot concerned is less than EUR 80,000 for goods or services or EUR 1 million for works, and the aggregated value of the lots does not exceed 20% of the aggregated value of all the lots into which the proposed procurement has been divided,[39] is a rather bold decision when it comes to corruption. This provision, aimed to facilitate complex and multi-layered procedures process contracting authorities acting in bad faith with the opportunity to split lots so that 20% of the most promising and expensive procurements to go directly into the hands of prese-lected contractors. Again in a purely transparent and even legitimate manner…

Unsubstantiated Implementation of a Negotiated Procedure Without Prior Publication of a Contract Notice

Which legal provisions are breached?

 (i) EU rules – Article 32 Directive 2014/24/EU and Article 50 Directive 2014/25/ EU,[40] (Article 31 Directive 2004/18/EC)[41]

---

[38] As is the Bulgarian legislative decision.

[39] Art 5(10) Directive 2014/24/EU. In Bulgarian legislation – Art 21(6) New PPA.

[40] Art 32 Directive 2014/24/EU and Art 50 Directive 2014/25/EU set out the possible cases where negotiated procedures without prior publication can be used; these are very limited and are consistent with the desire of the European legislator outlined in the preamble to Directive 2014/24/EU: 'In view of the detrimental effects on competition, negotiated procedures without prior publication of a contract notice should be used only in very exceptional circumstances. This exception should be limited to cases where publication is either not possible, for reasons of extreme urgency brought about by events unforeseeable for and not attributable to the contracting authority, or where it is clear from the outset that publication would not trigger more competition or better procurement outcomes, not least because there is objectively only one economic operator that can perform the contract. This is the case for works of art, where the identity of the artist intrinsically determines the unique character and value of the art object itself. Exclusivity can also arise from other reasons, but only situations of objective exclusivity can justify the use of the negotiated procedure without publication, where the situation of exclusivity has not been created by the contracting authority itself with a view to the future procurement procedure.

Contracting authorities relying on this exception should provide reasons why there are no reasonable alternatives or substitutes such as using alternative distribution channels including outside the Member State of the contracting authority or considering functionally comparable works, supplies and services.

Where the situation of exclusivity is due to technical reasons, they should be rigorously defined and justified on a case-by-case basis. They could include, for instance, near technical impossibility for another economic operator to achieve the required performance or the necessity to use specific know-how, tools or means which only one economic operator has at its disposal. Technical reasons may also derive from specific interoperability requirements which must be fulfilled in order to ensure the functioning of the works, supplies or services to be procured.

Finally, a procurement procedure is not useful where supplies are purchased directly on a commodity market, including trading platforms for commodities such as agricultural products, raw materials and energy exchanges, where the regulated and supervised multilateral trading structure naturally guarantees market prices'.

[41] Art 31 Directive 2004/18/EC: 'Contracting authorities may award public contracts by a negotiated procedure without prior publication of a contract notice in the following cases: (1) for public

(ii) National legislation – eg Article 79 et seq.[42] and Article 164 et seq.[43] New PPA

The amendment in the new rules is a step in a positive direction, as this type of infringement is obviously common for most Member States and the European legislator has taken restrictive measures within the new legislative framework which severely limit the cases where a negotiated procedure without prior publication/ prior call for competition is possible. This approach is expected to have a positive effect on this type of infringement by restricting the opportunities for using a negotiated procedure without prior publication for corrupt purposes. There is nevertheless a tendency for contracting authorities to be particularly creative when they have to prove, for example, unforeseeable emergency measures to justify the use of a lighter procedure, regardless the number of restrictive rules.

What is the essence of the infringement? A negotiated procedure without prior publication cannot be adopted freely and applied by contracting authorities at their own discretion as it involves limited application and can only be lawfully applied in cases where the imperatively enumerated conditions of the EU rules (transposed directly in to the national legislation) are satisfied.

However, controlling bodies continue to come across numerous illegal negotiated procedures.[44] In most cases the legal provisions are applied incorrectly or speculatively, namely the option for a negotiated procedure where, due to the need to take urgent action brought about by the occurrence of an extraordinary event, the time limits for the conduct of an open procedure cannot be complied with. In most cases the need for such an award is not a direct and immediate effect of an extraordinary event, but is rather caused by inadequate planning or deliberate postponing of the procedure to justify negotiation without prior publication at the last possible moment.

Procedures where the concluded contract will be implemented over an extended period are also regarded as unlawfully negotiated procedures based on urgency, given that the 'urgent' needs of the contracting authority, the resolution of which such an opaque procedure has been applied, will not be met in the immediate future but

---

works contracts, public supply contracts and public service contracts: (a) when no tenders or no suitable tenders or no applications have been submitted in response to an open procedure or a restricted procedure, provided that the initial conditions of contract are not substantially altered and on condition that a report is sent to the Commission if it so requests; (b) when, for technical or artistic reasons, or for reasons connected with the protection of exclusive rights, the contract may be awarded only to a particular economic operator; (c) insofar as is strictly necessary when, for reasons of *extreme urgency brought about by events unforeseeable* [emphasis added] by the contracting authorities in question, the time limit for the open, restricted or negotiated procedures with publication of a contract notice as referred to in Art 30 cannot be complied with. The circumstances invoked to justify extreme urgency must not in any event be attributable to the contracting authority [...]' etc.

[42] Regulating the use of negotiated procedures without prior notice.

[43] Regulating the use of the negotiated procedures without prior publication of a contract notice.

[44] This comment is made based on Bulgarian control authority practice before the entry into force of the New PPA and before the new procurement package rules were implemented in practice.

instead, after an extended period. A similar infringement (similarly motivated by contracting authorities) is observed in cases where the competitive dialogue is selected instead of a negotiated procedure without prior notice. This approach, however, is rather more specific and is hence used less frequently by contracting authorities.

With the New Procurement Directive rules, this option for award without publication remains one of the few opportunities to justify such disregard of the stricter rules and in accordance with the Preamble to Directive 2014/24/EU quoted above, the justification provided by the contracting authority in such cases will be insisted on much more rigorously, so that it can be clear that '[t]he circumstances invoked to justify extreme urgency shall not in any event be attributable to the contracting authority'.[45] It remains to be seen how this strictness, as transposed into national legislation, will be obeyed so that a difference is felt by contracting authorities and the 'frivolous' use of this option to select a desired contractor will be, at least to a large extent, thwarted.

Are transparency rules breached? Yes. The notice for the respective procurement is not published, while at the same time the time frame is considerably narrowed; competition is hence restricted, since the rules inherent to the legal procedure applicable in the specific case (usually an open procedure) are not applied.

What corruption loopholes are opened? Corruption arises primarily because, as commented above, the scheme leads to a significant restriction to competition and the selection of a corrupt/bribing candidate is facilitated, and also because the candidate itself can modify the contract parameters to its own advantage (nontransparently, during the negotiation phase) and thus negotiate much more favourable (to it) terms under the pretext that the contracting authority has urgent needs. The bribery, kickbacks or other means used to induce the contracting authority to organise the procurement in this manner can enter play at a much earlier stage, prior to the Announcement Phase, with the contracting authority delaying to the last moment the planning (determination of needs) in order to 'justify' the procedure as being urgent and unforeseeable.

The above three main types of infringements at the Choice of Object (and procedure selection) Phase are still characterised by a relatively common occurrence: they are observed mainly with respect to small contracting authorities with low administrative capacity and financial resources. A percentage of the infringements uncovered are of course ones which are made purely due to a lack of understanding of the complex legislative rules and do not represent corrupt intent.

These departures from legitimate procedure usually comprise a large proportion of the infringements detected by control bodies, but this can also be attributed to their relative easy detectability and observability (precisely for the fact that in most cases the transparency principle and the legislative rules have not been observed *en masse*), in which they differ from the types of infringements reviewed below. The characteristics of the infringements set out above allow for the secondary conclusion that their frequency can also be put down to the exceedingly inconsistent prac-

---

[45] Art 32(2)(c) Directive 2014/24/EU; Art 32 and Art 50(d) Directive 2014/25/EU.

tice of the authorities providing *ex post* control (for instance, Member States such as Bulgaria), which in some cases is overly restrictive even in the absence of a significant infringement in terms of its consequences. Against this background, as will be shown in the analysis below, 'grand' corruption in the higher levels of authority and lobbyist activities in the conduct of 'attractive' public procurement procedures remain undetected and far more difficult to prove, despite the almost non-existent infringement of publicity and transparency rules.

In view of these observations, the infringements from this group are more typical of countries such as Bulgaria which suffer a lack of efficient control over the procurement process and which observe legality compliance only. Nevertheless, a high prevalence of such infringements is not unusual in other Member States either.[46] As a basis for comparison of the frequency of occurrence of this type of infringement in Europe (with respect to the Regional Development and Cohesion funds projects in particular) the data provided by the Annual Public Procurement Implementation Review 2012 is a useful reference:

> The categories of 'absence of tendering or award of contract based on an inappropriate tendering procedure' and the 'award of supplementary contracts without competition' cover 34% of all the procurement-related errors detected in the audits. The inappropriate tendering procedure chosen is, naturally, the negotiated procedure. This infringement accounts for 65% of the errors. Cancellation of public procurement procedures and direct award (or negotiation without publication) of the main contract without sufficient reasons is the source of 16% of infringements. Artificial splitting of the contract is the error found in 14% of the cases and incorrect specification of the predominant aspect for 'mixed' contracts and, thus, application of an inappropriate procedure in 5% of the cases.[47]

5.3.2   Announcement Phase

Setting Very Short Time Limits for Tender Preparation

Which legal provisions are breached? EU rules – Article 47 Directive 2014/24/EU and Article 66 Directive 2014/25/EU.[48]

The New Procurement Directives define much shorter time limits (in some cases up to 50% shorter than previous time limits) for procurement awards, in order to

---

[46] Account must also be taken of the instances of incorrect application of the law due to a lack of understanding or misinterpretation during selection procedure.

[47] Commission (EU), 'Annual Public Procurement Implementation Review 2012' SWD(2012) 342 final, 9 October 2012, 36. Commission (EU), 'Annual Public Procurement Implementation Review 2013' SWD(2014) 262 final, 1 August 2014, does not provide such statistics; hence, the data discussed is that for 2012.

[48] Art 47(1) Directive 2014/24/EU: 'When fixing the time limits for the receipt of tenders and requests to participate, contracting authorities shall take account of the complexity of the contract and the time required for drawing up tenders, without prejudice to the minimum time limits set out in Articles 27 to 31.' Art 66(1) Directive 2014/25/EU provides for the same content.

speed up processes and reduce procedure-related costs.[49] It is unclear, however, whether this reduction of time limits will not also result in decreased bid quality and restricted competition. Such pressure on participants could also increase the number of the infringements discussed here.

What is the essence of the infringement? This type of infringement is one of the most common and the easiest to detect. Perhaps because of that, according to the Bulgarian control authorities, it falls into the category of unsubstantial legal violations, ie those which do not result in financial loss.[50] According to the PFIA: 'Infringements of public procurement legislation of a procedural nature which do not result in violation of the principles of publicity and transparency; free and fair competition, equality and non-discrimination were established [...] These infringements relate to failure to observe the set deadlines, failure to submit information subject to promulgation in the Public Procurement Register [...].'[51]

This analysis should not go unchallenged. Reducing deadlines may indeed, in some cases, comprise a negligible infringement, easily detected by the control authorities. At the same time, it must be expressly distinguished from deliberate reductions which aim to favour a specific future participant, which naturally are far more difficult to prove. In some cases the deadlines for submission of tenders for more complex procurements (such as those in the field of power engineering or construction works) are insufficient for potential candidates to prepare well-grounded and reasonable proposals. Deadlines exceeding those set out in the law would be sometimes necessary. According to the complaints received and inspections made by the control bodies, a favoured candidate will quite simply have the tender documentation at its disposal prior to the opening date for purchase of the documentation and consequently have sufficient time to prepare. The fact that this infringement is all too common 'comes to show that granting preference to a specific performer [...] can be carried out by reducing time limits or accepting documents submitted after the set deadline'.[52]

Are transparency rules breached? No. There is no legal mechanism to monitor whether a candidate has advance knowledge of the contents of tender documents. The hypothesis does not even define an administrative violation in this context, and the time limits provided by national law are observed but are set at the very mini-

---

[49] Recital 80 Directive 2014/24/EU: 'In order to make procedures faster and more efficient, time limits for participation in procurement procedures should be kept as short as possible without creating undue barriers to access for economic operators from across the internal market and in particular SMEs [...] Therefore, provision should be made for reducing the minimum time limits in line with the rules set by the GPA and subject to the condition that they are compatible with the specific mode of transmission envisaged at Union level'.

[50] The number of procedural violations (including those where time limits were not observed) in 2013, according to PFIA's report, was 599, ie 24 percent of the total number of audited procurements.

[51] *Report on the activity of the Public Financial Inspection Agency for 2012* (Sofia: PFIA, 2013) 11.

[52] Above (n 13) 29.

mum: this does not result in a lack of transparency. Notices are promulgated on time and sent to the OJEU (where applicable) and are published on the official website of the contracting authority (eg on the 'buyer's profile'). Publicity and transparency requirements have thus been observed, the documentation is in perfect order and, at a first glance, competition in the sector is not restricted.

What corruption loopholes are opened? The favoured (corrupt) candidate/tenderer is provided the opportunity to familiarise itself with details of the tender before all the other candidates/tenderers, which gives that candidate a very real chance of submitting the most suitable bid, while other candidates must meet the artificially reduced time limits. Shortening time limits can allow other infringements for corrupt reasons, as will be reviewed below. For example, ambiguous or 'tailor-made' requirements which can result in confusion and which could put off other potential tenderers may be imposed, while the preferred contractor will have all the details settled in advance and will be ready with the bid. In this case, it is again the contracting authority or its employees which are bribed beforehand to concede to the corrupt scheme.

Because such infringements are difficult to detect, no objective conclusion could be made whether they are common in many Member States. However, according to the data from the Eurobarometer report for 2015 'Companies that have not taken part in a public tender or procurement procedure were asked whether it was for specific reasons. [...] Nine percent of companies say the deal seemed to be done before the call to tender, while 8% said the deadlines were too tight and impossible to meet [...].'[53]

Lack of Coordination Between Documents

Which legal provisions are breached? Article 48 et seq. Directive 2014/24/EU and Article 67 et seq Directive 2014/25/EU.[54] The New Procurement Directives do not materially modify the content of the notice but introduce an additional option for the sub-central contracting authorities, which instead of publishing an pan-European notice will be able to publish a prior information notice indicating that the contract will be awarded without further publication of a call for competition and inviting possible participants to express their interest to receive direct information regarding the procedure. The effect of this option is yet to be seen.

What is the essence of the infringement? The manifestations of this type of infringement may be numerous and quite varied in terms of the different ways in which lack of coordination and precision in participation documents is achieved:

  (i) the tender notice does not contain all the elements on the basis of which eligibility is assessed, with those elements, or a portion of them, being listed only in the tender documents;
 (ii) the tender notice fails to indicate all the selection criteria, including minimum requirements, regarding the economic and financial standing of the candidate or

---

[53] Above (n 10).

[54] These are the rules on advertising and transparency, and in particular on the content of notices.

tenderer and/or the technical capabilities and qualifications required where the contracting authority makes such requirements, or fails to indicate all the documents to be submitted as proof of such financial and technical capabilities;

(iii) there are inconsistencies between the requirements set out on different pages of the contract documentation;

(iv) there are inconsistencies and/or contradictions between the instructions to tenderers and the document templates attached, or technical errors in the numbering of documentation attachments; or

(v) there are inconsistencies between the public procurement contract clauses and those contained in the draft contract attached to the contract documents.

Are transparency rules breached?   Where the infringement is connected with information which has not been reflected in the notice but only in the supplementary documentation, then transparency rules might be considered breached because only those candidates who express deeper interest in participating and review the full documentation set will receive additional information which, if reflected in the notice, could have broadened the pool of competitors. Realistically, these potential candidates who have made up their minds with respect to the participating in the procedure only on the basis of the announcement suffer, from a lack of information. This is particularly true for participants in public procurement who are non-residents. They have basic access to the notice as published in the OJEU, but to gain an idea of the detailed requirements of the procedure such candidates must first (in most cases) translate all the documentation.

However, if a lack of coordination and discrepancies are detected in the remaining documentation only, then transparency has not been violated to such a significant extent because the notification and publication process for the procurement has been successfully completed. The information published in the notice is publicly available; where it causes candidates and tenderers to reach ambiguous and contradictory conclusions they have the option to ask additional questions of the contracting authority on any unclear issues or to choose to appeal on those aspects. In some Member States (as is the case in Bulgaria), however, such an appeal will not result in the suspension of the procedure in most cases and this is discouraging for them.[55]

What corruption loopholes are opened?   Usually, control authorities would define this type of infringement as common and formal. The truth is that some of these infringements may indeed be classified as insignificant and/or technical errors. Moreover, contracting authorities which organise a large number of similar tenders often fail to carry out a thorough check of all the documentation (due to insufficient administrative capacity) and these are frequently prepared using a 'copy–paste' approach, with additional information being added indiscriminately to the contract documents or to the notice itself. Against this backdrop of easily detected infringements (and of all the other types discussed so far), the opportunities for corruption

---

[55] As discussed in Chap. 4, except for appeals of the final act appointing a contractor, appeals of actions or inactions by the contracting authority do not have a suspensive effect, although suspension of the procedure may be requested, separately from the appeal procedure, from the CPC, which rules on a case-by-case basis.

which such an inaccurately prepared procurement can create – with the desired candidate being instructed in advance on how to prepare its bid – should not be overlooked, however. Although in dealing with such procurements, it is often a fair assumption that the documentation is deliberately vague and too chaotic, such deliberate violation of rules is difficult to prove and therefore one cannot calculate statistically how often it occurs. It can definitely be concluded, however (again only on the basis of practice), that in countries with greater incidence of bribery in the sector, such as Bulgaria, this method is used to achieve corrupt ends.

In addition, this type of infringement can exist alongside infringements in the definition of selection criteria, as described below.

Inclusion of Selection Criteria and/or Technical Specifications Which Unreasonably Restrict Participation in the Procurement or Offer an Advantage to One of the Tenderers/Candidates

Which legal provisions are breached?

(i) EU rules – Article 58 Directive 2014/24/EU, Article 77 Directive 2014/25/EU[56,57]

(ii) National law – eg Articles 2(2) and[58] 49[59] of the New PPA

---

[56] These provisions regulate the selection criteria and qualification system requirements to be followed by both standard and utility sector contracting authorities so that all candidates and/or participants are treated equally and not discriminated against.

[57] Relevant ECJ practice with respect to contracting authority requirements, which reinforces and adds to the above comments, can be found in: (1) Joined cases C-226/04 to C-228/04 *La Cascina Soc. Coop. arl.* [2006] ECR I-0147, stating that the procedural conditions need to be clearly defined in advance and made public and to apply to all candidates; (2) C-218/11 *Észak-dunántúli Környezetvédelmi és Vízügyi Igazgatóság (Édukövízig) and Hochtief Construction AG Magyarországi Fióktelepe v. Közbeszerzések Tanácsa Közbeszerzési Döntőbizottság*, ECLI:EU:C:2012:643, shows that the ECJ held that a contracting authority may require a minimum level of economic and financial standing to be demonstrated by reference to particular aspects of a company's balance sheet. And this cannot be disregarded solely because it relates to an aspect of the balance sheet where there may be differences between the legislation of member states; (3) C-278/14 *SC Enterprise Focused Solutions SRL v. Spitalul Judeţean de Urgenţă Alba Iulia*, ECLI:EU:C:2015:228, stating that the contracting authority could not amend the technical specification in respect of an element of the contract, regardless of whether or not the element referred to in the specification was still in production or available on the market etc.

[58] Art 2(2) New PPA: 'By awarding public procurements the contracting authorities cannot restrict competition by including conditions or requirements that give undue advantage or unreasonably restrict the participation of businesses in procurement and which do not comply with the subject, the cost, complexity, quantity or volume of public procurement.'

[59] Art 49(1) New PPA: 'The technical specifications must afford equal access for candidates or tenderers to the procedure for awarding of the procurement and not to create unjustified obstacles award in competition; (2) The technical specifications may not contain a specific model, source or a particular process that characterises the products or services offered by a particular potential

Further to the currently known methods for the selection of participants and determination of technical specifications, the New Procurement Directives introduce several additional options which will not only help all the participants in the procedure but will also contribute to a significant decrease of this type of infringement, where it affects selection (eligibility) criteria requirements: (a) the recognition of the European Single Procurement Document (ESPD), consisting of an updated self-declaration as preliminary evidence replacing the certificates issued by public authorities or third parties confirming that the relevant economic operator meets the relevant selection criteria[60]; and (b) use of the e-Certis system which aims 'to facilitate the exchange of certificates and other documentary evidence frequently required by contracting authorities'.[61] In addition to achieving a significantly higher level of standardisation of the documents required for the selection, this will also help distribute the responsibility for the submitted evidence of suitability between the contracting authority and the contractor, which may in turn play a positive role in forestalling the unduly detailed requirements set out by some contracting authorities. Still, only time will tell whether these changes will be negated by corrupt practices, bearing in mind that the weakness of the ESPD is that the contracting authority verifies the authenticity of what has been stated after the contractor has been selected (in most cases), and only with regard to the selected contractor. If it turns out that the selected contractor fails to meet what has been declared in the ESPD, then the next one in line will have to be selected (if the current rule in this respect is retained) which could allow, for example, related-party schemes or bid rigging, as will be analysed below.

What is the essence of the infringement? In each public procurement award procedure, the contracting authority is entitled to set the minimum level of requirements concerning the tenderers' characteristics. Compliance with these requirements would serve as a guarantee that the tenderers which meet them have the capacity to ensure quality implementation of the contract. These requirements of economic and financial standing, technical capacity and tenderer qualifications have been identified by national and EU legislation under the aggregate term 'selection criteria'.[62] They must be as specific as possible and must conform to the individual subject matter of the public procurement, its complexity, scope and value.

In addition, the contracting authority also defines the technical specifications to be met by the bid itself, depending on the specific subject of the procurement. As opposed to the selection criteria, where specific documents and certificates are required to evidence the capacity of candidates, here the contracting authority

---

contractor or trademark, patent, type or specific origin or production with the effect of favouring or eliminating certain persons or certain products. Exceptionally, when the subject of the procurement is impossible to be described sufficiently precise and intelligible […] such indication would be allowed, where the words 'or equivalent/s' must be compulsory added'.

[60] Art 59 Directive 2014/24/EU.

[61] Recital 87 Directive 2014/24/EU.

[62] Or 'eligibility criteria'.

describes certain quantity, quality and other parameters and professional characteristics which it regards as absolutely essential for proper contract implementation.[63]

Naturally, the definition of technical specifications provides much greater opportunities for the contracting authority to prepare 'tailor-made' documentation.[64] The
specification of overly detailed technical characteristics has considerable potential
for corruption compared to other types of violations and infringements. For example, the characteristics of the 'required' piece of equipment may be listed in such
detail that only one particular type of equipment will comply, or the characteristics
of the construction materials used by a particular construction company are
described etc.

In addition to being one of the schemes most conducive to corruption, this type
of procurement manipulation is also very difficult for controlling bodies to detect
due to the highly specialised details of the specification. As Søreide (2002) notes,
'[t]he size and the complexity of the project or product in question are the most
important factors explaining differences in motivation and opportunities for grand
corruption [...] The more high technology involved, or seemingly involved, the
more attractive the project will be to the potential beneficiaries. This kind of 'mys-
tification' reduces the risk of being criticised for paying too much. (Moody-Stuart
exemplifies: *'How many people can say whether a particular fighter aircraft should
have cost $21 million rather than $23 million?').*'[65]

If the above conclusions are applicable for more or less all Member States, in
countries with weak economies, where the temptation to engage in corrupt practices
is greater, there are certain additional 'peculiarities' which further impede the detection of this type of corrupt manipulation. The example of Bulgaria illustrates this
below:

Usually, the main control bodies (PFIA and the NAO in Bulgaria) have insufficient financial and administrative capacity.[66] Control or appellate authorities can
only rarely afford to hire narrow (and thus more expensive) experts who are able to
analyse the complexity of the procurement in such detail as to establish discriminatory
conditions.[67] Pedantic observance of legality compliance is therefore usually

---

[63] These two different infringements which are manifested either in connection with the selection
criteria and/or the technical specifications are reviewed jointly because they have the same result,
namely restriction of competition in the procedure and facilitated selection of the 'favoured'
candidate.

[64] Recital 74 Directive 2014/24/EU draws particular attention to the fact that 'technical specifications should be drafted in such a way as to avoid artificially narrowing down competition through
requirements that favour a specific economic operator by mirroring key characteristics of the supplies, services or works habitually offered by that economic operator. Drawing up the technical
specifications in terms of functional and performance requirements generally allows that objective
to be achieved in the best way possible'.

[65] T Søreide, 'Corruption in Public Procurement: Causes, Consequences and Cures' (2002) Chr.
Michelsen Institute Development Studies and Human Rights Report R 2002: 1, 11.

[66] The CPC, as the Bulgarian first instance appellate authority, uses experts more frequently or
otherwise resorts to sending letters of inquiry to leading specialists in specific fields, but these do
not always ensure satisfactory results.

[67] In 2014 a particular public procurement for the 'Supply and warranty service of motor vehicles'
came to the public's attention. Because in this case there is a wider circle of experts familiar with

imposed, namely control which describes the various documents which tenderers may be required to provide as evidence of compliance with the selection criteria.[68] Consequently, the detection rate for such infringements is relatively small. For 2014, for example, in Bulgaria 'the contracting authorities under 36 public procurements were found to have set conditions which offer an advantage or unjustifiably restrict the participation of tenderers in the relevant procedures'[69] out of a total of more than 2400 procurements.

Precisely because of the above restrictions on the functions of control bodies, in the cases of exceedingly detailed and restrictive technical specifications, responsible bodies monitor very superficially whether the legally required wording 'or equivalent' is found at the end of the description without, however, examining the respective criteria themselves.

It should be noted with respect to manipulations of the selection criteria themselves that these are relatively easy to detect and hence less frequently used for 'grand' corruption. This type of infringement usually involves:

(i)   inclusion of requirements for turnover in such volume as bears no relation to the estimated value of the procurement;
(ii) introduction of restrictive requirements towards individual parties within an association/consortium, for example the requirement that each member of the association/consortium must individually meet the minimum eligibility requirements for general turnover/specific turnover or number of contracts completed, instead of the consortium as a whole;
(iii) restricting potential tenderers by introducing requirements for specific experience connected to a specific source of funding; or requirements for specific

---

the subject matter and there was no need for an expert opinion as to whether the technical requirements contained discriminatory conditions, the specifics of the technical requirements presented themselves all too clearly. A curious detail is that the contracting authority is the State Agency for National Security (a national body specialising in the detection of 'grand' corruption). By means of notice No 01666–2014-0003, dispatched for publication by the PPAgency, the contracting authority sought to purchase 84 motor cars to the estimated value of BGN 3,000,000 (approx. EUR 1,533,861) with the express instructions that: 'Upon preparation of their bids, participants must strictly adhere to the requirements to the vehicles, as set out in the technical specifications for the respective lots'. The technical requirements then proceed to set strict parameters per vehicle, for example: at least 300 horsepower 3.0 litre petrol engine, four-wheel drive, minimum 70 l fuel tank capacity, maximum CO_2 emissions of 235 g/km and exact parameters as to width and length. Naturally, only a very specific type of luxury car matches these parameters and this car was only offered by the desired candidate. In practice, all of the vehicles under the different lots were described in similar detail and, of course, as expected, the desired candidate won the contract. So far, however, except for the very vocal media response and the reaction of the CPCCOC that the procurement would be noted containing irregularities, there has been no reaction from control bodies, nor has there been any reference to the Prosecutor's office.

[68] eg appropriate statements from bankers or copy of a professional liability insurance policy; the annual financial statement or any of the constituent parts thereof; a statement of the overall turnover and of the turnover in respect of the supplies, services or works etc.

[69] *Report on the activity of the Public Financial Inspection Agency for 2014* (Sofia: PFIA, 2015) 14.

quality certificates which are in no way connected to or necessary for procurement implementation;

(iv) limiting the opportunities for participation of sub-contractors;

(v) some contracting authorities use 'parasitic' criteria which have no relevance to the subject matter of the public procurement. The purpose of this practice is to introduce a maximum number of criteria which are then assessed subjectively, in favour of one of the tenderers at the expense of other, more accurate and clearly measurable criteria. Such parasitic criteria are for example the phrases 'quality design of the tender' or 'clear vision for the development of the sector', widely quoted by control bodies as poor practice.

Case law in Bulgaria has over the years imposed a constant parameter with regards to certain more specific conditions regarded as discriminatory,[70] which have however already acquired wide popularity. Contracting authorities now tend to avoid them, becoming instead increasingly inventive in devising terms of reference which only narrow specialists in the respective field could possibly detect the presence of corrupt and restrictive mechanisms.

Are transparency rules breached? No. The notice is usually rigorously prepared without any technical errors; it is duly announced, sent to OJEU and uploaded on the webpage of the contracting authority (where applicable) in compliance with the requirements of the national legislation and the relevant EU legislation. In its subsequent phases, the procedure observes all publicity requirements.

What corruption loopholes are opened? As Rose-Ackerman (1999) notes: 'Whenever regulatory officials have discretion, an incentive for bribery exists'.[71] In this case, the inclusion of restrictive selective and technical conditions significantly impedes competition. The corrupt result is achieved by introducing considerable requirements which do not correspond to the complexity of the procurement or requirements which are overly detailed, to the advantage of a specific tenderer. Contracting authorities prepare and word the tender documents and the participation conditions in such a way that will allow the contract to be obtained by a specific candidate. All these cases result in the elimination of competitive bids and the award of the contract to the desired party. In this type of corrupt scheme, like those discussed already, the contracting authority has selected the desired contractor (and has already been bribed or promised certain benefits) at a much earlier stage, and by the time the procurement documentation is prepared and the Announcement Phase has been reached, the contracting authority is already deeply involved in the corrupt scheme.

---

[70] CPC Decisions 531–2007 and 1136–2007 declare the criterion 'number of subscribers of the mobile operator at the date of tender submission' as discriminatory; CPC Decision 983–2007 defines the criterion 'number of roaming agreements concluded' as discriminatory in some cases; and CPC Decision 39–2007 declares the requirement that each participant must indicate a list of main construction contracts performed in the country and other EU states over the preceding 5 years as discriminatory etc.

[71] S Rose-Ackerman, *Corruption and government* (New York: CUP, 1999) 18.

Apparently, this is one of the infringements in the procurement process which results in manifestations of corruption and which occurs most frequently in most Member States. The benchmark countries in this book are no exception.[72] The New Procurement Directives do not specifically provide for any innovative or different way to address this problem. These issues are therefore expected to remain unresolved in affected countries such as Bulgaria, despite the new legislative framework, and other (national) solutions should be sought.

Mixing Up Selection and Contract Award Criteria[73]

Which legal provisions are breached?

(i) EU rules – the principles of non-discrimination and proportionality in line with the New Procurement Directives, as well as the relevant ECJ practice, as discussed below.

(ii) National law – eg Article 70(12) New PPA[74]

What is the essence of the infringement? Selection criteria and contract award criteria must be distinguished. Selection criteria, as already commented on above, are the minimum criteria tenderers must meet for them to be able to participate in a procedure. Contract award criteria, on the other hand, refer to the quality of the offer itself. Such criteria and their relative weight must be directly linked to the subject matter of the public procurement with respect to quality, price, technical merit, aesthetic and functional characteristics, characteristics related to environmental protection, running costs, warranty after-sales service and technical assistance, delivery date etc.[75] In addition, the award criteria should be interpreted in the same way throughout the entire procedure.[76]

Furthermore, '[c]ompliance with the selection criteria set out by the contracting authority under a specific procedure must be assessed by the committee solely with a 'yes' or 'no' […] [It] cannot be subject to gradation. For this reason both the tenderer evidencing compliance with only the minimum level required by the contracting authority, and the tenderer who significantly exceeds these requirements should be admitted to further participation in the procedure'.[77]

---

[72] As also evident from Fig 4 above.

[73] ie in the cases where the selected criteria is 'the most economically advantageous tender', but only the lowest price is assessed.

[74] Art 70(12) New PPA: 'Contracting authorities may not include selection criteria as indicators of evaluation of tenders'.

[75] Art 67 Directive 2014/24/EU.

[76] See Case C-19/00 *SIAC Construction Ltd.* [2001] ECR I-07725, para 43.

[77] M Katsarova, 'Most common infringements in the award of public procurements established by National Audit Office' (2010) <http://212.122.184.197/files/_bg/statia-Petev-naru6enia_2010. doc> accessed 24 April 2016, 4.

Contracting authorities, however, wrongly assume that certain elements of the selection criteria can be used to evaluate the offer itself if those elements have not been quoted expressly as a selection requirement to the tenderers in the same procedure.

Prior to 2009, Bulgarian legislation did not contain explicit prohibitions regarding these criteria. Following the judgment in *Lianakis AE and others v Dimos Alexandroupolis*,[78] however, an amendment was introduced to bring matters into line with European practice in the field of public procurement by prohibiting the blending of selection and award criteria. The practice of the appellate bodies in Bulgaria conforms to European practice on this point.[79]

Contracting authorities need to apply minimum requirements as criteria to enable them to sift out inexperienced and poorly-prepared participants; in any case, pre-set conditions must not grant an advantage to, or limit the participation of, certain candidates.

Are transparency rules breached? Again, as in the above cases, this infringement does not concern the principles of publicity and transparency. All potential participants in the procedure are equally familiar with the conditions and may appeal them if they choose. All procurement publication requirements have been observed. The tenderers which applied to participate were provided with identical information.

What corruption loopholes are opened? Candidates which meet the selection criteria but which do not have the capacity to meet the evaluation criteria are nevertheless admitted to the subsequent phases. Based on the *'primus inter pares'* principle, candidates are assessed almost solely on the basis of selection criteria; this not only infringes the law but also frees contracting authority to select candidates completely subjectively – choosing candidates which were clearly unable to present the necessary technical or quality requirements to meet the needs of the contracting authority. This type of infringement allows corruption precisely in those cases where the brib-

---

[78] Case C-532/06 *Emm. G. Lianakis AE, Sima Anonymi Techniki Etaireia Meleton kai Epivlepseon and Nikolaos Vlachopoulos v Dimos Alexandroupolis et al.* [2008] ECR I-251.

[79] See eg CPC Decision No 420 of 28 April 2009 under File No 180/26.2.2009; CPC Decision No 499 of 26 May 2009 under File No 286/21.4.2009; CPC Decision No 510 of 26 May 2009 under File No 207/10.3.2009; CPC Decision No 513 of 28 May 2009 under File No 303/6.4.2009; CPC Decision No 613 of 23 June 2009 under File No 379/29.4.2009; CPC Decision No 713 of 14 July 2009 under File No 398/11.5.2009; CPC Decision No 723 of 16 July 2009 under File No 426/19.5.2009; CPC Decision No 749 of 23 July 2009 under File No CPC-500/12.6.2009 etc. CPC Decision No 765 of 23 July 2009 under File No CPC-574/2.7.2009 maintains that 'it is not possible, at the tender evaluation phase, to request a piece of equipment which must meet mandatory technical specifications and at the same time to evaluate compliance with these requirements. This is so because if a piece of equipment is offered which does not fully comply with the mandatory technical specifications, then the tender submitted by the respective tenderer should already have been eliminated at the phase of evaluating compliance of the offers with pre-announced conditions and should not have been admitted to evaluation and ranking. In this sense the introduction of an indicator which assesses compliance with technical requirements, an aspect which should be subject to the previous phase in the work of the committee, results in complete inapplicability and redundancy of such an indicator within the evaluation methodology'.

ing candidate is clearly unfit for the purposes of the procurement and where the documentation has been prepared in such a way as to allow that candidate nonetheless to receive points under some of the selection criteria (as per the relevant assessment formula), so that the selection will be 'by the rules'.

The incidence of such infringements has been overcome in most Member States due to strict and clear legislation. Bulgaria is an example of the opposite, because the legislation applicable before the transposition of the New Procurement Directives was burdensome and quite complex to implement, despite the transparency and publicity which ensures. Following the application of the ESPD and the e-Certis obligations under the New PPA, as noted above, it might be expected that this type of infringement and the corruption loopholes it opens to be reduced. However, the new national legislation introduced is far from being more understandable and flexible than before and only practice will reveal whether the new EU tools will be of any help.

Infringement of, and Changes in, the Evaluation Methodology[80]

Which legal provisions are breached?

 (i) EU rules – Recital 45 of the Preamble to Directive 2014/24/EU[81]
(ii) National legislation – eg Article 70 et seq. New PPA[82]

What is the essence of the infringement? The infringement in this case involves two separate problematic aspects. *Firstly,* these are cases involving ambiguous, incorrectly formulated bid assessment methodology. *Secondly,* the actions of the expert committee are also problematic, as they use/change the assessment methodology in breach of the law.[83]

The methodology for tender evaluation is expected to contain clear guidance and a specific evaluation range. The adopted rating scale must conform to the needs of the contracting authority and the need to select a contractor, and must be applied strictly and consistently with respect to all participants. For this reason and in accordance with legal rules, the contracting authority (in most cases in the various Member States) appoints an evaluation committee. This committee should comprise of individuals with the necessary professional qualifications and practical experience in accordance with the subject matter and complexity of the procurement. The committee must be able to apply the guidance provided in the methodology. It gives a reasoned expert opinion on the various elements subject to evaluation based on its

---

[80] ie under 'the most economically advantageous tender' criteria.

[81] According to Recital 45 Directive 2014/24/EU 'Award criteria and their weighting should remain stable throughout the entire procedure and should not be subject to negotiations, in order to guarantee equal treatment of all economic operators'.

[82] These are the articles in the new legislation which provide for all the requirements connected with award criteria and evaluation indicators.

[83] In this respect see also Case 496/99 *Commission v. Italy (Succhi di Frutta)* [2004] ECR I-3801.

own experience and also on the basis of standards, rules and convention in theory and practice.

In Bulgaria, it should be stressed that in performance of its obligations the committee acts as appropriate and its decisions are not subject to judicial or other control.[84] Bulgarian legislation naturally also prohibits arbitrariness and discriminatory evaluations by the evaluation committee, but this prohibition remains to a great extent *nuda* in the absence of subsequent control and counteraction activities. Control bodies monitor whether the committee has certain motives which coincide with the proposal made by the respective tenderer. The selected methodology and the evaluation of the committee, however, do not fall within their discretion,[85] and this was reproduced in the New PPA.

Common manifestations of infringements based on the contents of the assessment methodology and its application are as follows:

(i) In many cases the methodologies for evaluation of tender proposals set out specific formulas. The elements of these formulas, however, are assessed arbitrarily; they are not given a quantitative expression but are evaluated solely by means of a qualitative criterion which depends on the opinion of the evaluation committee. The absence of predefined correspondence between the rating given by the committee (most commonly expressed in points) and the tender indicators is a common reason for disputes and conflicts between contracting authorities and contractors;

(ii) Also commonly, the indicators are formulated without reference to the objective circumstances on which the number of points awarded should depend, or there is no clear and specific guidance on how the indicators are assessed, which creates conditions for arbitrary evaluation.[86] Unlawful conditions for tenderer elimination are introduced which ignore bids which meet the requirements for award of the public procurement and which should have been ranked.

(iii) Although the contracting authority has the freedom to determine the weight of the individual criteria, cases where the 'price' component was weighted under 50% (40 or 30%) in the final evaluation can usually be regarded as corrupt.

(iv) The contracting authority sets in the applicable methodology only the relative weight of the indicators (for example 50 points to be awarded under the 'war-

---

[84] Such control usually occurs at the level of the contracting authority's decision (if appealed), as the committee makes a recommendation to the former.

[85] For example, CPC Decision No 519 of 8 May 2012: 'The points awarded on behalf of the committee appointed by the contracting authority and more specifically the exact number thereof under the different sub-indicators is subject to the discretion of the committee and comprises an assessment of appropriateness. The control activities of the CPC constitute a review of legality and are aimed to assess whether the evaluation performed by the committee is motivated and whether it complies with the methodology adopted by the contracting authority and the requirements set out by the latter'.

[86] This is also the context of the *Report on the activity of the Audit Office of the Republic of Bulgaria for 2012* which states as follows: 'The efforts of contracting authorities to define clear and accurate instructions on tender evaluation are insufficient which poses the risk of arbitrariness on behalf of tender committees', 16.

ranty period for the procurement' indicator) without specifying how the maximum and minimum number of points are to be awarded. No rating or grading scale or additional clear instructions are provided. Thus the assessment rests solely on the subjective opinion of the evaluation committee;

(v) The evaluation methodology and the evaluation formula are changed in the course of submission of tenders under the respective public procurement.[87] This violates the main principles of equality and non-discrimination, and free and fair competition.

Are transparency rules breached? Except in the cases where the evaluation methodology is modified in the course of the procedure, there is no actual breach of transparency obligations because the methodology is announced in advance by all legal means, and candidates/tenderers are able to study and respectively challenge it before the appellate authorities if they find it abusive. Abuse of the evaluation methodology, however, is not easily detectable on the one hand, and moreover, such an appeal would not have suspensive effect on the procedure in the case of the Bulgarian example (as discussed above).

What corruption loopholes are opened? In the case of corrupt practices, evaluation criteria and formulas are either *too complex and intricate* with the aim of obstructing detection of manipulative factors, or *too vague and ambiguous*, allowing the evaluation committee to justify its arbitrary decision more easily. With this type of violation involving serious corruption risks, control bodies often find it difficult to identify discriminatory and restrictive elements, and infringements remain undetected. In addition, the infringement opens up the opportunity for bribery/kickbacks affecting the intermediary element – the evaluation committee. Consequently, the artificial weight attributed to a specific evaluation criterion and/or the behaviour of the committee, coordinated in advance, predetermines the outcome of the procedure to the advantage of the desired/corrupting future contractor.

In relation to the above, Pashev, Neshev and Indjova (2009) have rightly opined that '[t]he most serious risk of corruption following ranking is the reduction of the quality parameters of the tender or their gross disregard, even changes in price conditions. This allows the supplier who has provided the bribe to be ranked on the basis of most advantageous price or the most economically advantageous offer because the latter is aware that these parameters only aim to eliminate competition and have little relevance to the actual performance thereafter'.[88]

The analysis of infringements at the Announcement Phase reveals that this phase in the award procedure is exceedingly open to corruption mechanisms of all sorts – from the use of seemingly insignificant parameters in the tender notice to serious manipulation of the entire procurement, by setting highly professional and overly

---

[87] This infringement subtype systematically occurs at the Announcement Phase (as already discussed), but because infringements of the evaluation methodology are reviewed in this section, it is considered here as well.

[88] K Pashev and K Marinov (eds), *Reducing the risks of corruption and introducing good practices in public procurement management* (Sofia: Governance Monitoring Association and Economic Policy Institute, 2009) ch 1 (K Pahev, G Neshev, A Indjova), 54–55.

complicated technical requirements or using a complex or multilayered methodology to evaluate candidates and tenderers. Despite the publicity achieved through promulgation of the required documentation and proper formal completion of all the standard documents, corrupt models here are rife. Not accidentally, most of the infringements related to corruption interference surveyed by Eurobarometer[89] are from this phase of the award and are found in every Member State.

In Member States which experience a high incidence of manifestation of corruption in the award process, these infringements are additionally facilitated both by the fact that they are difficult to detect, and due to the absence of quality *ex ante* control. Even when detected, the administrative penalty applied in Bulgaria for example – a fine with a maximum limit of up to BGN 10,000 (approx. EUR 5113)[90] – evidently does not have a sufficient deterrent effect. The option of judicial review of the acts or omissions of the contracting authorities at this phase of the procedure is also not considered as a sufficiently effective and dissuasive remedy due to the additional time required for such proceedings and the statutory possibility of the award procedure continuing during such proceedings.

With regards to infringements at the Announcement Phase, the changes following the transposition of the New Procurement Directives deserve special attention. The European legislator, after numerous discussions and vacillations,[91] resolved that the award criteria will now be only one – the 'most economically advantageous tender'.[92] What has happened in practice is that the above criteria has absorbed the 'lowest price' criteria, which is also applicable, but which must now be bound (in most cases) with the use of a cost-effectiveness approach – such as lifecycle costing – and which may include the best price-quality ratio. 'Member States may provide that contracting authorities may not use price only or cost only as the sole award criteria or restrict their use to certain categories of contracting authorities or certain types of contracts'.[93] The motives of the European legislator for this change, regarded by some authors as purely cosmetic,[94] arise from the concern that 'public

---

[89] Above (n 10).

[90] All administrative penalties were almost halved with the New PPA because contracting authorities could now only be natural persons.

[91] See Commission (EU), 'Modernisation of EU Public Procurement Policy Towards a More Efficient European Procurement Market' (Green Paper) COM(2011) 15 final, 27 January 2011, 37; European Parliament, 'Resolution of 18 May 2010 on new developments in public procurement' (2009/2175(INI); European Parliament, 'Resolution of 25 October 2011 on modernisation of public procurement' (2011/2048(INI)); Opinion of the European Economic and Social Committee (EESC) on the European Commission's Green Paper on the modernisation of the public procurement rules and the Green Paper on expanding use of e-procurement [2011] OJ C191/84.

[92] Art 67(1) Directive 2014/24/EU: 'Without prejudice to national laws, regulations or administrative provisions concerning the price of certain supplies or the remuneration of certain services, contracting authorities shall base the award of public contracts on the most economically advantageous tender'.

[93] Art 67(2) Directive 2014/24/EU.

[94] S Arrowsmith, *The Law of Public and Utilities Procurement – Regulation in the EU and UK* (vol 1, 3rd edn, London: Sweet and Maxwell, 2014) 737.

procurers often have to prioritise legal certainty above policy needs and, given the pressure on public budgets, frequently have to award the contract or service in question to the cheapest offer rather than the most economically advantageous tender; [...] this will weaken the EU's innovative base and global competitiveness; [...] the Commission [*has*] to remedy this situation and to develop strategic measures to encourage and empower public procurers to award contracts to the most economical, highest-quality offers'.[95] Accordingly, regardless of the fact that the option remains for the main but not exclusive criteria to be the price, 'the most economically advantageous tender' becomes the preferred criteria.

From an anticorruption perspective, however, and particularly in view of the comments on infringements at the national level in Member States with issues like Bulgaria, this EU decision is hardly the best possible approach. The above analysis of infringements and indeed the entire present chapter indicates that the more complicated and complex a procurement is the more corruption loopholes it opens – especially at the selection methodology level, at the technical specifications level and at the evaluation committee assessment level. Practice reveals that where the criteria is 'the lowest price', the opportunities for manipulation – especially of types which control bodies find hard to detect – are significantly reduced. Therefore, the Bulgarian legislator has correctly decided not to use the option provided by the New Procurement Directives to exclude entirely the use of the pure 'lowest price' criteria. Future practice will tell whether this sub-criteria will be used with the same frequency as previously and whether the observation in this paragraph will remain true in the future in some Member States; practice will also reveal the resourcefulness of contracting authorities to manipulate tenders.

5.3.3   Procedure Conduct Phase

Unjustified Cancellation or Continuance of Procedure on Behalf of Contracting Authorities

Which legal provisions are breached?

(i) EU rules – Article 55 Directive 2014/24/EU[96] (the EU rules provide only that contracting authorities must inform the participants of their decision as soon and as correctly as possible);

(ii) National legislation – eg Article 110 New PPA (the cases in which the contracting authority may terminate the procedure are explicitly enumerated)[97]

---

[95] European Parliament 'Resolution of 18 May 2010 on new developments in public procurement' (2009/2175(INI) 4.

[96] Art 41 Directive 2004/18/EC.

[97] Art 110 et seq New PPA determines the cases in which the contracting authorities (i) are obliged to terminate a procedure by a reasoned decision (eg where not a single tender has been submitted; where none of the tenders conform to the terms and conditions as announced in advance by the

What is the essence of the infringement? In certain cases stipulated by law, the contracting authority is obliged to cancel the procedure.

In the example of Bulgaria the legislator has allowed for several scenarios which permit the contracting authority a margin of discretion. The procedure *may* be cancelled when only one tender or application has been submitted, or when only one candidate or tenderer has been admitted, or when only one offer complies with pre-set conditions; there are other situations as well which (regardless of the fact that there is no illegal action) restrict the competitive choice of the contracting authority. The contracting authority is provided with the discretion to select one of two possible courses of action: to cancel or to continue the procedure. If cancelation of the procedure is chosen, the contracting authority may open a new public procurement award procedure with the same object, but only after entry into force of the termination decision.

There are many cases in which the contracting authorities may decide *to cancel the procedure* at any of its different phases. The grounds cited are, for example, lack of available funding, or non-compliance of the candidates or their offers with valid requirements. A poor practice, and one which indicates corrupt intent, is termination of the procedure when the favoured candidate stops having realistic prospects of obtaining the contract. At the same time, the contracting authority, not being obliged to cover the costs incurred by candidates by that point – for the tender preparation, the acquisition of the required bank guarantee, the purchase of tender documents etc. – has nothing to lose (except time) if the tender is cancelled.

> When all the instruments [...] fail to secure victory for the predetermined supplier, the contracting authority may cancel the procedure justifying its decision with either lack of funding or non-compliance of submitted tenders with the terms of reference. In most cases there are no clear arguments to such decisions and 'unwitting' tenderers are left only with the expenses incurred for their application and a significantly diminished desire to participate 'as per general rules' next time. The negative experience from participation in fraudulent tender procedures contributes to restrict competition and widens the circle of companies willing to participate in public procurement tenders through bribery.[98]

The opposite scenario should also be highlighted, namely when *the procedure is not cancelled* despite there being grounds for cancellation. In most cases a corrupt procedure is not terminated solely because advantage for the pre-selected performer is sought. In this case the contracting authority makes use of the legal option to continue the procedure despite the absence of competition and to award the contract to the only remaining candidate which 'fits' the requirements or which has submit-

---

contracting authority; where all tenders which comply with the terms and conditions as announced in advance by the contracting authority, exceed the financial resources which the said authority can ensure etc); or (ii) may terminate a procedure by a reasoned decision (eg where only one tender has been submitted; or where only one candidate complies with the requirements etc).

[98] Above (n 88).

ted an offer, as the case may be. This practice not only reveals strongly corrupt motives but also runs counter to the concept in EU legislation that the contracting authority has the option to terminate the procedure on the least suspicion at the state of the candidates precisely for the purpose of ensuring maximum competition (in the subsequent procedure implementation) and participation only by those candidates with the necessary characteristics.[99]

Are transparency rules breached? No. The tender documents are meticulously prepared, made publicly available and are at the disposal of all candidates/tenderers. Offers are opened in a public procedure. All other measures guaranteeing the transparency of the contracting authority actions are taken in accordance with the relevant type of procedure.

What corruption loopholes are opened? In this case the infringement itself and the corruption loopholes it opens tend to blend in most cases, since the termination or the use of the legal opportunity to continue the procedure are employed precisely with the aim of achieving corrupt ends. This type of infringement would not exist on its own (or at least would not pose such a threat to society, if it concerned non-provision of information by the contracting authority or inappropriate selection motivation) if the relevant corrupt intent were not also there.

As discussed above, cancellation is often used as a desperate measure when none of the other available corrupt mechanisms are able to bring about victory for the preferred supplier, contractor or service provider. In the contrary case, when a procedure is not terminated despite the statutory requirements for such a step being met, the contracting authority usually endeavours to 'save' the procedure and validate the procurement, again with the aim of securing the contract for its favourite.

---

[99] In this connection, the ECJ in its preliminary ruling dated 11.12.2014 in Case C-440/13 *Croce Amica One Italia Srl v Azienda Regionale Emergenza Urgenza (AREU)*, ECLI:EU:C:2014:2435, ruled that derogation from the principle of the finality of findings of criminal liability as expressed in Art 45 Directive 2004/18/EC is possible and that '[a]rticles 41(1), 43 and 45 of Directive 2004/18/EC of the European Parliament and of the Council of 31.3.2004 on the coordination of procedures for the award of public works contracts, public supply contracts and public service contracts must be interpreted as meaning that, where the conditions for the application of the grounds for exclusion set out in Art 45 are not fulfilled, that article does not preclude the adoption by a contracting authority of a decision not to award a contract for which a procurement procedure has been held and not to proceed with the definitive award of the contract to the sole tenderer remaining in contention to whom the contract had been provisionally awarded'. National contracting authorities are thus given the option *per argumentum a fortiori* to terminate procedures with one remaining candidate where there are concerns regarding the personal characteristics of the said candidate (even without an effective judgment).

Participation and Award to 'Related Parties'. Conflict of Interest.[100] Bid Rigging

Which legal provisions are breached?

(i) EU rules – the principles of fair and loyal competition as set out in the New Procurement Directives; Article 57(4)(d) Directive 2014/24/EU[101];

(ii) National law – eg Articles 101(11),[102] 54(1) item 7[103] and 55(1) item 3[104] New PPA.

What is the essence of the infringement? The infringement consists of the unlawful existence of different 'connections'[105] between participants in the procedure which limit competition.

Three types of 'relationships' can be distinguished in this context to illustrate the subject of this type of infringement:

The first type can be labelled '*unlawful (vertical) relations*'. This concept covers the relationships between contracting authority and a future participant in the procedure – the candidate. Unlawful relationships create avenues for corruption and conflicts of interest and are consequently prohibited by the law by means of the statutory provision quoted above. In the case of Bulgaria, this type of infringement is also mainly committed by the patrons of municipalities and certain agencies, usually in awards to municipal companies. Construction, services and supply contracts

---

[100] Directive 2014/24/EU now provides a definition to 'conflict of interests' as part of the package of anticorruption legislative measures which the New Procurement Directives envisage, according to which, where such conflict cannot be prevented, it can serve as grounds for possible exclusion of the participant: Art 24 – 'Member States shall ensure that contracting authorities take appropriate measures to effectively prevent, identify and remedy conflicts of interest arising in the conduct of procurement procedures so as to avoid any distortion of competition and to ensure equal treatment of all economic operators. The concept of conflicts of interest shall at least cover any situation where staff members of the contracting authority or of a procurement service provider acting on behalf of the contracting authority who are involved in the conduct of the procurement procedure or may influence the outcome of that procedure have, directly or indirectly, a financial, economic or other personal interest which might be perceived to compromise their impartiality and independence in the context of the procurement procedure'.

[101] Art 57(4)(d) Directive 2014/24/EU provides that contracting authorities may exclude or may be required by Member States to exclude from participation in a procurement procedure any economic operator 'where the contracting authority has sufficiently plausible indications to conclude that the economic operator has entered into agreements with other economic operators aimed at distorting competition'.

[102] Art 101(11) New PPA: 'Affiliates cannot be independent candidates or participants in the same procedure'. Definitions of affiliates and affiliate undertakings are provided in the supplementary provisions to the New PPA – §2(44) and (45).

[103] The provision determines the 'conflict of interest' as a mandatory ground for exclusion.

[104] The provision determines 'bid rigging' as ground for exclusion which is used at the contracting authority's discretion.

[105] Including agreements which are not based on the exercise of control between the parties.

are awarded to related parties,[106] which can exercise control over the contractor either by means of participation in ownership or participation in management bodies.

The second type of connection which creates a risk of corruption can be defined as '*unfair (horizontal) relations*'. This term refers to participation in the procedure by one or more candidates/tenderers which are related between themselves and collude to obtain the contract at a higher price.[107]

> The mechanism of participation of related parties in a competition or tender consists in their offering different prices and other terms and conditions. The winner among them is the one offering the lowest price or best comprehensive indicators under the 'most economically advantageous tender' criteria. This candidate will subsequently decline the contract [...] The tender will then be awarded to the next related party but at a higher price or more unfavourable conditions for the contracting authority.[108]

In addition, the third type of relationship is again 'horizontal', along the candidates/participants axis, but does not arise from the exercise of control but rather from the establishment of '*concerted practices*'[109] (ie bid rigging) between them. Bid rigging in public procurement has attracted the attention of Member States authorities in earnest in the last years because it was found that this is a method for large scale restriction of competition and manipulation of the results of tenders and public procurement procedures in the course of which Member States lose considerable funds. According to the New Procurement Directives, bid rigging may now serve as a ground for exclusion of candidates from a public procurement procedure.[110]

Are transparency rules breached?   The publicity and transparency rules applicable to the notice, the type of procedure selected and the conduct of the procedure are

---

[106] Depending on the definition of related parties in the relevant national legislation.

[107] The use of subcontractor-related parties may also be defined as a subcategory of this type of manipulation.

[108] B Danev, K Kolev and S Todorova (eds), *Monitoring public procurements. Common infringements and corruption practices* (Sofia: Bulgarian Industrial Association 2005) 16.

[109] eg according to Art 15 (1) the Bulgarian Competition Protection Act, (*Закон за защита на конкуренцията*, SG 102/28.11.1998, as amended) the following are prohibited: 'all types of agreements between undertakings, decisions by associations of undertakings as well as concerted practices of two or more undertakings having as their object or effect the prevention, restriction or distortion of competition on the relevant market, such as those which: 1. directly or indirectly fix prices or other trading conditions; 2. share markets or sources of supply; 3. limit or control production, trade, technical development or investment; 4. apply to certain partners dissimilar conditions for equivalent transactions, thereby placing them at a competitive disadvantage; 5. make the conclusion of contracts subject to acceptance by the other party of supplementary obligations or to the conclusion of additional contracts which, by their nature or in accordance with commercial usage, have no connection with the subject of the main contract or to its performance. (2) Any agreements and decisions referred to in paragraph (1) shall be null and void'.

[110] See above (n 101).

usually not breached. In the horizontal types of relationship between candidates/ participants, transparency is by no means impaired as the contracting authority is not part of the circle of perpetrators and is usually meticulous as to advertising and publicity of the tender and its own actions. In vertical relationships which also result in conflicts of interest between participant representatives and the contracting authority, it is possible that transparency principles may be breached as the agreement between those involved in the bribery/kickback could have been established as early as the procurement Announcement Phase, or additional information could have been withheld from other participants in the course of the subsequent procedure phases.

What corruption loopholes are opened? All types of relatedness open up corruption loopholes during the Procedure Conduct Phase, as follows:

Unlawful relations cause conflicts of interest and distort the market, but do not necessarily result in substantial financial losses for the contracting authority, since the latter does not always benefit from such corrupt schemes, except eg in cases where funds are diverted towards municipal companies.

Unfair relations and *Bid rigging* can also exist as independent infringements which are not related to corrupt schemes, and can be combined with another of the infringements discussed previously, involving bribing of the contracting authority so that a more complicated corrupt scheme can be implemented which includes all the participants in the procedure and pursues the selection of a pre-determined contractor. However, these infringements create serious risks of considerable additional costs being paid 'from the taxpayers pocket' for the same activities, which results in an ineffective procurement procedure and private gain for the winning supplier, contractor or service provider. Moreover, these two connections along the horizontal axis are much more difficult to detect, especially bid rigging, bearing in mind that control bodies in public procurement generally focus on the actions or omissions of contracting authorities and not so much on those of participants.[111]

Unreasonably Favourable Offers

Which legal provisions are breached?

(i) EU legislation – Article 69(3)(2) Directive 2014/24/EU,[112] Article 84(3)(2) Directive 2014/25/EU; The New Procurement Directives differ from the Procurement Directives in the social commitment of the new rules, namely that contracting authorities are now obliged to reject a tender where they have estab-

---

[111] In Bulgaria bid rigging can only be reviewed by the CPC as part of a procedure separate from the normal appeal procedure initiated upon receipt of a complaint or of the CPC own motion.

[112] Art 69(3)(2) Directive 2014/24/EU: 'Contracting authorities shall reject the tender, where they have established that the tender is abnormally low because it does not comply with applicable obligations referred to in Article 18(2)'.

lished that the tender is abnormally low because of non-compliance with obligations in the fields of environmental, social and labour law;

(ii) National legislation – eg Article 72 New PPA.[113]

What is the essence of the infringement? The infringement involves elements of the public procurement which are also used as evaluation indicators. This creates conditions where they may be inflated by candidates without any significant benefit to the contracting authority. Classic examples in this respect are those in which (a) candidates/tenderers extend the proposed warranty service period beyond all measure (proposing, for example, a period of 40 or 50 years) or (b) reduce the execution period in order to obtain the contract, although the time period they have set is completely unrealistic. In such cases the assessment committee usually acts at its subjective discretion and is not obliged to eliminate such a tenderer.

The legislative provisions may also be circumvented if all or most tenderers introduce, by colluding, similar unrealistic proposals (eg in bid rigging, as discussed above).

Complex public procurements with complicated constituent elements make the detection by control bodies of artificially enhanced offerings (in such a great numbers) very difficult. In such cases 'it must be established, for each parameter of the proposal which can receive a numerical expression, what proposals were made by all other tenderers in the open procedure, these must be then compared and only then it can be identified whether a specific offer proposes, under a certain parameter, 30%[114] more favourable conditions than other tenders'.[115]

---

[113] In accordance with the New PPA when a proposal in a participant's tender related to cost or expense which is subject to evaluation is more than 20% more favourable than the average of the proposals of other participants for the same evaluation indicator, the contracting authority requires detailed written justification of its formation to be provided within 5 days of receiving the request. The justification may refer to: (a) economic characteristics of the manufacturing process of the services or of the construction method; (b) the technical solutions chosen or any exceptionally favourable conditions for participants for the provision of products or services or the execution of the construction; (c) originality of the proposed decision by the participant in relation to the works, supplies or services etc. The justification can only be rejected and the participant excluded from the procedure when the evidence is not sufficient to justify the proposed price or cost. In addition, the contracting authorities do not accept offers where the price or costs offered are more than 20% more favourable than the average of the relevant proposals in other bids because they do not comply with relevant rules and regulations on environmental protection, social and labour law, collective agreements and/or provisions of international environmental, social and labour law. Finally, the contracting authorities do not accept offers where the price or costs offered are more than 20% more favourable than the average proposals in other bids because of state aid received when the participant cannot prove within the relevant period that the aid is compatible with the internal market. No legal definition of 'abnormally low tender' is provided.

[114] Previous versions of the PPA stipulated a percentage difference of 30%.

[115] Decision No 698/26.3.2013; Administrative Court, Burgas, panel XIII, Judge Evtimova.

Are transparency rules breached? Again, as with the other infringements at the Procedure Conduct Phase, this type does not breach the principle of transparency as all requirements for the assurance of publicity and equal access to identical information for all candidates/participants have been duly observed.

What corruption loopholes are opened? 'More favourable' offers allow a tenderer which at least at first glance was selected by the contracting authority precisely because it offered the best value for public funds, to obtain the contract through unfair means. By bribing the contracting authority, the candidate justifies its abnormally low/favourable offer in accordance with the law; the contracting authority accepts this justification as sufficiently persuasive, and the candidate becomes the selected contractor. The undefined and ambiguous phrasing of the Directives (in both the old and the new procurement package) such as 'originality of the work' or 'any exceptionally favourable conditions available' which allow the contracting authority to decide not to eliminate the candidate also facilitates this type of corrupt scheme, which eliminates other candidates and ensures the painless selection of the desired candidate. In the long run, the 'successful tenderer' is not only unable to meet the indicators set out in its own offer, but is often unable to complete the contract.

As has been observed, some of the infringements at the Procedure Conduct Phase are easier to detect due to the significantly larger document flow and also the requirement for justification of evaluation committee decisions, while others require serious analysis of the case and its context by the control bodies. Appellate and control authorities should be able to prove lack of motives or purely perfunctory motivation for challenged decisions, but only upon appeal of the decision by the contracting authority itself. What is most noteworthy, however, is the conclusion (similar to that made regarding the Announcement Phase) that infringements at this phase are carried out against the background of adequate publicity and transparency, which is ensured throughout the entire process of submission of the tenders, their opening and evaluation. The majority of these infringements result in a considerable loss of public funds, caused not only by the contravention of legal rules but mainly because of the involvement of corrupt schemes in their perpetration, which automatically precludes the protection of public interest.

The statistical assessment of how often this kind of infringement occurs in one or another Member State is difficult precisely for the reasons listed above. Accordingly, this type of infringements, necessarily implying serious corrupt intent, should be considered in the determination of the functions of all supervisory bodies at local level, which should pursue not only palliative measures (based on publicity) to limit it.

5.3.4   Contract Implementation Phase

Unwarranted Amendments in the Course of Implementation of Public Procurement Contracts

Which legal provisions are breached?

(i) EU rules – the New Procurement Directives codify *Pressetext*,[116] Article 72 Directive 2014/24/EU sets out the possible scenarios for contract modification[117];

(ii) National legislation – eg Article 116 New PPA[118]

---

[116] Case C-454/06 *Pressetext Nachrichtenagentur GmbH v Republik Österreich (Bund), APA-OTS Originaltext-Service GmbH, APA Austria Presse Agentur registrierte GmbH* [2008] ECR I-4401.

[117] Art 72(1) Directive 2014/24/EU provides that '[c]ontracts and framework agreements may be modified without a new procurement procedure in accordance with this Directive in any of the following cases: (a) where the modifications, irrespective of their monetary value, have been provided for in the initial procurement documents in clear, precise and unequivocal review clauses, which may include price revision clauses, or options. Such clauses shall state the scope and nature of possible modifications or options as well as the conditions under which they may be used. They shall not provide for modifications or options that would alter the overall nature of the contract or the framework agreement; (b) for additional works, services or supplies by the original contractor that have become necessary and that were not included in the initial procurement where a change of contractor: (i) cannot be made for economic or technical reasons such as requirements of interchangeability or interoperability with existing equipment, services or installations procured under the initial procurement; and (ii) would cause significant inconvenience or substantial duplication of costs for the contracting authority. However, any increase in price shall not exceed 50% of the value of the original contract. Where several successive modifications are made, that limitation shall apply to the value of each modification. Such consecutive modifications shall not be aimed at circumventing this Directive; (c) where all of the following conditions are fulfilled: (i) the need for modification has been brought about by circumstances which a diligent contracting authority could not foresee; (ii) the modification does not alter the overall nature of the contract; (iii) any increase in price is not higher than 50% of the value of the original contract or framework agreement. Where several successive modifications are made, that limitation shall apply to the value of each modification. Such consecutive modifications shall not be aimed at circumventing this Directive; (d) where a new contractor replaces the one to which the contracting authority had initially awarded the contract as a consequence of either: (i) an unequivocal review clause or option in conformity with point (a); (ii) universal or partial succession into the position of the initial contractor, following corporate restructuring, including takeover, merger, acquisition or insolvency, of another economic operator that fulfils the criteria for qualitative selection initially established provided that this does not entail other substantial modifications to the contract and is not aimed at circumventing the application of this Directive; or (iii) in the event that the contracting authority itself assumes the main contractor's obligations towards its subcontractors where this possibility is provided for under national legislation pursuant to Art. 71; (e) where the modifications, irrespective of their value, are not substantial within the meaning of paragraph 4. Contracting authorities having modified a contract in the cases set out under points (b) and (c) of this paragraph shall publish a notice to that effect in the OJEU. Such notice shall contain the information set out in Annex V part G and shall be published in accordance with Art. 51'.

[118] The provision of the national legislation transposes fairly precise the wording of Directive 2014/24/EU.

What is the essence of the infringement? Because amendments to concluded public procurement contracts are generally understood to be a strictly regulated exception, infringements in the form of 'annexed contracts' have significantly dropped in number in all Member States. Nevertheless, control bodies continue to come across cases in which the grounds for modification of the contract conditions are unjustifiably used or '[o]ften contract amendment is not formalised by means of addendums or additional agreements but simply regarded as a fact. For example, inspections often establish cases in which the contractor has invoiced, and the contracting authority has subsequently paid, higher unit prices than initially agreed (this being observed most often in the supply of foodstuffs) or cases in which contract implementation extends over a period of time exceeding the one initially agreed between the parties, with the knowledge but not the opposition of the contracting authority (and often without any delay damages being sought)'.[119] A similar infringement can also be perpetrated by signing a contract presumably on the basis of an existing framework agreement but with significantly modified conditions compared to those set out in the framework agreement.

Because control bodies are able to detect amendments to existing contracts relatively easily (on the basis of existing payment documents), corrupt practices have shifted in recent years towards infringement in the course of contract performance itself. In the case of complex supply and construction works contracts, measuring the compliance of actual performance against the offer and the contract is much more difficult and often requires expert investigation at the instigation of the control and appellate authorities. Precisely for this reason, the New Procurement Directive rules codifying *Pressetext* seem to stand little chance of being completely effective against corruption, since verbal agreements cannot be regulated and remain outside the scope of the rules.

With respect to Bulgaria, despite the numerous supplements and amendments to the legislation in this respect, as well as the proposals in the New PPA which extend the *ex ante* control over contracts subject to amendment (as discussed in Chap. 4 and although in some particular cases only), the actual implementation of public procurement contracts remains beyond the view of the legislator and of the control institutions in this Member State (the legislator regards these relationships as commercial in nature and therefore not subject to a special regime).

> This is valid for the private sector and also for the public sector if we assume that the contracting authority cannot have mercenary motives to waive the rights given to it under the contract, ie if we assume that there can be no corruption following contract conclusion, which, indisputably, is an unrealistic assumption.[120]

Are transparency rules breached? Yes, although the answer to this question is not unambiguous. Formally (except in the pure case of 'annexed contracts' in violation of the law), transparency *vis-à-vis* third parties has not been infringed because the

---

[119] Above (n 77) 5.
[120] Ibid.

procurement as a whole and its separate elements and documents are publicly available, and all the participants can make themselves acquainted with their contents. Verbal arrangements between the contracting authority and the contractor, however, often remain unverifiable, while compliance with the principle of transparency at this stage is considerably diluted by pedantic debates about whether public procurement rules are actually applicable in this case or whether general commercial rules should apply under which transparency is not required.

What corruption loopholes are opened? Judging from the analysis of recent case law in Bulgaria, verbal arrangements are indeed most common, introducing amendments to the initially agreed price, extending the period of validity of the contract (in the absence of any statutory grounds for such extension)[121] or negotiating an undocumented agreement between the contracting authority and the contractor for under-budgeted or incomplete performance, with the purpose of allocating unspent resources between the two parties. Due to the absence of subsequent quality control, such practices are hard to prove and expose. Given the insufficient capacity of the control bodies in this Member State, as well as their financial limitations, it is uncertain whether the legislative changes transposing the New Procurement Directives and widening their control will simply remain 'on paper', with control bodies failing to detect a significant number of modifications to contractual parameters, especially those which concern 'grand' corruption and usually require a much more thorough and comprehensive analysis.

Further, although the new system facilitates the modification of contracts in cases where this does not affect their volume and price significantly, it should be recognised at the same time that the new hypotheses leaves fairly wide scope for interpretation and frees the authorities to justify their failure to reprocure and to allow the corrupt continuation of contracts which prefer the old contractor.

Pashev et al. (2006) make an addition to the above situations in which this type of infringement occurs by considering the behaviour of future contractors at the tender submission stage.[122] In their opinion the bribing party will submit a tender quoting a much lower price compared to the level of quality proposed (to justify 'selection' by the contracting authority) in the full knowledge that the quality will not be a decisive factor during the subsequent contract performance.

Infringements at the Contract Implementation Phase can be brought under the common umbrella of 'unjustified amendments', although the various manifestations can in this case also be numerous: a) the contracting authority pays for goods, services and construction works at prices higher than the national average; b) the contractor invoices the contracting authority for activities which have not been performed; c) the contracting authority fails to make use of available remedies in the

---

[121] In this context, see Decision No 101/27.6.2013, Administrative Court of Gabrovo, Judge G Kosev; Decision in Criminal case No 123/27.6.2013, Regional Court of Veliko Tarnovo, Judge P Tsankov; Decision in Criminal Case No 1269/11.11.2011, Lovech Regional Court, Judge G Marinova.

[122] Above (n 6) 33–34.

event of poor performance and fails to seek agreed liquidated damages etc. Again, as in the previous two phases, violation of transparency rules is not the focus of these manifestations and corrupt mechanisms require much more profound control than the simple, formal requirement for publicity.

Such corrupt behaviour is observed in most Member States, and the comparison of the figures provided in Table 5.1 above shows that Bulgaria suffers twice as much from such behaviour as Germany and Austria. Although these are only figures based on the perception of the people interviewed,[123] the comparison of these two Member States in the following chapters, and the completely different effects achieved by their control bodies' activities, answers to some extent why there is such a great difference in the incidence of this type of infraction.

Finally, the definition used by Wensink and Maarten de Vet (2013) applies in full force to this type of infringements, namely that '[v]ery often, corruption is a hidden offence, with – in most instances – no obvious victims, damage and with most importantly, two or more parties involved that have everything to gain by being silent and acting discreetly'.[124]

5.4 One Verdict, Among … Few

To illustrate all of what has been discussed so far, it is worth mentioning one emblematic Bulgarian case from 2010 which is even more famous for finally resulting in a conviction in early 2014 (following appeal to all instances), than because of the characteristic of the case itself. Nevertheless, the infringements are typical of the conduct of the procurement process in Bulgaria and shed light on the corrupt practices there far more clearly than pure theory can alone.

5.4.1 Background

In 2009 a Bulgarian municipality[125] announced a public procurement procedure for the supply of engineering services for improved drinking and waste water infrastructure under Operational Programme 'Environment 2007–2013'. The municipality was represented by Mr. T (mayor of the municipality). An expert committee was appointed, chaired by Mr. C (a former municipal official). Tenders were submitted by candidates 'K', 'P' and 'D'. On the basis of the committee's report which eliminated candidates 'K' and 'P', the contracting authority chose candidate 'D' as contractor, with an offer of over BGN 28 million (or over EUR 14 million). Following announcement candi-

---

[123] See above Fig 4.

[124] Above (n 3) 58.

[125] Dulovo municipality.

date 'D' as the chosen contractor,[126] candidate 'K' appealed the decision before the CPC, alleging a conflict of interest.[127] The appeal suspended contract implementation. CPC failed to find violations in the procedure. Accordingly, *ex ante* control over the public procurement was brought to an end.[128] Much later, in 2011, and only after candidate 'K' alerted OLAF to the case, the Bulgarian Prosecutor's Office decided to initiate criminal proceedings which were also motivated by political reasons (Mr C was a Member of Parliament). Ultimately, after several years and court instances, the criminal proceedings were concluded with an effective sentence issued by the Supreme Court of Cassation. This can, somewhat cautiously, be declared as a precedent, against a background of very limited detection of corrupt practices in public procurement resulting in conviction and sentencing.[129] Mr. T and Mr. C were convicted of abuse of office and imprisoned.[130]

5.4.2   Infringements Found

Inclusion of Requirements Which Unreasonably Restrict Participation in the Procurement and/or Offer an Advantage to One of the Tenderers

The procedure was initiated and approval was granted to the relevant documentation and the public procurement notice, which listed the selection criteria including minimum requirements as to the economic and financial standing of the candidate or tenderer, and its technical capabilities and qualifications, which however did not correspond to and were not coordinated with the complexity of the subject matter and the scope of the procedure. Candidates were required to provide evidence of the necessary technical equipment for performance of the works but there was no further specification as to what such equipment should include although the practical implementation of the procurement would require significant amounts of high quality technical equipment. No reference was made to the minimum number of machines and facilities either. This formulation of the requirement was so vague and

---

[126] It should be noted that the main line of business of candidate 'D' was bus service and repair and not construction work and also that the company was managed by Mr. T's brother.

[127] Which conflict of interest was later confirmed by the Criminal court, as noted below.

[128] There is no information pointing to any appeal of the case having been lodged before the SAC, nor of any alert to the PFIA, related to the procurement in question, nor is there information of whether the procurement was included in the PFIA's or the NAO's control plans.

[129] Especially compared to other Member States, where the judiciary pays much more attention to this area, as will be discussed in the following chapters.

[130] Mr. T was sentenced to 5 years deprivation of liberty and 6 years disqualification from holding or being appointed to public office. Mr. C was sentenced to 4 years deprivation of liberty and 5 years disqualification from holding or being appointed to public office – Sentence dated 12 December 2011 in Criminal Case No 5760/2010, Sofia City Court, Criminal Department, panel XXIV.

general that it was as good as omitted. The possibility of a subjective evaluation of the 'necessary' equipment was deliberately left open.

Further, no requirement for proof of turnover from construction activities was required but only information on the candidate's general turnover – thus the contracting authority could not assess whether the tenderer has the necessary potential to complete the contract. This left a loophole for non-specialised companies with no experience in construction, such as tenderer 'D', to obtain the contract.

Tenderers were required to submit references (letters of recommendation) from at least three contracting authorities as proof of business reputation but there was no requirement for these recommendations to match the subject matter of the procurement. Also, a requirement was made for the tenderer to have at its disposal the funds (own and borrowed) necessary for the realisation of the contract, and as evidence of such funds, the candidate was required to submit a bank reference indicating financial stability but no reference was made as to the minimum sum guaranteed by such a bank reference.

Infringement of, and Changes to, the Evaluation Methodology

The tender evaluation methodology, approved through the tender documentation, was deliberately changed. The approved methodology provided that bids would be evaluated to ascertain the most economically advantageous tender. Three factors would be taken into account: (a) implementation period, (b) warranty period and (c) proposed price. Each factor would be evaluated using a separate mathematical formula. Instead of applying the evaluation methodology for the three indicators as announced in advance, the contracting authority introduced a new, subjective criterion to the implementation period – 'inadmissibility and unreasonableness'. Furthermore, tenders were not evaluated at all under the 'warranty period' factor.

Unjustified Elimination of Tenderers and Continuing the Procedure with Only One Candidate

An unreasoned selection decision was issued and unreasoned findings in the evaluation committee's report were adopted, in which the 'time limit for contract performance' factor was viewed as a basis for elimination although no requirement for a minimum period had been set. Tenderer 'D' was thus ranked first and selected as contractor for the procurement, despite 'D's' tender failing to meet the requirements set out in advance by the contracting authority,[131] and although the said tenderer had

---

[131] (i) The certificate of registration in the Central Register of Professional Builders submitted with the offer does not meet the requirements of the contracting authority as set out in the tender notice; (ii) the submitted professional liability insurance for the respective group and category of construction works does not meet the requirements for a minimum insurance amount for construction works of the type stipulated in the procurement; (iii) the list of own and hired technical equipment,

proposed a longer implementation period and shorter warranty period than the other two candidates.[132] For no obvious reason, this decision eliminated the other candidates who fully complied with the preliminary conditions. The obligation on the contracting authority to terminate the procedure given that the bid submitted by the only remaining candidate – tenderer 'D' – failed to meet the preliminary conditions was not observed. In addition, the court found sufficient evidence that the preferred company 'D' supported the financial and economic interests of one of the defendants' brothers.[133]

A contract for the sum of BGN 28,876,258 (approx. EUR 14,780,709) net of VAT was nevertheless concluded. The municipality undertook to pay this sum to the contractor 'in order to secure financial gain for 'D' which would in turn result in a substantial loss to the municipal budget of BGN 11,132,025 (approx. EUR 5,698,080). This sum comprised the difference between the price offered by 'D' under the contract and the actual value of construction and mounting works at market prices at the time, and also serious injury to the reputation of and trust in the local administration'.[134]

The court found the defendants guilty of those and several other infringements,[135] having committed a number of offences under the Bulgarian Criminal Code.[136]

The above case is a very typical example of a scheme for siphoning off funds from the municipal budget, which comprises several different violations aimed at ultimately securing (a) benefits for the contracting authority, represented by the mayor; (b) benefits for the committee chairman, who was bribed to act in the interests of the winning candidate; (c) benefits for the winning candidate firm which not

---

construction machinery and mechanisation does not contain the required documents evidencing origin and ownership of the same.

[132] Candidate 'K' offered an implementation term of 400 days and 50 years' guarantee, candidate 'P' – 540 days for implementation and a 50-year guarantee. The winner, candidate 'D', offered to complete the contract in 1004 days and only 15 years' guarantee. Despite this, one of the committee's members – a hydro-melioration expert – ruled that the offers of candidates 'K' and 'P' were unrealistic and the committee prepared a report proposing elimination of those two participants from the competition.

[133] 'An official who violates or does not fulfil his official duties, or exceeds his authority or rights with the purpose of obtaining for himself or for another benefit or to cause somebody else damage which can cause major harmful damages, shall be punished by imprisonment of up to 5 years [...]. If the act has caused substantial consequences or it has been committed by a person who occupies an important official position the punishment shall be imprisonment of one to 8 years, whereas the court can also rule [...]'. Judgment of 12 December 2011 in Criminal Case No 5760/2010, Sofia City Court, Criminal Department, panel XXIV.

[134] Ibid.

[135] According to the judgment: 'The criminal activities of the two defendants reveal a high level of organisation and conspiracy. These activities have also drawn and involved other municipal administration officials. The potential pecuniary and non-pecuniary damages which would have been incurred by the municipality [...] are huge. All this demonstrates an exceptionally high degree of threat to society on behalf of both the offence and the perpetrators themselves'.

[136] Article 282(2) item 2, with reference to Article 282(1), and with reference to Article 20(2) Criminal Code (*Наказателен Кодекс*, promulgated SG 26/2.4.1968, effective as of 1 May 1968, as amended).

only won a contract at a value much greater than the realistic price but is further unable to fulfil its contract obligations. This set of violations, conflict of interests and corrupt techniques resulted in a considerable financial loss for a relatively poor municipality and also seriously compromised the administrative apparatus at municipal level.

Another important conclusion of relevance to the analysis performed in this book is that of all the infringements of legislation in the said procurement procedure, transparency is the least affected. The requirements made of candidates were clearly announced and promulgated. The notice, although ambiguously formulated and allowing quite a broad interpretation of the needs of the contracting authority, was not appealed. The change in methodology in the middle of the procedure does, indeed, violate the publicity principle but in reality, the scheme which eliminated the other candidates turned almost entirely on the decisions of the corrupt committee and not on concealed information or information incorrectly presented to the candidates. Competition was restricted at the Procedure Conduct Phase, thus allowing the award to move forward and the only remaining participant to waltz through the selection process to be selected as the contractor.

5.5 Findings and Future Challenges

5.5.1 Relevant Conclusions

The list of infringements occurring in the course of the four phases of public procurement procedures can always be supplemented with other types of corrupt practices and specific infringements of the respective national law or combinations thereof,[137] depending on the type of procedure selected or the exact phase in which they occur. The conclusions, however, would not significantly differ from those already drawn above.

By analysing the different types of infringements and their occurrence in the course of public contract award and performance, a number of findings ring true.

Against the background of the complicated bureaucratic procedures imposed by the example national legislation in compliance with the Procurement Directives and also with the New Procurement Directives, most infringements which open up loopholes for corruption are, at the same time, meticulous in terms of observing publicity and transparency principles. In this context, a large portion of seemingly impeccable procedures turn out to be precisely those in which 'grand corruption' is perpetrated, with the subsequent loss of significant financial resources.

Of course, in addition to purely economic harm to society, corruption in the field of public procurement results in severe restriction of competition in that sector. As the above examples show, the actual contract price can be lowered and the bribe

---

[137] See V Nusheva, V Marinova, I Georgiev and L. Toneva (eds), *Corruption offences in the award of public procurements in Bulgaria* (Sofia: Transparency International Bulgaria, 2007).

securing favourable treatment for the supplier, contractor or service provider can take the form of incomplete performance or performance of poor quality. According to theory '[s]urplus income generated by the lack of competition, although more visible for each individual transaction is hard to calculate at macro level. If we assume that such income is allocated equally between the parties in a corrupt transaction, this would mean that loss for the budget would constitute approximately double the amount of bribes in the field'.[138]

The analysis in this chapter reveals that most Member States suffer from infringements motivated by corruption mostly at the Announcement Phase. Nevertheless, for some Member States the administrative part of the procedure is regarded as being of greater significance than the subject matter of the procedure. This view reflects strongly how control over the award and execution of public procurement contracts is carried out in such countries (eg Bulgaria). Control bodies only monitor the strict observance of the law and of the specific set of documents required by contracting authorities. The lack of human financial resources in the control bodies hinders the detection of sophisticated corrupt schemes, including deliberately convoluted technical requirements or intricate evaluation methodologies. Given the lack of control over the subjective evaluations of the evaluation committees, these infringements often remain invisible. Well-contrived manipulation mechanisms can also be implemented at subcontractor level or at the level of associations between several enterprises, which makes detection an even greater challenge.

Søreide's (2002) observations are very much to the point here: 'some elements important to understand the risk of corruption in public procurement are: The *amount of money* involved, the *complexity* of the technology involved, the *urgency to acquire* the goods or the *immediacy* of the project, as well as the *discretionary authority* among the public officials'.[139]

Finally, a verdict, such as the one examined, is too rare an outcome to be able to serve as a deterrent to corrupt schemes in the case of Bulgaria. In reality, the fiscal damage, restriction of competition, market distortion and the discouragement of the majority of candidates from wishing to participate in public procurement procedures cause damage to this Member State which cannot be compensated only through the imposition of sanctions, unless these sanctions are able to ensure reduced corruption in the sector.

5.5.2 New Legislative Decisions – New Corruption Loopholes

The above conclusions are made based on the relevant practice so far, as well as through investigation of the provisions of the new procurement package, which somewhat complement the palette of infringements. With each new legislative framework however come, along with the expectations that it will overcome the

---

[138] Above (n 6) 28.
[139] Above (n 65) 13 (emphasis added).

painfully familiar problems of the previous system, suspicions that some of the new rules will lead to the opening of other corrupt loopholes and opportunities for manipulation.

Under the New Procurement Directives there are several legislative proposals which are deliberately stressed in this chapter because even if sufficient practice to conclude definitely on them is lacking, their theoretical base already points to the possibilities for their application in bad faith. For countries still failing to fight corruption in the sector, these concerns are better identified as early as possible. They help in the detection of one additional conclusion, slightly removed from the focus of this book – namely, that once again there is a major weakness in the framework of European legislation which attempts to carry solutions from successful practice in various economically stable and growing Member States over without considering whether these solutions are also suitable for other, less developed states. This conclusion is clearly reflected in the next two chapters as well.

Reserved Awards[140]

Reserved contracts represent an European proposal which has proved its social worth. However, this institution enables '*reverse discrimination*' and provides opportunities for corruption.

In Bulgaria the first attempt to regulate reserved contracts was made in 2014, before the full transposition of the New Procurement Directives in the New PPA. What has happened in the year and a half since clearly shows that this privilege has often been used completely manipulatively. The number of companies registered as employing disabled people has doubled in a few months,[141] as the regulation provided that an ordinary candidate may not be preferred over such companies by the contracting authorities, even if there are objective doubts that they will not execute the procurement satisfactorily. A lighter regime for such reserved procurements is also envisaged. Some improvements have now been made in the New PPA,[142] but the question remains whether these privileges would be used for bona fide purposes only.

---

[140] Art 77 Directive 2014/24/EU: 'Member States may provide that contracting authorities may reserve the right for organisations to participate in procedures for the award of public contracts exclusively for those health, social and cultural services […]'

[141] According to the register kept by the Agency for Persons with Disabilities register in Bulgaria for the period since 2005 to date, there are a total of 223 specialised companies registered, 96 (or 44%) of which were registered from the beginning of 2015. More is available from <http://ahu.mlsp.government.bg/portal/se/> accessed on 26 April 2016

[142] New PPA, Art 12, where under Art 12(7) 'In the procedure for the award of reserved procurement can participate also other candidates, but their offers shall be considered only if no accepted offers of persons under par. 1 [ie in general, companies, using more than 30% disabled or disadvantaged people in their staff]'

Preliminary Market Consultations[143]

In the hands of the contracting authorities this tool will definitely contribute to the announcement of far more adequate and feasible procurements which meet the needs of the particular institution and/or company, but which also conform with market realities. Nevertheless, what also needs to be accomplished is (a) that these consultations are not used for the preliminary selection of candidates, and (b) to ensure that the consultant does not participate in the procedure where the criteria for it are drafted so discriminatorily that they precisely require the market consultant's selection. This requires very precise legislative solutions to ensure the absence of any advantage (also achieved by corrupt means) for the consultant instructed.

The regulation the New PPA, after transposition of the new EU rules, is not bad at first glance, but some 'gaps' are already visible. For example, again for the purposes of absolute transparency, the Bulgarian legislator has opted for publication in the buyer's profile of all information exchanged in connection with the preparation of the procurement and the market consultations, and if this is impossible, an indication in the buyer's profile of where this information may be obtained. However, the oral (eg over the phone) agreements between the contracting authorities remain untraceable and confidentiality on the part of the consultant is also not ensured and requested. Accordingly, the possibility of prior distribution and/or use of the information on the structure and designation of the procurement could be a magnificent bargaining chip or a means for indirectly winning the related award.

Self-Cleaning Mechanism[144]

Using this mechanism will definitely attract the majority of economic operators who will now be able to rehabilitate themselves before the contracting authorities. However, the prerequisites for this new for some Member State tool, eg for Bulgaria,

---

[143] Art 40 Directive 2014/24/EU: 'Before launching a procurement procedure, contracting authorities may conduct market consultations with a view to preparing the procurement and informing economic operators of their procurement plans and requirements. For this purpose, contracting authorities may for example seek or accept advice from independent experts or authorities or from market participants. That advice may be used in the planning and conduct of the procurement procedure, provided that such advice does not have the effect of distorting competition and does not result in a violation of the principles of non-discrimination and transparency'.

[144] Art 57(6) Directive 2014/24/EU: 'Any economic operator that is in one of the situations referred to in paragraphs 1 and 4 may provide evidence to the effect that measures taken by the economic operator are sufficient to demonstrate its reliability despite the existence of a relevant ground for exclusion. If such evidence is considered as sufficient, the economic operator concerned shall not be excluded from the procurement procedure.

For this purpose, the economic operator shall prove that it has paid or undertaken to pay compensation in respect of any damage caused by the criminal offence or misconduct, clarified the facts and circumstances in a comprehensive manner by actively collaborating with the investigating authorities and taken concrete technical, organisational and personnel measures that are appropriate to prevent further criminal offences or misconduct.

are expressed so broadly that along with the contracting authorities' ultimate discretion to decide whether to remove a candidate or not, some pessimists, such as the author of this book, can already see 'great opportunities' for corruption and the whitewashing of poor performers.[145]

The relevant provisions of the New Procurement Directives have been adopted generally, literally permitting rehabilitation where the possibility presents itself – eg where the candidate can prove that all facts and circumstances have been clarified comprehensively 'by actively collaborating with the investigating authorities and has taken concrete technical, organisational and personnel measures that are appropriate to prevent further criminal offences or misconduct'[146] – which is already arousing ridicule in most law-enforcing bodies, since proving such 'righteous' actions is practically impossible, but instead opens the doors wide for interpretations and chicanery. Further, the secondary legislation applicable in Bulgaria has attempted to clarify the above cited provision by adding the explanation that to prove these circumstances the relevant candidate should provide the contracting authority with a 'document issued by the relevant competent authority to confirm the circumstances described'.[147] This 'clarification' has made the provision even vaguer.

This mechanism is discussed in detail in the following chapters and through the prism of states who applied it long before the entry into force of the new rules. In any event, as already discussed, not every single mechanism will be suitable to all Member States just because it has yielded good results in some. For states with problems similar to those of Bulgaria, it is already clear that this will either be yet another provision which allows the discretion of the contracting authority to be bought, or another rule which will remain stillborn within the law. Of course it can count the legislation to regulate 'the documents and deadlines, so the procedure to be technically feasible and to ensure that it will not lead to the unjustified degree of subjectivity in its implementation',[148] but it is still early for such hopes.

These examples of legislative decisions from the new legal framework that could lead to new possible infringements and further – to fresh corruption, have yet to be refuted, nor indeed have they been observed as such in practice. Whatever actually

---

The measures taken by the economic operators shall be evaluated taking into account the gravity and particular circumstances of the criminal offence or misconduct. Where the measures are considered to be insufficient, the economic operator shall receive a statement of the reasons for that decision.

An economic operator which has been excluded by final judgment from participating in procurement or concession award procedures shall not be entitled to make use of the possibility provided for under this paragraph during the period of exclusion resulting from that judgment in the Member States where the judgment is effective.'

[145] For Germany and Austria the self-cleaning mechanism is not new and was in use before the new EU rules to be adopted. This is explicitly discussed and analysed in the subsequent chapters.

[146] Art 56(1)(3) New PPA.

[147] Art 4(1)(2) Regulation for Implementation of the New PPA.

[148] I Stoyanov *The second PPA – Analytical review of the key points of the Regulation for implementation of the Public Procurement Act* (2016) 3 ZOP+ 8.

occurs, their timely outlining could form the basis for future amendment of the various national legislation in the Member States, so as to head off the loopholes for corruption they represent, because there will be more examples, which used with unlawful intent, could occur against a background of the otherwise complete transparency of the procedures in which they are found.

Bibliography

B Danev, K Kolev and S Todorova (eds), *Monitoring public procurements. Common infringements and corruption practices* (Sofia: Bulgarian Industrial Association 2005)

C Dahlström, 'Bureaucracy and the different cures for grand and petty corruption' (2012) University of Gothenburg, QoG Working Paper Series No 2011:20

I Stoyanov *The second PPA – Analytical review of the key points of the Regulation for implementation of the Public Procurement Act* (2016) 3 ZOP+

K Pashev, A Dyulgerov, G Kaschiev, *Corruption in Public Procurement – Risks and Reform Policies*, (Sofia: Center for the Study of Democracy, 2006)

K Pashev, *Controlling corruption in public procurement: Indicators for assessing policy impact* (Sofia: Governance Monitoring Association, 2009)

K Pashev and K Marinov (eds), Reducing the risks of corruption and introducing good practices in public procurement management (Sofia: Governance Monitoring Association and Economic Policy Institute, 2009) ch 1 (K Pahev, G Neshev, A Indjova)

M Katsarova, 'Most common infringements in the award of public procurements established by National Audit Office' (2010) <http://212.122.184.197/files/_bg/statia-Petev-naru6enia_2010.doc> accessed 24 April 2016

S Arrowsmith, *The Law of Public and Utilities Procurement – Regulation in the EU and UK* (vol 1, 3rd edn, London: Sweet and Maxwell, 2014)

S Rose-Ackerman, Corruption and government (New York: CUP, 1999)

S Stoychev, *Corruption Violations in Public Procurement in Bulgaria* (Sofia: Transparency International Bulgaria, 2007); and Transparency International <www.transparency.org/whoweare/organisation/faqs_on_corruption/2/> accessed 24 April 2016

T Søreide, 'Corruption in Public Procurement: Causes, Consequences and Cures' (2002) Chr. Michelsen Institute Development Studies and Human Rights Report R 2002: 1

V Nusheva, V Marinova, I Georgiev and L Toneva (eds), *Corruption offences in the award of public procurements in Bulgaria* (Sofia: Transparency International Bulgaria, 2007)

V Lazarov, representative of the National Association of Municipal Employees in Bulgaria, *Corruption in public procurement costs taxpayers an estimated 1.3 billion leva* (interviewed on 17 October 2008) <www.mediapool.bg/koruptsiyata-v-obshtestvenite-porachki-kostva-13-mlrd-leva-na-danakoplattsite-news144808.html> accessed 24 April 2016.

W Wensink, J. Maarten de Vet et al, *Identifying and Reducing Corruption in Public Procurement in the EU* (Brussels: PwC, Ecorys, with support from Utrecht University, 2013)

Chapter 6
The German Procurement System –
A Successful Battle Against Corruption

> *'She, not even as large, all in all, as an egg hitherto,*
> *Envious, stretched, swelled, strained, in her zeal*
> *To match the beast in overall size,*
> *Saying, 'Sister, lend me your eyes.*
> *Is this enough? Am I not yet there, in every feature?'*
> (Jean de La Fontaine
> 'The Frog Who Would Be as Big as an Ox')

6.1 Benchmarking Mechanism

As the basic idea of this book is to distinguish the failures of public procurement practices and rules which rely mainly on transparency to combat corruption and to emphasise other effective methods to tackle this phenomenon, the choice of benchmark Member States is not an end in itself, but must be consistent with the national characteristics of the legislation of these states and the links between them. When the closest legislative decisions and the basis on which a branch of the law evolves are highlighted, the distinctions and controversial practices stand out more easily, and the benchmark acquires a didactic character, particularly when used to construct conclusions applicable to a wide range of legislation.

Since the Bulgarian legislation in the public procurement field has been found to be unsatisfactory in terms of corruption prevention, the countries whose legislation would be used for benchmarking were selected with the aim: (a) to develop proposals which are actually usable and applicable in Member States with issues like those of Bulgaria, and (b) to draw general conclusions to build a more flexible legislative framework in such states, appropriate to reducing the losses in procurement procedures caused by corruption.

Choosing the methodology to apply to select the countries with which Bulgaria should be compared in order to highlight better practices turned out to be a real challenge because although the goal is to identify practices suitable for more than one Member State, the analysis would only be trustworthy if it commented on concrete legislation and compared Bulgaria to countries specifically and logically linked with that Member State and not by speculating with examples in general. Various criteria have been used to select the benchmark countries in order to establish a

© Springer International Publishing AG 2017
I. Georgieva, *Using Transparency Against Corruption in Public Procurement*,
Studies in European Economic Law and Regulation 11,
DOI 10.1007/978-3-319-51304-1_6

meaningful and reasoned rationale for locating them on the same plane as a country with corruption issues and poor procurement legislation.

One of the first reference points was the level of corruption in the countries concerned (adopting the highly popular CPI used by TI, despite its limitations).[1]

Another important reason for the choice made was the *status quo* of the public procurement award system in three respects: *first*, its efficiency in the country concerned; *second*, the rules in place to limit manifestations of corruption in the field (other than excessive publicity and transparency requirements); and *third*, the extent to which certain aspects of this system could be pinpointed as good practices and could serve to resolve problems in other Member States. An attempt has been made to determine which examples could be borrowed (in their entirety or at least in part) despite the obvious differences in the economic and social environment between the different countries.

A significant reason for the choice made was the existence of historical and substantive similarities with the Bulgarian legal system. Perhaps, however, it would have been easiest to opt for Scandinavian countries as brilliant examples of corruption limited to a negligible minimum.[2] Yet the methodology of benchmarking against 'the best example' is not the most suitable for this work, since the application of achievable quantities and systems relatively familiar to the Bulgarian legal system seemed more appropriate, to avoid La Fontaine's 'frog effect'. As admitted in theory: '[a]mong the world ranking of the countries with lowest levels of corruption in Europe are Denmark, Sweden, Finland and Switzerland. [I]n order to supplement the experience of other European countries in the process of public procurement management, the experience of countries which, to a larger extent, are closer to the economic realities in Bulgaria must also be taken into account'.[3]

From a historical perspective an attempt was made to identify the national legislation forming the basis of Bulgarian public and commercial law from the late nineteenth century[4] onwards – the period when Bulgaria's legal system was conceived, a time characterised by radical reorganisation of public and social structures from a feudal to a more Western type.

All things considered, the countries which came closest to matching these requirements and concepts for a meaningful benchmark analysis appeared to be Germany and Austria: the grounds for the choice of each will be further elaborated in the relevant chapters.

---

[1] Bearing in mind the limitations of the CPI, as already discussed in Chap. 3 of this book.

[2] Similar investigations have already been undertaken for Bulgaria, eg *Manual of good practices in the public procurement field and concession appealing*, (Sofia: Bulgarian Competition Protection Commission, 2009); K Pashev and K Marinov (eds), *Reducing the risks of corruption and introducing good practices in public procurement management* (Sofia: Governance Monitoring Association and Economic Policy Institute, 2009); K Pashev, 'Reducing Corruption Risks and Practices in Public Procurement: Evidence from Bulgaria' (2009) Paper presented at the First Global Dialogue on Ethical and Effective Governance Amsterdam, etc.

[3] K Pashev and K Marinov (eds), *Reducing the risks of corruption and introducing good practices in public procurement management* (Sofia: Governance Monitoring Association and Economic Policy Institute, 2009; ch VI), 134.

[4] The period of the restoration of the Bulgarian state after being part of the Ottoman Empire for five centuries is known as the 'post-liberation period'. Historically this period runs from 1879 to 1920.

The present chapter examines Germany as a subject of comparison and outlines the advantages of the German legal system in the public procurement field which could be suitably modified and adopted by Member States like Bulgaria to prevent corruption.

6.2   Why Germany?

6.2.1   Legislative Similarities

The first point to be made in this respect is to outline the legislative analogies between Germany and Bulgaria. Both legal systems belong to the continental (Romano-Germanic) legal family which suggests a large number of fundamental similarities: a single foundational legal instrument (the Constitution/*Grundgesetz*), abstract legal formulas for all legally significant cases, subordination of law enforcement to statutory law and the absence of a precedent system typical of the Common-law world. Further, both countries are Member States of the European Union and are thus required to conform – regardless of the socioeconomic and political-historical differences – to the requirements and policies of European law. On the other hand, the German legal system is also historically connected with the foundation of the Bulgarian post-liberation legal system – the organisation of commercial relations is the result of reception mainly from the German civil code (*Bürgerliches Gesetzbuch*),[5] and the resemblance between the two systems is evident even in modern legislation. A large number of Bulgarian legal theorists of the past century were students of German jurists and followed the German example in their works.[6]

6.2.2   Corruption Level

The most important factor justifying the choice of Germany is of course the level of corruption. For 2015, according to TI's CPI, Germany came tenth out of a total of 168 countries with a score of 81.[7] According to the National Integrity System Report for Germany,[8] despite the fact that the general German population regards corruption as a serious problem for the country, in fact only about 2% of those surveyed admit to having been forced to pay bribes. This is a significant aspect when benchmarking the two countries, because obviously, the perceptions of citizens of the existence of corruption in Germany and the actual situation do not match, as opposed to the situation in Bulgaria, where public perceptions is in fact a reflection close to the actual frequency of corruption in different spheres of public significance.

---

[5] First developed in 1881, effective as of 1 January 1900.

[6] Prof Lyuben Dikov (1895–1973), Dr Petar Dzhidrov (1876–1952), Prof Konstantin Katsarov (1898–1980), etc.

[7] Transparency.org. (2015) <www.transparency.org/cpi2015> accessed 25 April 2016.

[8] *National Integrity System Report Germany 2012 (short version).* (Berlin: Transparency International Deutschland, 2012) 19 et seq.

In connection with the level of corruption in Germany and the obviously positive measures undertaken in the public procurement field, a very indicative source is the statistical data contained in the First EU Anti-Corruption report with respect to public procurement in Germany:

> In the area of public procurement, according to the 2013 Eurobarometer business survey, 20% of those who participated in public procurement procedures in the past three years reported that they were prevented from winning because of corruption (EU average: 32%). Almost all negative practices in the context of public procurement are perceived to be less common than the EU average. Respondents in Germany reported tailor-made specifications for particular companies in 48% of cases (EU average 57%). Collusive bidding was reported to be a widespread practice by 54% of the respondents (EU average 52%). Conflicts of interests in the evaluation of bids were noted by 47% of respondents (EU average: 54%) and 43% reported to unclear selection or evaluation criteria (EU average 51%).[9]

For the sake of an objective review, it should be explained that regardless the fact that corruption levels in the public procurement field in Germany appear negligible when compared to the situation in Bulgaria, Germany also suffers from gaps in corruption prevention which affect the public's perception of corruption in the country. Germany's federal structure, the different levels of government in the various regions and the differences in award procedures at local level all play a role in this context. Therefore, generalising about corruption levels in Germany is not the best approach. According to a study made by the Max-Planck Foundation[10] and to the analyses of the Federal Criminal Police Office (*Bundeskriminalamt*) covering 2010–2011, the largest number of corruption cases, greatly exceeding corruption levels in other districts, were detected in North Rhein-Westphalia.[11] This situation was addressed in the period after 2012, and the total number of corruption offences dropped by 10% from 1528 to 1373, which is the lowest level of corruption for the previous five years (since 2008).[12] Of course, it must not be forgotten that North Rhein-Westphalia is one of the largest regions in Germany, and consequently one of the first in terms of economic and industrial development. Competition is therefore much more intense than in other regions. Accordingly, even if the higher levels of corruption appear somewhat shocking, they could be regarded as proportionate to the level of business development in the region.

The below figures from Globaleconomy.com[13] could facilitate comparison with corruption levels in Bulgaria for the last decade (Figs. 6.1, 6.2 and 6.3).

---

[9] Commission (EU), 'First EU Anti-Corruption Report', Annex 5 – Germany; COM(2014) 38 final, 3.

[10] L Hensgen, *Fight against corruption in the Danube region: A study of regional best practices*, (Max Plank Foundation for International Peace and the Rule of Law, Sankt Augustin: Konrad Adenauer Stiftung, 2013) 32.

[11] Ibid – 'More than 22,800 single corruption offences and bribery in the course of trade were registered in two large investigations alone, namely against employees of an automaker and against civilian employees of the British Army of the Rhine, as well as against their respective contractors'.

[12] *Korruption – Bundeslagebild 2012* (2012) Bka.de <www.bka.de/nn_193376/DE/Publikationen/JahresberichteUndLagebilder/Korruption/korruption__node.html?__nnn=true> accessed 25 April 2016, 3.

[13] TheGlobalEconomy.com, 'Compare countries, compare economies, compare indicators' (2015) <www.theglobaleconomy.com/compare-countries/> accessed 25April 2016.

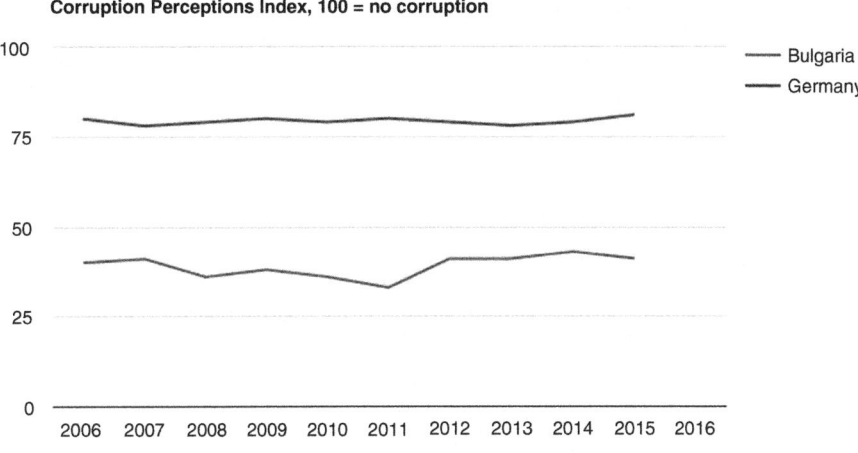

Source: The GlobalEconomy.com, World Bank

Fig. 6.1 Movement of the CPI (2006–2016)

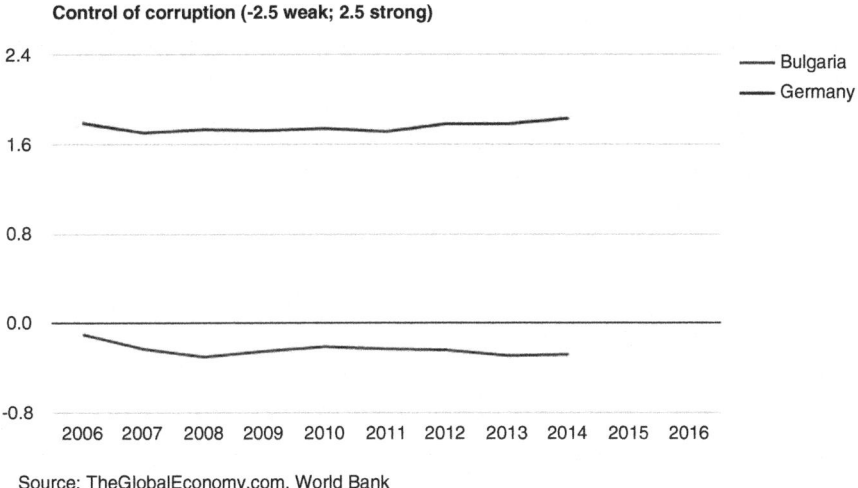

Source: TheGlobalEconomy.com, World Bank

Fig. 6.2 Control over corruption (2006–2016)

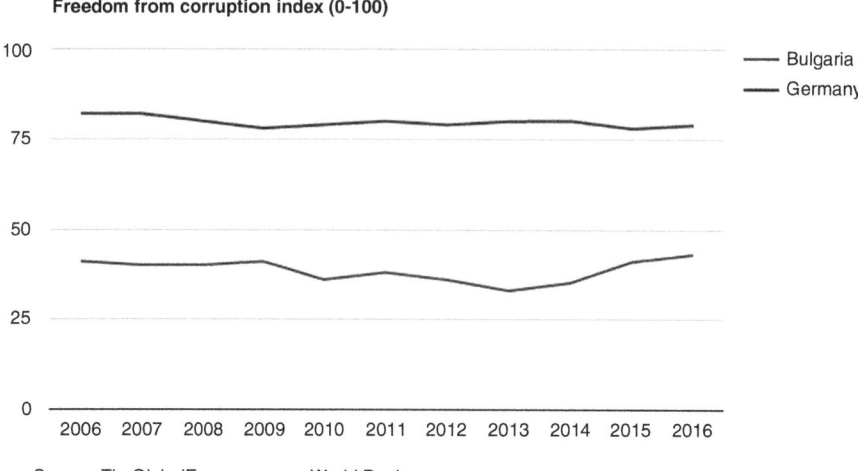

Freedom from corruption index (0-100)

Source: TheGlobalEconomy.com, World Bank

Fig. 6.3   Freedom from corruption (2006–2016)

6.2.3   Public Procurement System

The next factor concerns the public procurement system.[14] The legislative decisions underlying the main parameters and specifics of the German legal system in the public procurement field reveal several fundamental characteristics (in addition to the more detailed analysis and specific features identified below) which would have a favourable effect on the Bulgarian public procurement award system, provided they are properly implemented and harmonised with the Bulgarian reality. These are, *firstly*, the fact that legislation strives to align itself as closely as possible to European requirements without overburdening bidders with obscure and overabundant rules;[15] *secondly*, that the language of regulations is clear, concise and precludes ambiguous interpretation; and *thirdly*, the presence of streamlined and efficient control and appellate authorities.[16]

---

[14]Again, as a matter of statistics, the fact that the public procurement sector in Germany forms around 17% of national GDP and thus has a serious impact on the economic welfare of the country should be noted. The annual volume of public procurement in Germany is huge. According to the Annual Procurement Review 2011 of the European Bank for Reconstruction and Development (p 14 and Annex 3) the awards made by country of origin of the tenderers, presented by contract type for 2011 for Germany are as follows (i) work contracts – EUR 9,800,809; (ii) supply and installation contracts – EUR 2,202,692; (iii) goods – EUR 201,337; and (iv) consultancy services – EUR 59,430. The total value of procurement contracts for Germany in 2011 is EUR 12,264,268.

[15]Also considering the fact that a major part of the EU procurement legislation is strongly influenced by the German legislation itself. Therefore, some procurement package parameters which are new to other Member States are well known and used in practice in Germany.

[16]In choosing to consider Germany, it is impossible to ignore the work of CPCCOC and the BORKOR Project, discussed in Chap. 4, in the field of reducing corruption in the award of public procurement contracts in Bulgaria. In the formulation of its anti-corruption methodology and the

6.2.4   Socioeconomic Differences

There are of course clear socioeconomic distinctions between Germany and Bulgaria. Naturally, when comparing the legislative systems, good practices and efficient methodologies between two countries, account must be taken of their obvious differences, not only in terms of legal characteristics but also in terms of their cultural and lifestyle characteristics. By using some of the National Integrity System Reports conclusions for Germany and Bulgaria[17] as reference points, the main parameters of the two countries which characterise the differences in government and economic status and the perceived reliability and security of the system can be summarised as follows:

Germany: (a) The central political institutions operate effectively, the political system is stable and civil rights in Germany are not compromised; (b) economic activities in the country have been able to establish sustainable prosperity and a high standard of living; (c) a functioning and stable network of social services and social assistance is in place; (d) Germany has the fourth highest gross national product in the world behind the USA, Japan and China; and (e) there is a consistently high level of trust in the police and the justice system.

Bulgaria: (a) The continuing reforms in Bulgaria have yet to earn back the trust of the people in institutions; (b) considerable public funds have been invested in strengthening the public integrity of institutions – there is sufficient institutional capacity but the public investment of funds has as yet not resulted in improvements in integrity and anticorruption; (c) most of the public institutions are not cost-efficient and public resources are spent in vain; (d) the law enforcement bodies (prosecutors and the police) are unable to generate significant public trust and are often criticised by European partners; and (e) the judiciary enjoys a high level of independence and autonomy in law. However, the judiciary's practice does not inspire trust and confidence in the institution in Bulgaria.

The figures from Globaleconomy.com[18] demonstrate, without the need for further analysis, the disparities between the two countries on several fundamental parameters: economic growth, GDP, government costs, administrative efficiency and regulatory quality (Figs. 6.4, 6.5, 6.6, 6.7 and 6.8):

---

elaboration of a model to counter corruption in the public procurement field, the CPCCOC has endorsed the German model – similar to one of the German online platforms (the 'V-Model') for the detection of corruption gateways and related to certain elements of German legislation.

[17] Above (n 8); *National Integrity System Assessment – Bulgaria Country Report 2011* (Sofia: Transparency International Bulgaria, 2011).

[18] TheGlobalEconomy.com, 'Compare countries, compare economies, compare indicators' (2015) <www.theglobaleconomy.com/compare-countries> accessed 25 April 2016.

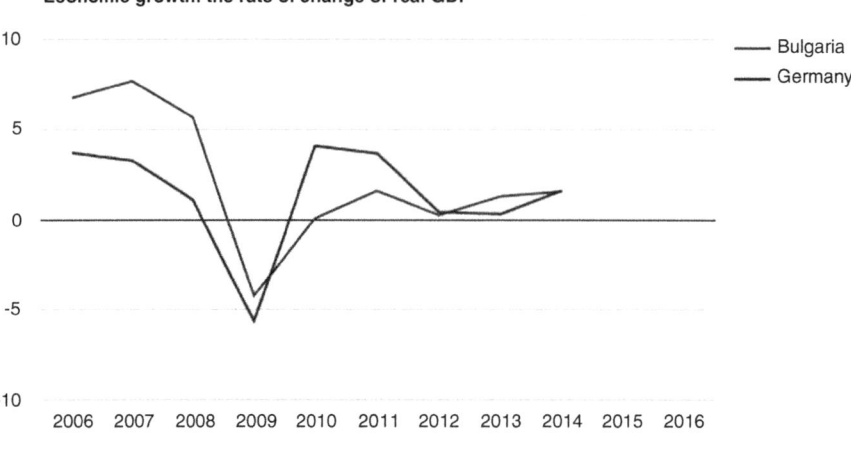

Fig. 6.4 Changes in economic growth (2006–2016)

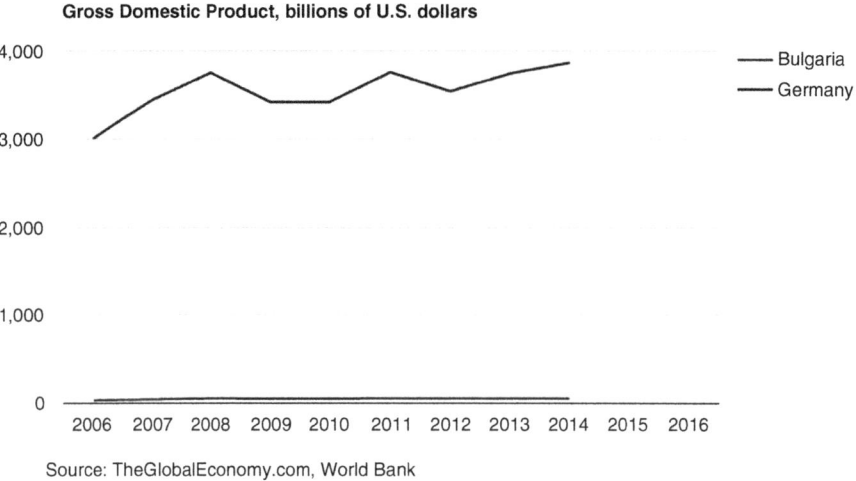

Fig. 6.5 Gross Domestic Product (2006–2016)

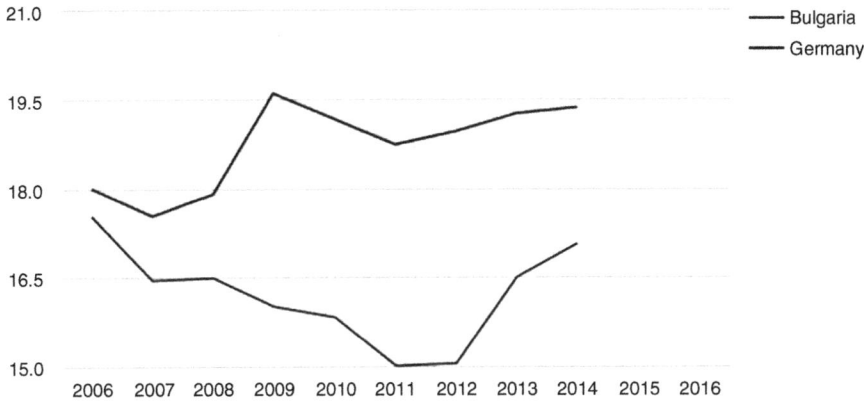

Source: TheGlobalEconomy.com, World Bank

Fig. 6.6 Government spending (2006–2016)

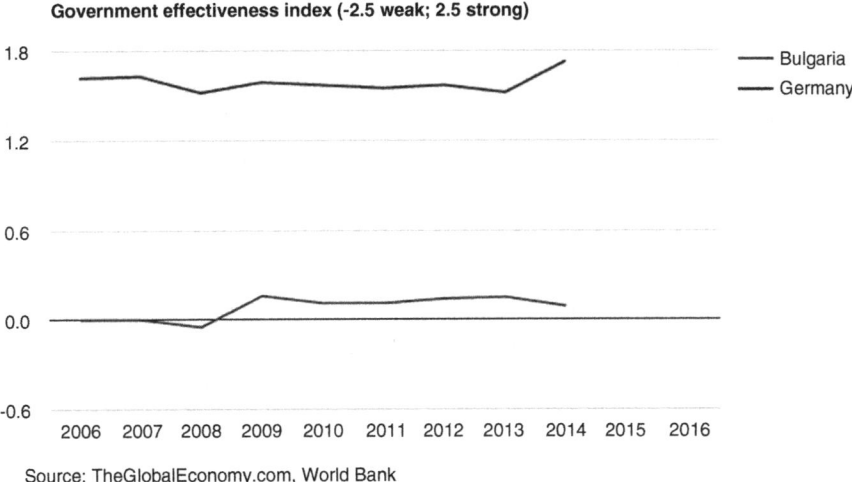

Source: TheGlobalEconomy.com, World Bank

Fig. 6.7 Administrative efficiency (2006–2016)

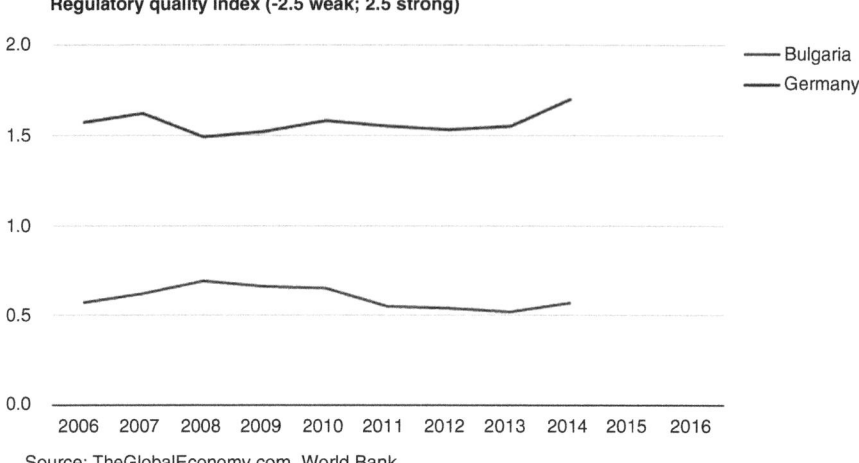

Source: TheGlobalEconomy.com, World Bank

Fig. 6.8 Regulatory quality (2004–2014)

6.3 Main Characteristics of the German Public Procurement System – Applicable Legislation

As an EU Member State, Germany is subject to EU public procurement law. The New Procurement Directives were transposed into German legislation on time – the Regulation for an Act for the Modernisation of Public Procurement Law (*Verordnung zur Modernisierung des Vergaberechts*, VergRModVo) was approved by a regulation of the Federal Council in 2016,[19] with the text of the Act for the Modernisation of Public Procurement Law (*Gesetz zur Modernisierung des Vergaberechts*, VergRModG) being promulgated earlier same year.[20]

German public procurement law is, as is the case in other Member States, artificially divided into two clearly distinguished parts – legislation applicable *above* and legislation applicable *below* the thresholds. This is one of the most significant differences from the Bulgarian model which in this respect tends to be more restrictive (and thus resembles the Austrian model, as will be discussed in the next chapter). This is, however, not necessarily a positive feature of Bulgarian law. Given that Bulgaria is also a Member State, the same European legislation and thresholds apply. However, according to the PPA and now the New PPA, there are also national thresholds which need to be observed. The restrictive rules of the Bulgarian framework are not completely applicable to procurements below the national thresholds.

The main applicable legislative acts which regulate procurement awards above the EU thresholds in Germany are presented in Part IV of the Act against Restraints

---

[19] 18 March 2016.

[20] BGBl. I S. 203/23.2.2016, Federal Gazette I 26 August 1998, p. 2546, as amended.

of Competition (*Gesetz gegen Wettbewerbsbeschränkungen*, GWB), now amended by the VergRModG and the German Ordinance on the Award of Public Contracts (*Vergabeverordnung*, VgV), which is amended by the VergRModVo.[21] The more specific rules governing the utilities sector are found in the Ordinance on the Award of Public Contracts by Utilities (*Verordnung über die Vergabe von Aufträgen im Bereich des Verkehrs, der Trinkwasserversorgung und der Energieversorgung*, SektVO),[22] also amended with the VergRModVo.

The German legislator has used the opportunity to further tweak its legislation through the transposition of the New Procurement Directives and has also simplified it and concentrated into fewer regulations than before.[23] The change is considered one of the biggest in the public procurement field in the last decade. The requirements at EU legislation level are to a great extent being implemented through the GWB.

> It appears, however, that the material changes compared to the current legal situation (and the corresponding practical impact of the amendment) will not be significant because in many areas principles of public procurement case law (of the ECJ) which already exist and are applied in practice are being codified without any major changes – for example the self-cleaning mechanisms […], the provisions on contractual changes and legal consequences […] or the regulations on public-public forms of cooperation which do not require a call for tenders […] The fact that the principles set out by case law to date in these areas are now being expressly regulated and defined is, however, sensible and welcome in view of the increased legal certainty which this creates.[24]

Under the German model, invitations to tender must be issued whenever the value of a contract equals or exceeds the relevant EU threshold. Below the EU thresholds only certain restricted procurement legislation provisions apply.[25] Tender notices are published nationally only. In both cases (below or above EU thresholds), bearing in mind the decentralised federal structure of Germany, the specific laws, rules and manuals of each of the sixteen *Bundesländer* have to be observed, since there are contracting authorities and purchasers (for a particular district) at each separate federal level.

The present work focuses on the fundamental rules of the GWB (with its respective amendments concerning the transposition of the new procurement package, as

---

[21] BGBl. I S. 321/22.2.1994, as amended.

[22] BGBl. I S. 3110/23.9.2009, as amended.

[23] The Procurement Regulation for Public Works (*Vergabe- und Vertragsordnung für Bauleistungen*, VOB/A) has now shortened, with most of its provisions being shifted to the GWB and VgV; the Procurement Regulation for Public Supplies and Services (*Vergabe- und Vertragsordnung für Leistungen*, VOL/A) and the Procurement Regulations for the Award of Independent Contractor Services (*Verdingungsordnung für freiberufliche Leistungen*, VOF) have been repealed and their provisions are now incorporated in the GWB and VgV.

[24] F Raddatz, 'Modernisation of public procurement law – will this impact the healthcare industry?' (2015) Noerr.com <www.noerr.com/en/press-publications/News/modernisation-of-public-procurement-law.aspx> accessed on 25 April 2016.

[25] The budgetary laws of the federal, state and local governments, as well as the relevant part of the VOB/A are, however, mandatory.

adopted in the VergRModG) and the relevant special ordinances and acts which apply to the whole country. The individual acts of the various *Bundesländer* fall outside the focus of the work because they can only serve as a representative sample for the *Land* concerned but not for the comprehensive state policy in the sector.[26]

6.4   Main Principles. Transparency Obligations

The basic principles of German public procurement law are logically the same as those stipulated in the Procurement Directives and now the New Procurement Directives applicable throughout the EU – competition, non-discrimination, transparency, equal treatment, proportionality and the right to judicial review.

Given that Part IV of the GWB is 'the flagship in German procurement law',[27] and that after harmonisation with the new procurement package it consist of even more basic rules, literally pasting in the EU rules, the main principles of public procurement above the thresholds are found in this act.[28] The GWB (VergRModG) extends the principles of the New Procurement Directives with exact requirements with respect to awards to 'skilled and efficient (suitable) undertakings'.[29] The right of the participants in the awarding process to ensure compliance of the procedure with all public procurement rules is also stipulated as a general principle of German public procurement legislation. Last but not least, a principle which demonstrates the specificity of German procurement legislation is the consideration and protection of the interests of medium-sized companies,[30] which as a policy, almost completely reproduces the legislative decisions underlying the provisions of the New Procurement Directives.[31]

With respect to the transparency principle in particular, there are some material rules dealing with publicity and openness throughout the entire procurement process. However, as a whole, the transparency rules are remarkably simplified and

---

[26] The rules for the award of concessions (*Verordnung über die Vergabe von Konzessionen*) and the public procurement regulation on defence and security (ie *Vergabeveroednung Verteidigung und Sicherheit*) will remain beyond the scope of this work, with the exception of some sporadic references aiming to highlight the general rule.

[27] M Burgi, 'Public Procurement Law in the Federal Republic of Germany: Annual Report' IUS Publicum <www.ius-publicum.com/repository/uploads/09_02_2012_9_43_Burgi.pdf> accessed 25 April 2016, 5.

[28] The fundamental procurement principles are enshrined in §97 GWB (VergRModG).

[29] §122(1) GWB (VergRModG).

[30] Aside from the primary legal protection system for above-thresholds awards, enforceable protection can also be provided by §19 and §20 GWB and the Act Against Unfair Competition (*Gesetz gegen unlauteren Wettbewerb*, Federal Gazette 3 March 2010, as amended), which are applicable in the case of abuse of a dominant position or unfair commercial practices (such as bid rigging) under the German Civil jurisdiction. Finally, Art 3 of the German Basic Law (*Grundgesetz*, Federal Gazette 23 May 1949, as amended) must also be observed, according to which every bidder must be treated equally by the executive branch to which awarding agencies generally belong.

[31] The mandatory/preferable splitting of public procurements into lots with the purpose of awarding each lot to a different SME, as per §97(3) GWB (now §97(4) GWB (VergRModG)), fully corresponds with Art 46 Directive 24/2014/EU.

generalised. There are a variety of well-developed online platforms which publish information on completed tenders.[32] The information is usually limited to basic data such as the contracting authority, the bidder, the type of procedure, the subject and scope of the services, and the contract period.[33] In fact, the GWB refers to 'transparency' only once, in Part IV on the general rules on public procurement, where the main principles are set out. This remains a trend in the new GWB (VergRModG), where the general rule of GWB is expressed as follows:

> The procurement contracts and concessions would be awarded through competition and transparent award procedures.[34]

According to the VergRModVo, the VgV now deals with the main rules on transparency, provision of information and the maintenance of buyer's profiles by the contracting authorities (specific rules should be provided in the secondary legislation of the separate districts).[35]

> The contracting authority shares its intention to award a public contract or to conclude a framework agreement through a contract notice.[36]

> Contract notices, preliminary information, notices and notices on contract changes [...] shall be forwarded to the Publications Office of the European Union by electronic means. The contracting authority must be able to prove the date of dispatch [...] Notices may be published at national level only after the acknowledgment of receipt of the notice by the Publications Office or 48 hours after confirmation of receipt of the notice by the Publications Office of the European Union. The publication may contain only information contained in the notices sent to the Office for Publication of the European Union or published on a buyer's profile. In the national publication the date of submission to the Office of Publications of the European Union or the date of publication on the buyer's profile must be indicated.[37]

An example of a somewhat more detailed approach to legislative rules for transparency is the provision of the VgV which discusses the creation of a 'buyer's profile' in accordance with the option provided by the New Procurement Directives:

> The contracting authority may also set up a buyer profile on the Internet. It contains the disclosure of preliminary information, details about planned or ongoing award procedures, award notice or repealed procurement procedures and all other related to the award information such as contact point, address, e-mail address, telephone and facsimile numbers of the contracting authority.[38]

In comparison to the Bulgarian procurement legislation which overflows with transparency rules and obligations (see Chap. 2 above), the German approach is

---

[32] For example, www.bund.de – the Federal Government's tender platform – e-Allocation, e-Vergabe and others.

[33] In this sense see also 'Public procurement in Germany: overview, Country Q&A' (2013) Us.practicallaw.com <http://us.practicallaw.com/8-521-5162> accessed 25 April 2016.

[34] §97(1) first sentence GWB (VergRModG).

[35] In accordance with §113 GWB (VergRModG).

[36] §37(1) VgV (as amended by the VergRModVo).

[37] §40 (extracts) VgV (as amended by the VergRModVo).

[38] §37(4) VgV (as amended by the VergRModVo).

rather more basic and constructive. The applicable legislation does not pay excessive attention to detailed norms describing each and every single document and/or step which must be published and made available on several different types of platforms and/or media. The idea here (as with all other principles) is rather to stick to the New Procurement Directive's requirements and to ensure a clear and transparent approach to the audit of public expenditure in practice and not just in the letter of the law.

Even where more detailed transparency provisions exist, these are left to the discretion of contracting authorities. The issue of the creation of a 'buyer's profile' and the information to be uploaded has been resolved in a diametrically opposite manner to that adopted by Bulgaria. As already noted in Chap. 2, the creation of a 'buyer's profile' is mandatory for all contracting authorities in the country, while the information required to be published includes at the beginning almost the entire dossier for each public procurement. As the legislator noted that this imperative requirement for an 'absolute transparency' further inconveniences the work of the contracting authorities while its anticorruption effect remains in the realm of wishful thinking, the New PPA has now limited the list of documents to be uploaded on the buyer's profile somewhat, but its use remains mandatory.

Viewed in its entirety, the public procurement system in Germany and the anticorruption measures it undertakes confirm the impression that the effective fight against corruption in the field is not integrally connected to the level of publicity secured throughout the process. According to German legislation, the core rule related to transparency in the award process is the lawful publication of the notice (or invitation, respectively) for the tender. Clearly, legal rules aim to achieve maximum competition in the award serve as a natural corrective to any attempts to engage in corrupt practices. The remaining documentation, including the procurement contract, is not required to be published and promulgated, as long as all the rules applicable to the award of the specific type of procurement have been observed.

The different approaches adopted by the two countries when setting the publicity and transparency obligations in the award of public procurement contracts supports the view that an increase in the number of transparency rules does not necessarily result in a decrease in corruption in the award process, as has already been commented above. Germany is a perfect example in this respect, given the significantly lower levels of corruption in the country. The specific legislative measures applied by Germany for the prevention of and in the fight against corruption in public procurement are discussed below, along with good practices in this field which could be of advantage to countries with similar issues to Bulgaria's.

6.5   The Integrity Pact as a Tool to Optimise Transparency and Curb Corruption

In the context of ensuring sufficient publicity and transparency in the award process, another parallel between Germany and Bulgaria is that TI has introduced its instrument against corruption in the sector in both countries, namely the Integrity Pact.

The results of the pilot implementation of the Pact in Bulgaria in 2012 were discussed in Chap. 4. Germany saw the introduction of a similar Integrity Pact in 2004 in connection with a multi-million procurement for the Berlin Schönefeld Airport Project. The discussion of the Bulgarian experience revealed that the model has its positive characteristics, but also too many poorly functioning elements, which, according to the analysis provided in Chap. 4, limit the opportunities for its additional monitoring functions to achieve appreciable anticorruption results. The main criticism was levelled at the incentive of registering in the White List those participants in the respective procedure which observed the Pact provisions and made no attempts to distort the imperative rules during procurement procedures. The absence of significant sanctions is a considerable drawback of the Bulgarian model of the Pact, all the more so because the national 'specifics' of corruption in Bulgaria cannot justify the sole application of the incentive aspect of the Pact.

The German example in the application of an Integrity Pact reveals the very opposite policy – 'In case of breach of the Schönefeld Airport Integrity Pact, the liquidated damages clause is set at three per cent of the contract value, up to an amount of EUR 50,000. In addition, the authority is entitled to exclude the bidder from the bidding process (and in case of serious violations, also from future bids). This amount is increased to the equivalent of five per cent of the contract value (without a monetary ceiling) if the contractor violates any of the provisions of the Integrity Pact after the contract award. In this case, the authority may cancel the contract and, in the case of serious violation, may exclude the contractor from future bidding processes'.[39]

Such sanctions have a much more motivating and disciplinary effect against attempts to undermine the public procurement by corrupt actions. The German model of the Integrity Pact is thus much more successful and fits the essence of Bulgarian reality much better. This combination of publicity, constant control by an independent entity at each phase of the award process, and the strict sanctions provided could constitute a valid prescription against bribing participants in public procedures in countries suffering severe corruption loopholes like Bulgaria. Of course, the whole concept is for the Pact to be applied sporadically, to isolated procedures, and thus no comprehensive treatment of the problem could be expected, but at least for socially significant projects of exceptionally high value, such a considerably more restrictive draft of the Integrity Pact would be very appropriate.

As demonstrated in previous chapters,[40] the fight against corruption in public procurement systems such as the one in Bulgaria needs to have a clear punitive and restrictive character in order to be effective. Practice has clearly shown that prevention and optional provisions only serve to facilitate the introduction of inoperative mechanisms, such as maintaining data on offending contractors or the encouragement of individual positive practices. Such measures do not yield satisfactory results but only

---

[39] J Olaya, 'Case study: the implementation of an Integrity Pact in the Berlin Schönefeld Airport Project' (Transparency International, 2010).

[40] And especially in view of the cultural and historical grounds for corruption in Bulgaria, as explored in the first chapters.

serve to 'throw dust in the eyes' of the control exercised by the EU over public procurement award and implementation, and corruption levels in the country.

6.6   Contracting Authorities Under GWB

The contracting authorities in the German federal structure under the GWB (VergRModG) are:

1. regional or local authorities as well as their special funds;
2. bodies governed by public law
3. associations whose members fall under (i) or (ii);
4. natural or legal entities from the private sector, as well legal entities form the public sector, distinct from (ii) in certain specific cases (eg engineering and construction of hospitals, sports, recreation or leisure facilities, schools, universities or administrative buildings) being subsidised by more than 50 percent;
5. natural or legal entities under private law which operate in the fields of drinking water, energy supply or transport (ie utilities), having been granted special or exclusive rights by a competent authority;
6. works concessionaires.

This list of possible contracting authorities fully complies with the New Procurement Directives. At the level of public procurement entities, the basic German legislation in the field again demonstrates a close link to the main EU rules, refraining from superfluous 'creativity' in its legislative decisions. Conservative observance of EU law in the spending of public funds is ensured and the players in this part of the market are not needlessly burdened.

In addition to the categories of contracting authorities listed above, German law, once again in accordance with the EU rules, allows joint procurement by means of collaboration between two or more awarding authorities, although this is quite rare. Further, the use of central purchasers is widely practised in Germany (under the Procurement Directives) and this trend has continued with the transposition of the new procurement package which additionally promotes CPBs. The use of a public purchaser from or through which other contracting authorities acquire works, supplies or services is viewed in Germany also as an anticorruption weapon, as detailed below.

6.7   Procedures

In accordance with the New Procurement Directives, German public procurement law provides for all types of award procedures for tender awards above threshold values for classical and utility sector authorities.

However, as a general rule, the contracting authorities have until recently had to apply the open procedure unless otherwise allowed by the GWB.[41] Now, according to the new GWB (VergRModG), the contracting authorities may choose principally between the open and restricted procedures (as is also the case in Bulgaria), only using the other procedures where provided by law.[42] In theory, an incorrect choice of procurement procedure does not mean that an unsuccessful bidder will win a challenge in every case. 'For example, if the unsuccessful bidder is unreliable so that it is excluded from the procurement procedure in any case, there is no causality between the incorrect procurement procedure and the failure of the bid'.[43]

In contrast to other European countries, but quite similarly to Bulgaria, there is insufficient experience with award procedures under the competitive dialogue. Public-private partnerships in Germany are usually awarded using the negotiated procedure.

The use of the procedures available under the New Procurement Directives is almost the same in both countries.

However, the prevalence of the open procedure as an explicit rule under the German legislation was by definition a good anticorruption practice, praised by the author of this book. Although the idea of the German legislator to give more freedom and flexibility to the contracting authorities is logical, the open procedure ensures to the greatest extent that the award will not be influenced by subjectivity and that there will be no substantive changes to the preliminary goals of the respective contracting authority. Therefore, the prior German legislative regime seemed to be more satisfactory for Member States such as Bulgaria. The open procedure is also commonly used in Bulgaria, but there is no imperative requirement that this procedure should be followed as a priority. Consequently, negotiated procedures without a call for competition has been used to achieve corrupt aims in a number of cases (see Chap. 5). With the transposition of the New Procurement Directives, the opportunities for chicanery in the use of the negotiated procedure without prior publication are significantly limited, but it is nonetheless still a good idea to put to public debate the option for Bulgarian legislation (and other Member States with corruption issues) to give legal priority to the open procedure. This will, on the one hand, increase competition in the sector, which will inevitably obstruct the achievement of corrupt schemes related to the elimination of candidates and participants from the procedures. It is also a much more valid approach to safeguard the principle of transparency in the award process instead of endlessly inventing new rules which require the accumulation and repetition of information. A mechanism which requires contracting authorities to motivate and justify their using any of the lighter award regimes would serve to discipline contracting authorities and would have a distinct anticorruption effect. It is however possible to view such prioritisation of the open

---

[41] See §101(7) GWB.

[42] §119(2) GWB (VergRModG). By way of exception, an awarding authority subject to the SektVO (§13(2)) can choose freely between the open procedure, the restricted procedure, the negotiated procedure with a call for competition and the competitive dialogue.

[43] J Ellison and L Baudrihaye (eds) *International Comparative Legal Guides to Public Procurement 2014* (London: Global Legal Group Ltd, 2013) ch 10, 70 et seq.

procedure as encumbering and impeding bidders and running contrary to the desire for a more efficient and less burdensome award process. But if a balance can be found between a low administrative burden and the absence of additional bureaucratic obligations on contracting authorities, the preferred use of the open procedure could be 'absorbed' and organised in a manner similar to the one previously adopted in Germany to combat corruption.

6.8   Award Criteria

Unsurprisingly, award criteria under the German public procurement system are also fully harmonised with the EU requirements, without too many differences. Until the New Procurement Directives become operational, the awarding authorities were empowered to choose between awarding the contract on the basis of the 'most economically advantageous tender' or on the basis of the 'lowest price' alone. However, a German law national characteristic is the predominance of the 'most economically advantageous tender' even before the transposition of the new EU rules. In accordance with §127(1) GWB (VergRModG) again '[t]he economically most advantageous tender shall be accepted' as a rule. In the words of Burgi (2012), 'the price is not the only decisive criterion. But without doubt, the price is still the most crucial factor when deciding about the most economically advantageous tender'.[44]

Most frequently, contracting authorities use a combination of price and quality criteria to determine the most economically advantageous tender. In fact, sometimes lawyers forget even to mention 'the lowest price' as a possible criteria[45] (or now – sub-criteria) when describing the German public procurement system. However, such a criteria is of course permitted, and is used mainly in the utilities sector – there are a number of supply and service contracts where the lowest price could be the only possible award criteria (eg waste disposal services and public transport).

As observed in a comparative report from 2012:

> Interestingly, where quality criteria are used to determine the most economically advantageous tender, German judicial rulings call for greater disclosure of the criteria and sub-criteria on which quality will be assessed. It is not clear whether this results in greater weightings being attributed to design.[46]

From an EU perspective, prioritising the 'most economically advantageous tender' is clearly a good anticorruption measure, which broadens the scope of the criteria evaluated in the course of a procurement procedure and provides the opportunity for a

---

[44] See above (n 27) 6.

[45] eg A Hantschel and A Schlange-Schöningen, 'Public Contracts in Germany' (2010) Executive Agency for Competitiveness and Innovation (Leaflet) <www.een-ireland.ie/eei/assets/documents/uploaded/general/Public%20Contracts%20in%20Germany.pdf> accessed 25 April 2016.

[46] RIBA, 'Comparative Procurement: Procurement regulation and practice in Germany, Sweden and the UK' (2012) Report prepared by contributors from Burges Salmon LLP <www.architecture.com/Files/RIBAHoldings/PolicyAndInternationalRelations/Policy/PublicAffairs/2012/ComparativeProcurement.pdf> accessed 25 April 2016, 6.

more complex rating by the contracting authority. This approach was apparently taken into consideration during the preparation of the New Procurement Directives, where the 'lowest price' criteria is no longer available as a separate criteria, save where the most economically advantageous tender is identified on the basis of price alone.

The situation in Bulgaria is quite the reverse – before transposition of the new procurement package the 'most economically advantageous tender' was used more often by the contracting authorities than the 'lowest price' criteria, despite the fact that the then applicable legislation did not provide an explicit provision in that respect. As was discussed in the previous chapter, however, this is a negative trend given that the analysis of the most common infringements and corruption loopholes indicates that the 'most economically advantageous offer' criteria is used specifically for corruption incentives. The more complex and varied the criteria, the better the chance of selecting the 'pre-approved' candidate. That is why the amendment introduced into the New Procurement Directives is not particularly beneficial, given that in Member States combating corruption in the award of public procurements, like Bulgaria, barring the 'lowest price' (in its 'old and familiar' form) criteria could serve to further spread corruption, despite the fact that the amendment intends to achieve the very opposite.

In view of the above, Bulgaria has harmonised its model with the German one in the course transposing the common rules applicable to all Member States. However, given the 'national characteristics' of corruption in the country, the legislator has cleverly not precluded the possibility of the 'the lowest price' criteria being used as a sub-criteria, which is worth noting as a proper legislative solution. To eliminate the use of this criteria completely, as the New Procurement Directives allow,[47] would have a detrimental effect on Member States like Bulgaria, as the opportunities for creative corruption through the use of the 'most economically advantageous tender' could extend beyond recognition. It can thus be concluded that this is a decision of the Bulgarian legislator in the right direction and it is one of the few times where the legislator has appropriately considered the nation's characteristics and needs.

6.9 Appeal

The possibilities for award procedures to be challenged by unsuccessful bidders are viewed as the 'dichotomy' of the German public procurement system by some authors.[48] The review system only applies to contracts above EU thresholds.[49] The GWB (VergRModG) provides in §160, that:

> Every undertaking which has an interest in the contract and claims that its rights […] were violated by non-compliance with the provisions governing the awarding of public contracts

---

[47] Art 67(2) last paragraph Directive 2014/24/EU.

[48] See above (n 43).

[49] Below the EU thresholds, the system of protection for bidders is significantly weaker. Bidders are generally restricted to administrative complaints, where the remedies are limited to compensation for damages (if a legal provision was not complied with in the award procedure and the procurement contract was not awarded to the claimant).

has the right to file an application. In doing so, it must be shown that the undertaking has suffered a loss, or may be about to suffer a loss, in consequence of the alleged violation of provisions governing the awarding of public contracts.

There are two levels of review body: the public procurement tribunals (*Vergabekammern*) acting at first instance,[50] and the award senates at the Higher Regional Courts (*Oberlandesgerichte*) at second instance.

Generally, an interested party which is able to demonstrate a violation of rights must, as a first step, seek review from the awarding body, ie the contracting authority. The objection must be raised 'without undue delay',[51] which in effect means immediately (within a few days). If the objection is rejected by the contracting authority, the bidder has fifteen days in which to commence first instance proceedings. As a rule, an appeal before the public procurement tribunal suspends further implementation of the public procurement procedure.

The framework of appeal provided in Bulgarian legislation and reviewed in Chap. 4 does not in reality provide specific time or opportunity for contracting authorities to respond to an appeal. The appeal is instead sent directly to the first instance (ie the CPC) and within the time limits designated for the investigation of an appeal by the CPC, the contracting authority may react and correct errors, omissions and other defects in the procurement, where such are deemed to exist.[52] German legislation, on the other hand, allows contracting authorities much wider opportunities to react independently thus avoiding the unnecessary squandering of the resources of the appellate authority, and allowing the contracting authority to take individual responsibility for the public procurement at hand. In particular, where corruption is established, the contracting authority may well react in good time and not within the period of the investigation under the official appeal, which contributes to quicker resolution of any imperfections in the award (if of course this is possible, which may also depend on the phase of the procedure). This option, provided to the contracting authority along with the suspensive effect of the appeal, discussed below (at both first and second instance)[53] has a relatively stronger disciplining effect on the contracting authority and on other participants in the procedure and could constitute a useful approach to the appeal of procurement procedures in Bulgaria.

The automatic suspensive effect of the application for an award review in the form of a prohibition of the award, is an essential part of the remedies procedure under German law. 'If the public procurement tribunal informs the contracting entity in writing about the application for review, the latter must not make the award prior to the decision of the public procurement tribunal and before the expiry of the

---

[50] The awards chamber of the Federal Government at the Federal Cartel Office reviews public contracts awarded by the Federal Government, while the awards chambers of the separate *Bundesländer* have jurisdiction over the contracts attributable to the individual states.

[51] §60(3)(4) GWB (VergRModG) (the '*unverzügliche Rüge*').

[52] Art 121(8) PPA: 'The contracting authority may eliminate the violation until receiving the notification […] for completed investigations under the appeal by the Commission for Protection of Competition'.

[53] §160 GWB (VergRModG).

period for a complaint'.[54] An award in violation of this prohibition will be considered null and void.

This legislative solution, adopted in Germany, varies greatly from the Bulgarian situation, where – despite the numerous debates over and amendments to the PPA and the opportunity for this to be decided presented by the New PPA – there is no automatic suspensive effect, with the exception of appeals against the decision of the contracting authority announcing the contractor selected. This approach results in the conclusion of contracts despite concerns about infringements (unless the court grants the appellant suspension of the procedure for the period of the appeal, at its own discretion and after an explicit request by the appellant) and strongly discourages bidders to attempt to protect their rights before the respective control and appellate authorities. Consequently, the absence of an automatic suspensive effect also affects cases of procurement awards involving well-implemented corruption – the remaining bidders see no point in appealing against acts or omissions of contracting authorities because costs will inevitably be incurred during the appeal proceedings, and the entire process will be protracted indefinitely before any compensation can be obtained, even if the complaint is upheld. A significant proportion of unlawful public expenditure is thus not even challenged. Automatic suspensive effect is a very positive practice, especially as the GWB (VergRModG) provides sufficient guarantees that suspension of the procedure and delays in procurement implementation will not have a negative effect on the social and economic relations sought to be resolved.[55]

Currently, under the New PPA, only appeals against the final decision of the contracting authority have an automatic suspensive effect. The model adopted allows the decision selecting the contractor to enter into force only after all preceding contracting authority decisions have entered into force and have not been appealed, or, where appealed, where the dispute has been resolved. The appeal against the decision selecting the contractor thus suspends the procedure at the Procedure Conduct Phase (i.e. the contract conclusion). In all other cases appeals against the acts and omissions of the contracting authority do not have an automatic suspensive effect (although suspension of the procedure could be requested and possibly, but rarely, approved by the first instance of appeal, as discussed above). The Bulgarian contracting authority is thus able to protect its rights with regard to an appeal against the procedure within the first instance proceedings period, and then to proceed with the procurement itself, which could actually be finalised and the contract concluded while an appeal against the notification for the very same procurement is still under review. This is most

---

[54] §169(1) GWB (VergRModG).

[55] For example, §169(2) GWB (VergRModG) states that: 'The public procurement tribunal may allow the contracting entity […] to award the contract after the expiry of two weeks after the announcement of this decision if, taking into account all interests which may be impaired as well as the interests of the general public in the quick conclusion of the award procedure, the negative consequences of delaying the award until the end of the review outweigh the advantages involved. In its assessment, the public procurement tribunal shall take account of the interests of the general public that the contracting entity carries out its tasks efficiently. The public procurement tribunal shall also consider the overall prospects of the applicant to win the award in the award procedure. The prospects of success of the application for review need not be taken into account in every case'.

certainly imprudent. A much better organised anticorruption policy would require the adoption of a model similar to the German one, where the appeal can suspend a procedure at any phase and the contracting authority is first given the individual opportunity, within a short period, to respond to the appellant's claim and to rectify or to decline to rectify any shortcomings alleged.

This difference in the two approaches towards the option for direct contact with the contracting authority and the lodging of objections against its actions and decisions prior to referring the issue to an appellate body, as well as the different scope of the suspensive effect in the two systems arises from the options left open by Directive 66/2007/EC, which provides that 'Member States may require that the person concerned first seek review with the contracting authority. In that case, Member States shall ensure that the submission of such an application for review results in immediate suspension of the possibility to conclude the contract'.[56] The Bulgarian legislator has chosen not to avail itself of this additional opportunity, which, as has already been commented, could have a considerable anticorruption and instructive effect on all participants in award procedures.

In Germany it is only after an objection has been lodged with the contracting authority that the legal facility for the actual appeal before *the first instance* – the public procurement tribunals,[57] is occasioned. Each public procurement tribunal is competent to issue an order to stop a procedure (as is usual, as discussed above), to alter the status of the proceedings, to revise the decisions taken, or in some exceptional cases, even to intervene in the procedure[58] if the procedure is not suspended.[59]

Once an award has been made and the procurement contract has been signed, such award cannot be revoked.[60] The parties concerned may seek compensation by claiming damages against the contracting authority. This is yet another imperative measure which would most definitely have a 'sobering' effect in Bulgaria as well, causing the contracting authorities to succumb less readily to corruption. It assists interested parties seeking to protect their rights at the earliest possible moment, and indeed on the slightest suspicion of corrupt interference in the choice of the contracting authority. This also encourages internal control over the award process exercised by the contracting authority itself, which would, in this case consciously strive to avoid infringements in the procedure, because any appeals against its acts and actions would suspend the procedure. Moreover, where a contract has been concluded by means of a corrupt procedure, then the parties concerned can seek compensation. Bulgarian legislation of course also provides the option of claims for damages under general civil law.[61] This option is used, albeit increasingly rarely, and as has already been

---

[56] Art 1(5) Remedies Directive.

[57] §160(3)(4) GWB (VergRModG).

[58] §169(3) GWB (VergRModG).

[59] See also 'Report concerning the Study on Pre-Contract Problem-Solving Systems' (Copenhagen: The Danish Competition Authority 2002).

[60] §156(2) GWB (VergRModG).

[61] Pursuant to the Obligations and Contracts Act, SG 2/5.12.1950, as amended, and the Commercial Act, SG 48/18.6.1991; effective as of 1 July 1991, as amended.

analysed in the broader sense, the multitude of procedural rules and the absence of guarantees of a lawful conclusion to appeal proceedings often discourage interested parties from seeking to protect their rights at a later stage.

Last but not least, the GWB (VergRModG) has created another disciplining measure concerning appeals (once again on the basis of the general rules set out by Directive 66/2007/EC) and which also has an anticorruption effect. In several strictly defined cases (and as an exception to the rule that a contract, once concluded, cannot be annulled) the public procurement tribunal is competent to declare the procurement award to be ineffective *ab initio* (*Umwirksamkeit von Anfang an*).[62] Where the contracting authority failed to inform rejected bidders and wait for the conclusion of a contract or awarded the contract without including other candidates in the procedure and assuring a minimum level of competition, the contract may be deemed by the tribunal to be ineffective.[63] 'Thus, it can be concluded that an independent legal procedure has been established for primary legal protection in contract award matters'.[64]

Naturally, following the transposition of the Remedies Directive, the Bulgarian PPA and then the New PPA also adopted a similar measure but with several quite significant differences from the German model, which render the legal arrangement 'weaker' and the anticorruption effect much smaller. Caranta (2011) has observed that:

> The Directive allows Member States to choose whether the ineffectiveness operates retroactively or for the future only, and this both accommodates potential different approaches [...] Unsurprisingly given the novelty of the remedy, a number of Member States rather preferred to limit ineffectiveness to the proactive effects, even if this impacts the effectiveness of the remedy (the so called 'ineffectiveness light'). [...]. In other jurisdictions, however, ineffectiveness operates retroactively. This is the case for instance in France, Romania and in Germany'.[65]

Bulgaria has respectively chosen the lighter option by determining that concluded contracts are voidable in such cases.[66] Under Bulgarian law ineffectiveness can result in (a) nullity of the contract, but which can also be expressed in (b) its voidability: a loophole has been left for the correction/restoration of the challenged

---

[62] §135 GWB (VergRModG).

[63] German law differentiates between ineffectiveness and annulment. The difference is mainly that ineffectiveness provides the option for remedying the defect and is also applicable from a certain point in time onwards. Applicable is also ineffectiveness '*ex tunc*' or '*ab initio*', which, in practice, coincides with the general concept of 'annulment' – there is no option for remedies and effect is retroactive. Quite separately, ineffectiveness can be regarded as one of the possible remedies set out in Art 2d Remedies Directive, which has been transposed into the GWB (VergRModG).

[64] See above (n 43).

[65] R Caranta, 'The Comparatist's Lens on Remedies in Public Procurement' (2011) Istituto Universitario di Studi Europei ECLI Working Papers Series No 2011-1/2-ECLI <http://working-papers.iuse.it/wp-content/uploads/2011/08/2011-02-ECLI.pdf> accessed 25 April 2016, 9.

[66] Art 41b(1) PPA: 'The following contracts or framework agreements shall be ineffective in respect of the persons covered under Art 122i, para 1, where concluded: 1. Without a public procurement award procedure despite the existence of grounds for conduct of such procedure; 2. Upon legally non-conforming application of the grounds of Art 4, Art 12(1), Art 90(1), Art 103(2) or Art 119c(3)'. The provisions listed cover cases where the contracts concluded fall beyond the scope of the Act: unlawful conduct of negotiated procedure without prior notification, etc.

contractual relations. This means that the legislator has provided the option for contracts concluded without conduct of a public procurement procedure and in complete disregard of competition rules, as well as contracts concluded on the basis of unlawful application of the negotiated procedure without publication (again, harming the competition in the sector) not to be declared void. In fact, contracts with such severe defects[67] may be 'repaired' and continue to be effective between the parties (if ruled so by court).[68] This is definitely to the detriment of the anticorruption efforts in Bulgaria, where the issue of corruption is much more serious and poorly resolved than in Germany; which itself adopted the more restrictive model proposed by Directive 66/2007/EC, as discussed above.

Following an appeal to the public procurement tribunal, the decision may be challenged before the German Higher Regional Courts, acting at *second instance*. Appeal at the second instance again has a suspensive effect, this time with respect to the decision of the first instance body.[69] The Higher Regional Court has the competence to confirm the decision of the first instance or to overrule it. It is further possible to return the appeal to the first instance level and to oblige the respective public procurement tribunal to redecide the case with consideration of the instructions provided by the Higher Regional Court. Several hundred award review procedures are conducted each year under the GWB regime.[70]

6.10 Corruption in Public Procurement and the German Way to Combat It

6.10.1 Corruption Prevention Legislation

Germany is a signatory of the OECD Anti-Bribery Convention, UNCAC, and the Civil and Criminal Law Conventions against Corruption.[71] In addition, Germany is also a member of GRECO. However, Germany has not yet ratified UNCAC nor the

---

[67] Discussed in Chap. 5 as a common form of corruption aiming at the selection of a preferred candidate and elimination of the other participants in the procedure.

[68] With the new rules provided by the GWB (VergRModG), there are now some exceptions where ineffectiveness does not occur, eg the contracting authority considers that the contract without prior publication of a contract notice in the OJEU is permitted and would not be declared ineffective; the contracting authority has published a notice in the OJEU, with which it expressed its intention to conclude the contract etc. However, the disciplining effect discussed above is not reduced, in contrast with the Bulgarian approach.

[69] According to §173(1) GWB (VergRModG): 'The suspensive effect shall lapse two weeks after the expiry of the time limit for the complaint'.

[70] More general statistics indicate that around 17 percent of the applications before the public procurement tribunals were successful.

[71] Civil Law Convention on Corruption (adopted 4 November 1999) CETS 174; and Criminal Law Convention on Corruption (adopted 27 January 1999) CETS 173.

Civil and criminal law conventions,[72] and has been repeatedly criticised over the past decade by numerous international organisations for being 'a notorious laggard on implementing adequate anti-corruption measures'.[73]

Various German legislative acts deal with corruption offences: the main act is the German Criminal Code (*Strafgesetzbuch* – StGB).[74] It criminalises giving and receiving bribes in the public (§331–338) and private (§299–302) sectors. The main texts regulating corruption in public bids and in public administration (one of the types of corruption with a high percentage of incidence – around 35 percent over the last few years)[75] are §298 and §331 et seq StGB. §298 regulates criminal liability for restricting competition through agreements in the context of public bids and targets bidders who present an offer based on an unlawful agreement so as to influence the decision of the contracting authority. §331 et seq StGB regulate criminal liability for bribery in the public sector, where both the taking and giving of bribes are criminal offences.[76] Particularly serious cases of bribery of a public official can be punished by imprisonment for up to 10 years. In addition, the suppression of corruption at international level is dealt with by the International Bribery Act (*Gesetz zur Bekämpfung Internationaler Bestechung*)[77] and the EU Bribery Act (*EU-Bestechungsgesetz*).[78] There are also mandatory guidelines and regulations relating to the prevention of corruption in the public sector.[79]

---

[72] ie The Council of Europe Civil Law Convention on Corruption was signed by Germany 1999; The Council of Europe Criminal Law Convention on Corruption was signed by Germany 1999, The Additional Protocol to the Criminal Law Convention on Corruption of the Council of Europe was signed by Germany 2003 CETS 191.

[73] A Pulito, 'Germany the anti-corruption laggard' (2012) Academia.edu <www.academia. edu/2225981/Germany_the_anti-corruption_laggard> accessed 25 April 2016, 1.

[74] Federal Gazette I, p. 945, p. 3322/13.11.1998, as amended.

[75] Information taken from the official statistics of the German Federal Police Office (*Bundescriminalamt*) (2015) *BKA Startseite* <www.bka.de/DE/Home/homepage__node.html?__ nnn=true> accessed 25 April 2016.

[76] eg taking bribes (§331 StGB): 'It is a criminal offence if a public official demands, allows himself to be promised or accepts a personal benefit for himself or on behalf of a third party for the discharge of an official duty. 'Benefit' would be any advantage to which the public official is not legally entitled and is not necessarily pecuniary in nature'.

Taking bribes intended to encourage violation of official duties (§332 StGB): 'It is the aggravated form of the offence in section 331 and requires the performance of an official act that violates an official duty'.

Giving bribes (§333 and §334 StGB): 'Under §333 and §334 of StGB, promising and giving bribes to public officials is a criminal offence. §334 additionally requires the performance of an official act that violates an official duty'.

[77] Federal Gazette II 2327/1998, as amended.

[78] Federal Gazette II, p. 2340; III, p. 18888/10.9.1998, as amended.

[79] eg 'Guidelines of the Federal Government on the Prevention of Corruption within the Federal Administration' (*Richtlinie der Bundesregierung zur Korruptionsprävention in der Bundesverwaltung*) (2004) Bmi.bund.de <www.bmi.bund.de/SharedDocs/Downloads/DE/ Themen/OED_Verwaltung/Korruption_Sponsoring/Richtlinie_zur_Korruptionspraevention_in_ der_Bundesverwaltung.html> accessed 25 April 2016.

6.10.2 Anticorruption Strategies and Institutions

Funk (2014) has noted that a report by the OECD Working Group on Bribery in March 2011 characterised Germany as having assumed a 'leading position' in the investigation and prosecution of foreign bribery cases.

> Germany's enforcement has increased steadily and resulted in a significant number of prosecutions and sanctions imposed in foreign bribery-related cases against individuals.[80]

This, as will be explained in detail below, is precisely one of the keys to success in the fight against corruption which should most certainly be adopted by all countries. *Per argumentum a fortiori* this applies with full force to countries such as Bulgaria, which not only have a serious problem with corruption at all levels of government, but whose specific cultural and historical characteristics reveal an acute need for the adoption of effective, strict and 'condemning' measures against offenders.

Further, according to the Business Anti-Corruption Portal, German corruption strategies are commonly based on the Concept of Corruption Prevention and Combating adopted by the Standing Conference of Federal State Ministers and Senators of the Interior (IMK) in 1995. This nationwide anticorruption strategy outlines key concepts and goals in German corruption prevention, and its implementation is monitored through periodic reports to the IMK, submitted by the supervisory bodies in the federal states' administrative departments.[81]

The prosecution authority responsible for investigating corporate or business fraud is the competent Public Prosecutor's Office (*Staatsanwaltschaft*). At federal level, the Federal Criminal Agency (*Bundeskriminalamt*) and the relevant municipal authorities are also fundamental in monitoring and combating corruption at each institutional level.

Further, in Germany the function of the courts of auditors as controlling organs is well developed and very strong.[82] Financial audit is divided between the State Courts of Auditors, which examines the financial management of the states, and the Federal Court of Auditors (*Bundesrechnungshof*), which examines financial management at the federal level. Both institutions have budgetary autonomy, meaning that each individual State Court of Auditors adopts and implements its own budget and has its own external audit institution.[83]

---

[80] T M Funk, 'Germany's Foreign Anti-Corruption Efforts – Second-Tier No More' (2014) 1 *ZDAR* 24. Funk also cites the OECD Working Group on Bribery.

[81] Business-anti-corruption.com (2015) <www.business-anti-corruption.com/country-profiles/europe-central-asia/germany/initiatives/public-anti-corruption-initiatives.aspx> accessed 25 April 2016.

[82] As evaluated by Transparency International in the German NIS Report 2012 (above (n 8) 35). The human and financial resources of this institution were found to be appropriate to their duties and its governance was assessed as excellent.

[83] The structure of the Federal Court of Auditors, the appointment of its members and the procedures required for a decision to be reached are regulated by the Federal Audit Office Act (*Bundesrechnungshofgesetz*, Federal Gazette I, p. 160/5.2.2009, as amended) and supplementary

This organisation of *ex ante* efficiency control over public expenditure is exactly the reverse of what is observed in Bulgaria (in Chap. 4 of this book). As noted, the NAO in Bulgaria is the only comparatively independent institution (or at least is meant to be) which should in practice play a key role in the control of public procurement and serve as the main disciplinary non-judicial body, implementing violation prevention, including the prevention of corrupt activities of all kinds, in award procedures. The conclusions reached in Chap. 4, namely that the role and functions of the NAO as a control body need to be speedily enhanced (as opposed to what has been happening in reality over the last few years) are confirmed in practice by the German model. Germany has a well-developed and active system of Courts of Auditors, which are independent institutions with an anticorruption impact. Due to its division into districts, this system is also divided into several levels but performs, nevertheless, the same functions within the separate regions. Germany's model is thus quite dissimilar to the Bulgarian model, with its two different financial control bodies (PFIA and NAO), which though differently organised, in essence have a lot of overlapping activities.

The Federal Court of Auditors is a complex body comprising nine audit divisions and around 50 units. Each audit division is headed by senior audit directors and consists of several audit units and steering units. Audit decisions are adopted by panels made up of the senior audit director and audit directors. Panels of three members may also be formed in certain cases. If the three-member panel fails to reach agreement on a particular point, the issue is referred to the Senate, which is the supreme decision-making body of the Court of Auditors. This complex system of units is organised precisely so that these bodies can reach objective and independent decisions in the event of opposing opinions between panels or divisions.

The Federal Court of Auditors carries out annual audits on the activities and financial management of the entire German administrative apparatus and additionally is competent to examine bodies or other third parties outside the federal administration where these receive or handle federal funds.

Another fundamental and substantial difference between the main auditing bodies of Germany and Bulgaria can be found in the much wider rights enjoyed by the Federal Court of Auditors, which in many cases is not content to only establish and report infringements.[84] It may also issue instructions on how contracting authorities are to act and in practice it intervenes in the organisation of the award process. It also schedules a follow-up on how its recommendations have been applied at a later stage (the following audit year). According to an annual report of the Federal Court of Auditors, for example:[85]

---

provisions. The audit functions, objects, criteria and procedures are outlined in the Federal Budget Code (*Bundeshaushaltsordnung*, BGBl. I S. 1284/19.8.1969, as amended – BHO), the Budgeting Principles Act (*Haushaltsgrundsätzegesetz*, BGBl. I S. 1273/19.8.1969, as amended) and other specialised acts.

[84] The Bulgarian NAO also has sanctioning functions as part of its competence, which recent years have occasionally been removed than restored by the legislator within endless amendments to the relevant legislation (see Chap. 4).

[85] 'Annual Report on Federal Financial Management 2013' (Abridged English Version) <www.bundesrechnungshof.de/en/veroeffentlichungen/bemerkungen-jahresberichte-en/dateien/2013-annual-report> accessed 25 April 2016, 29.

> We found that the division [of the Foreign Office providers] in charge of procurement and contract awards frequently purchased items inefficiently and non-competitively by ordering them from particular manufacturers or suppliers with which it maintained long-standing business relationships. [...] Budgetary and procurement law require that contracting authorities procure goods and services efficiently under a formal procurement procedure, having special regard to open competition. The awarding of public contracts is particularly vulnerable to corruption. The Federal Government's Guidelines on Corruption Prevention call for preventive measures. One of them is to separate the awarding process from procurement planning functions and the specifications of the goods and services to be procured [...]
> We demanded that the Federal Foreign Office reorganise the procurement of furnishings and office equipment for its foreign missions, comply henceforth with budgetary and procurement law and take steps to mitigate risks of corruption. Furthermore, we suggested that suitable standardised products be procured more frequently either by means of blanket agreements or by having the needed items purchased locally by the respective foreign mission in order to achieve better bargains and save transport costs.

In addition, the Federal Court of Auditors focuses much more on efficiency control than is the case with the NAO. Anticorruption policies have a much stronger presence during audits and thus the functions of the main auditing body are much more meaningful than those of a purely verifying body, like the NAO.

Unfortunately, as was noted in the previous chapters, the NAO in recent years has become the object of far too many and far too contradictory political games, which have sullied its image and broken the anticorruption powers which should presumably be inherent to such an 'independent' auditing body. German practice definitely provides a positive example of the image that a Member States audit office, with an overall status similar to that of the Bulgarian one, should strive to acquire, if such a body is to be expected to fight corruption in public contracts and provide guidance as to efficiency. Bearing in mind, however, that the initial legal framework regulating the Bulgarian NAO was established with the active participation of experts from the German Federal Court of Auditors, following which the act was repealed and rewritten several times, all hopes for the reintroduction of Germany's good practices obviously remain entirely in the hands of the political class.

6.11   Successful Pillars to Raise Against Corruption in the Award of Public Contracts

As noted above, when a public tender criteria is the 'most economically advantageous offer', German law requires an increased level of transparency and disclosure. However, the transparency principle, although of great importance for the conduct of legal and enforceable procurement procedures, is not primarily focused on combating bribery. The whole strategy of the German public procurement system is rather aimed at limiting any attempts at abuse of power. The analysis in this book shows that the successful German procurement process rests on three main pillars combating corrupt efforts in the sector: *first*, adequate legislative decisions, providing clear and unambiguous rules; *secondly*, state-of-the-art procedures, including e-procurement and whistle-blowing systems which are in the process of development; and, *thirdly*, centralised awards (ie separation between the requisition and award entities).

6.11.1   Adequate Legislative Decisions Providing Clear and Unambiguous Rules

Several specific German public procurement regulations have already been noted above as having an impact on curbing corruption. The rules and/or restrictions discussed below (based on the New Procurement Directives but also expanded, where applicable) are explicitly constructed, or contain important elements to combat bribery and fraud in procurement awards.

(i) Under German public procurement law there are serious requirements as to the *suitability of bidders*. In conformity with the New Procurement Directives, candidates must demonstrate their expertise, economic and technical capacity and their reliability, by submitting proof and declarations as requested by the contracting authorities in the tender notice. Two-stage award procedures, such as the restricted procedures, contain a prequalification stage, where competitors allowed to submit bids are selected on the basis of best economic and financial standing and technical or professional expertise. After having submitted their bids, bidders are shortlisted and assessed on the basis of the award criteria. The primary means in the new EU legislation for dealing with corrupt candidates, namely their exclusion, is of course also part of the legal framework of Germany.[86]

Germany has established practice at the prequalification stage of preliminary 'filtering' of suitable candidates from unsuitable ones, which results in significant reduction in the workload of the bureaucratic machine at the candidate assessment and ranking stage. Prequalification means bidder suitability is verified within a public procedure which precedes the award procedure and is independent of the procurement in accordance with the definitive requirements introduced back in 2006 under VOB/A.[87] As proof of suitability (expert knowledge, capacity for work and reliability) registration on a publicly available list of the association for prequalification of construction undertakings (nationwide prequalification list) is admissible and may be requested directly by the contracting entity. Additional evidence relevant to the specific procurement may also be required. With the transposition of the new EU rules the ambition is for this prequalification list to be aligned to e-Certis and both systems to work together for a much easier procurement process.

---

[86] §123 and §124 GWB (VergRModG).

[87] The Federal Ministry of Environment, Nature Conservation, Building and Nuclear Safety introduced a new version of the guidelines for pre-qualification of contractors on 15 October 2015, which entered into force on 2 January 2016.

Germany has even developed a system of voluntary prequalification comprising of designated bureaus which conduct the prequalification and registration of applicant undertakings into the relevant register. In essence, Germany makes proper use of the opportunities offered by Article 52(1) Directive 2004/18/EC, which permits Member States, when assessing the suitability of candidates, to rely on official certification lists.[88] This opportunity makes life significantly easier for the Member States and ensures harmonisation of certificates. There is criticism in Germany as to how effective this procedure is, and whether it is overly expensive.[89] Ultimately, however, opinions are almost entirely unanimous that the implementation of the public procurement regime following previous implementation of the complex procedure of assessing candidate capacity is tremendously facilitated and allows contracting authorities to concentrate on evaluating the procurement award criteria.[90] Furthermore, the New Procurement Directives also support the German model, by focusing on simplifying the award procedures, with the phase dedicated to assessment of the tenderers' suitability being significantly facilitated by the implementation of e-Certis, as well as by providing the option to shift responsibility for verification of suitability to the respective participant or candidate, who is thereby enabled to submit a self-declaration as valid proof of suitability for participation in a particular procedure using the ESPD.

When considering the anticorruption effect of such a preliminary pre-registration, however, it is obvious that the proposal to follow the German model should not be discounted. Bulgaria is an example of a Member State which could profitably make use of the German pre-qualification model.[91] The analysis of the most frequent offences and corruption schemes made in this work reveals that despite explicit prohibitions, candidate selection criteria and candidate assessment criteria are often wrongly mixed up and/or used precisely for the selection of a previously agreed bidder. By transferring the evaluation of selection criteria into a separate stage, perhaps even performed by a separate entity independent of the contracting authority, this infringement could be completely precluded. Contracting authorities would be free to select only from among suitable bidders and, further, would not waste time reviewing documents intended solely to evidence the suitability of the candidates and not directly related to the subject of the procurement.

(ii) Related to the foregoing, and in view of the expected transposition of the New Procurement Directives, the 'self-cleaning' mechanism[92] is also borrowed

---

[88] ie lists maintained by certification bodies established in public and/or private law.

[89] In this sense see also C Sesterhenn, 'Erfolg durch Präqualifikation in Deutschland und Europa?' (2009) Seminar paper: 11th Interdisciplinary Conference of Construction Economics and Building Law in Hanover (*Seminarunterlagen zur 11 Interdisziplinären Tagung für Baubetriebswirtschaft und Baurecht, Hannover*) <www.semina.de/verlag/pdf/11_praequalifikation.pdf> accessed 25 April 2016, 72.

[90] Ibid.

[91] The next chapter will review the Austrian model which is not mandatory but also achieves positive results.

[92] As envisaged in Art 57(6) Directive 24/2014/EU.

from German law,[93] which is connected to the bidder's suitability but which also stands as an effective anticorruption measure from the German perspective. The idea is that in addition to the basic rule that public procurement law permits the exclusion of unreliable tenderers, the reverse option is also enabled where the tenderer takes effective measures to ensure that omissions do not recur in the future and provides sufficient proof to permit them to regain reliability and not to be excluded (at the contracting authorities' discretion). The participants are highly motivated to restore their reputations which means that their subsequent actions should be fundamentally averse to further acts of corruption. This mechanism was strongly criticised and discussed in connection with its implementation in the New Procurement Directives. In countries like Germany and Austria it proves its anticorruption effect, transferring responsibility to the candidates in procurement procedures and disciplining them to seek 'to clear their name' on their own initiative, in order to participate in further procedures. It is uncertain, however, whether this mechanism would have similar effects in all Member States. With respect to Bulgaria, or other countries with wide-spread corruption in procurement, where the very existence of discretion for a contracting authority inevitably opens loopholes for corruption, this is rather doubtful. 'Besides, when the assessment of 'self-cleaning' is made by the contracting authorities, there is also a risk that similar situations will be treated differently'.[94] The New PPA has already exactly duplicated the self-cleaning provisions of the New Procurement Directives. However, the provisions are absolutely not suitable for the Bulgarian reality and some parts are indeed not even possible in practice, eg the participant 'has exhaustively clarified the facts and circumstances, actively cooperated with the competent authorities and fulfilled specific prescriptions, technical, organisational and staffing measures by which to prevent new crimes or violations'.[95] This is neither feasible nor can actual compliance be demonstrated securely. The decision therefore remains at the sole subjective discretion of the contracting authority.[96]

(iii) Further, the *financial consistency* of the candidate is of particular importance for the German model. The applicable budgetary legislation must be observed in public procurement,[97] which means that the contractor must have access to sufficient funds for contract performance. This financial aspect has to be approved even prior to the award on the basis of the successful bid, and may lead to the cancellation of the award if the funds are not available. However, it

---

[93] The relevant before provisions were §6a(1)(3) VOB/A, §6EC(5) VOL/A, §4(8) VOF and §21(2) SektVO. Now the self-cleaning mechanism is provided in §125 GWB (VergRModG).

[94] Commission (EU) 'Minutes of the Meeting of the Commission Stakeholder Expert Group on Public Procurement' (2012) <http://ec.europa.eu/internal_market/publicprocurement/docs/expert-group/120925_minutes_en.pdf> accessed 25 April 2016, proposition of M Tanferma, 6.

[95] Art 56(1)(3)New PPA.

[96] There are additional comments on this point in the next chapter as well.

[97] ie the BHO and the separate regional or state budget laws.

is important to note that 'budget laws are only binding on the public administration but do not provide enforceable rights for the bidders'.[98] The principle of equal treatment[99] must naturally be complied with at all times. Once a candidate is considered as suitable, the candidate no longer needs to be tested in further procedures, unless indications justifying such a step arise at a later point.

(iv) The candidate must also have a clean record of honest trading and *not have participated in corrupt practices*. It should not be considered by the contracting authority and must even be excluded if it has participated in corrupt practices, bribery or fraud in Germany or abroad (which is fully consistent with the requirements of EU legislation).

Both Germany and Bulgaria have adopted provisions which prohibit the participation of candidates which have been a party to corruption, bribery and other similar offences.[100] The weight and application of these provisions, however, differ significantly:

In Germany, this legislative rule constitutes a significant obstacle and 'threat' to participants, because corruption proceedings are initiated speedily and resolved just as quickly, and as a final result, a court decision finding corruption could ruin the business and reputation of the potential participant.

The contrast with the example of Bulgaria is self-explanatory – the number of court proceedings which have actually been initiated, and especially those which have resulted in an enforceable sentence, can be counted on the fingers of one hand. Consequently, the current provision in the law is more or less a dead-letter in its essence and has neither material practical impact nor preventive effect.

The by now often-stated conclusion that a significant portion of Bulgarian provisions in the public procurement field (even those borrowed directly from the EU procurement package) fail to provide the required legislative and practical effects due to the existence of unfavourable secondary factors is also perfectly true in this instance. If speedy legal proceedings and a significantly higher rate of detection and sanctioning of corruption schemes occurred, and the relevant political will was also there, the preventive function and significance of these rules could be improved substantially. In this case the comparison with good practices again shows that the amassing of a theoretical reserve of legal rules as an end in itself, albeit borrowed from countries with proven experience in the field of combating corruption, is not and cannot be the only antidote for Bulgaria or other Member States sharing its levels of corruption.

---

[98] See above (n 43).

[99] The principle of equal treatment could also imply a transparency obligation, following Case C-470/99 *Universale-Bau AG, Bietergemeinschaft: (1) Hinteregger & Söhne Bauges.m.b.H. Salzburg, (2) Östü-Stettin Hoch- und Tiefbau GmbH v Entsorgungsbetriebe Simmering GmbH* [2002] ECR I-11655.

[100] Art 54 New PPA: 'The contracting authority shall exclude from participation in a public procurement award procedure any candidate or tenderer who or which: 1. has been convicted by an enforceable sentence, unless rehabilitated, of: [...]; (b) bribery under Art. 301 to 307 of the Criminal Code [...]'.

(v) *The aggregation and anti-avoidance EU rules* explicitly prohibit the avoidance of awards by using multiple contracts below the threshold: they have given rise to infringement proceedings against Germany. In *Commission v Germany*[101] the Court of Justice found that Germany had breached public procurement rules by artificially splitting a contract for planning services, which meant the financial thresholds for the application of the regulations were not triggered. Contracts whose value falls below the thresholds are not subject to the full procurement rules although the Treaty principles, such as transparency and equal treatment, and the TFEU's free movement provisions always apply. Such prohibited splitting, in addition to circumventing the award rules, also tends to open up corruption possibilities for the unchecked selection of the 'bribing candidate' (as discussed in Chap. 5). The analysis of *Commission v. Germany* exemplifies, however, not only the Court's view on the splitting of contracts and the correct interpretation of the Procurement Directive's rules; it also demonstrates one of the few cases of this kind of procurement infringement in Germany, and which was not actually intended to achieve corrupt ends, but was rather allowed mainly for budgetary reasons.

The parallel between the two countries' practices with regards to this type of infringement is of particular interest precisely for this reason. Splitting is quite a prevalent practice in Bulgaria: it is one of the easier types of infringement to detect. The contracting authority may become confused as to the nature of the required activities and may consequently divide them into several contracts. Only *ex post* control can establish whether the actual characteristics and value of the contracts are such as to require their consolidation into a single procedure and the application of the stricter rules on procurement awards. Although Germany, a Member State of

---

[101] Judgment of 15 March 2012 in Case C-574/10 *Commission v Germany* [2012] ECLI:EU:C:2012:145: In 2006 and 2007, the municipality of Niedernhausen appointed a local engineering company to renovate a hall. The renovation was to be conducted in a phases. The German authorities considered that the planning services for each phase constituted a separate services contract, the value of each contract falling below the financial thresholds. The ECJ alleged that Germany had artificially divided the contract in breach of public procurement rules: 'An almost arbitrary division of the contracts is contrary to the effectiveness of the directive. It would indeed often lead to values artificially falling below the threshold and thereby to a reduction of its scope of application. The Court notes in its settled case-law the significance of the directive on the award of public contracts for the free movement of services and for fair competition at European Union level. An arbitrary and subjective 'dismemberment' of uniform service contracts would undermine that objective. Budgetary reasons for the division into construction sections could also not justify an artificial division of a unified contract value. It is contrary to the objective of the European public procurement directives for a unified proposed purchase which is carried out in several stages purely for budgetary reasons to be considered solely for that reason to consist of several independent contracts and thereby to be prevented from coming within the scope of application of the directive. Art 9(3) of the directive indeed forbids such an artificial division of a unified proposed purchase. It must be concluded that the contracts in question constitute a unified proposed purchase, the value of which at the time of the contract award exceeded the threshold laid down in the directive. The contract should therefore have been the subject of a Europe-wide invitation to tender and awarded according to the procedure provided for in the directive. That is not the case and therefore the defendant infringed Directive 2004/18/EC'.

longer standing than Bulgaria, has its share of experience with infringements involving splitting procurements, in most cases the problem was rather that of a purely formal violation of public procurement rules and a restriction of competition and not necessarily corruption.

In stark contrast in Bulgaria splitting is used in the majority of cases precisely in order to circumvent the law and select a favoured candidate. Hence in the Bulgarian case splitting has far more serious repercussions and throws open the gates to bribery and violations from individuals in an official position: clear corrupt practices. In Germany the same infringement poses a much smaller public threat and occurs far less frequently. Of course, the argument that Germany, having been sanctioned following infringement proceedings, has become far more disciplined and responsible, can also be made.

(vi) Award procedures are based on the expectation that *no material changes will occur between the beginning of the process and the award of the contract*. This is underlined by a rule in German law (transposed correctly from EU legislation) which states that offers must not be changed after being submitted to the awarding authority.[102] Therefore, if the need for changes becomes apparent during a procedure, each situation must be considered thoroughly. Decisions must take account of the principles of non-discrimination, fair competition and transparency in particular. However, any changes in the final tender prior to the actual award of the contract run a very strong risk of falling foul of the principle of non-discrimination. Thus, material changes to final tenders are basically excluded at that stage.

(vii) The above applies in general with respect to *post-contract award changes*, but for different reasons. With regard to post-signature changes to procurement contract terms, German law sets out certain rules under the GWB[103] in compliance with the new EU rules. In fact, Germany strictly adhered to the possible departures from the rule, as set out in *Pressetext*[104] even before its codification in the New Procurement Directives, which means that it does not allow any other amendments to concluded public contracts.

Unlike Germany, one of the most common manipulations in the award of public procurement contracts in Bulgaria (as an example of a jurisdiction within which corruption occurs) is precisely the amendment of public procurement contracts which have already been concluded in accordance with applicable rules. Explicit rules restricting the possibility for contract amendment are provided in the New PPA.[105] The preliminary ruling in *Pressetext* is also taken into account by appellate authorities which monitor the lawful conduct of the procurement before the trans-

---

[102] An exception to this rule applies to negotiated procedures and the competitive dialog.

[103] §132–133 GWB (VergRModG).

[104] Case C-454/06 *Pressetext Nachrichtenagentur GmbH v Republik Österreich (Bund), APA-OTS Originaltext-Service GmbH, APA Austria Presse Agentur registrierte Genossenschaft mit beschränkter Haftung* [2008] ECR I-4401.

[105] Art 116 New PPA.

position. However, the lack of adequate control (although broadened with the New PPA) following contract conclusion in Bulgaria allows corrupt schemes to proceed almost unhindered because, as has been explained in previous chapters, a large proportion of corrupt schemes are implemented by oral agreements between the contracting authority and the contractors. These in reality introduce significant changes to the contract but the changes remain untraceable due to the lack of sufficient control over efficiency, to complement legality control. Only future practice will show whether the newly provided *ex ante* control over contract amendments in certain cases, as discussed in Chap. 4, will really significantly mark a departure from the situation as it has been until recently.

By way of summary, German rules and imperative norms could serve as a stepping stone for Member States lacking sufficient controls: drawing on this model, other legislations could introduce imperative restrictive and sanctioning norms against behind-the-scenes modifications to public procurement contracts. In this light, the Bulgarian legislative framework needs refashioning despite already having introduced the new procurement package. It is desirable also to consult on how legal norms regulating contract amendments following effective conclusion could properly be supplemented so that they can bring an end to the indiscriminate abuse of this practice, and in a separate vein – how control over contract implementation could be affected. Again, however, such a legislative change would be insufficient in the absence of the relevant will to observe imperative rules and prevent attempts at their circumvention.

6.11.2   Modernised and Facilitated Conduct of Procurement Procedures

Germany is acting in full compliance with the general EU policy to completely transition to e-procurement. Among the demands for transparency and reduced corruption in public procurement set out in the German NIS Report 2012, published by TI Deutschland,[106] were those for implementation of a central platform for mandatory publication of public tender procedures. Today this requirement is more or less a fact. German and EU tenders are centralised and accessible on several e-tender platforms – e-Vergabe, bund.de[107] and others. Some older systems such as 'BundOnline2005' also facilitate the centralised electronic procurement procedures in federal administration. Furthermore, there is a well-developed e-Governance sys-

---

[106] See above (n 8).

[107] bund.de is a partner of 'Deutschland-Online' – an e-government strategy which offers a secure gateway to the services and online information of the German federal administrations. Two years ago, the Ministry of the Interior started another government communication system – the so called De-Mail, which will enable and facilitate the exchange of electronic documents between citizens and public authorities over the internet. There also other initiatives aiming to digitalise the entire German administration.

tem which German citizens are free to use to carry out many administrative requirements. This reduces bureaucracy tremendously and enables the authorities to offer high-quality services in the shortest of time frames and at markedly decreased administrative costs.

In this respect, transposition of the New Procurement Directives will not confront Germany with the need to restructure its legislative system and allocate funds for the creation of electronic award platforms, as will be the case in Bulgaria, for example. The Federal Ministry for Economic Affairs and Energy and the Federal Ministry of the Interior have already started initiating conferences to inform the contracting authorities in all *Länder* about the new e-procurement requirements. There is also an effort at the federal level to move all business to a single federal e-platform.[108]

A key difference between the public procurement award models in the two other Member States studied here is precisely the development of electronic platforms. In Bulgaria electronic tenders are already a fact, but for the most part moving to full e-procurement is chimerical for the time being (a typical issue for all economically weaker countries). The CPCCOC and BORKOR projects (as reviewed in Chap. 4) were working towards the creation of electronic platforms for the promulgation, award and control of public procurement procedures in unison with the EU's ambitions for future e-procurement. Unfortunately, the Bulgarian state demonstrates negligible progress in this direction because of factors such as a lack of financial resources, lack of political will, and the constant postponement of the launch of e-government in Bulgaria.[109]

The development of e-procurement is one of the most significant factors in combating corruption, and states like Bulgaria will have to conform to European trends and the requirements of the New Procurement Directives to switch completely over to e-procurement by 2018 at the latest. The German example is invaluable in this respect, and BORKOR employs German experts who are attempting to introduce and reorganise a portion of the German model to meet Bulgarian needs. However, the creation of electronic award and control platforms should not be an end in itself. On the contrary, it is directly connected with matters such as urgent legislative changes, the training of officials, and a complete overhaul of the communication system between contracting authorities and participants, which are currently regarded as far too expensive and difficult for Bulgaria.[110]

---

[108] In addition, the Federal Ministry for Economic Affairs and Energy intends also to establish a new database on public procurements to provide reliable statistical information on the size of procurement awards, the number of procedures etc in conformity with §114 GWB (VergRModG).

[109] The latest development in this e-government strategy for the period 2014–2020 was the decision that Bulgaria needs to reach the average European level of e-government by 2020.

[110] To date (and before the transposition of the new EU legislation), the main excuse offered by the Bulgarian state is the lack of financial resources for the realisation of the BORKOR project or of any other project (if any exists) aiming to achieve the transition to electronic procurement. In addition, any project, including the BORKOR project, sooner or later falls prey to political games, nepotism and changes in governmental, which have so far in practice crushed all attempts at the development of e-procurement.

Overwhelmed by the anticipation of the New Procurement Directives and by the constant criticism of the rampant corruption in the sector, the Bulgarian legislator has adopted several measures to work towards the transition to e-procurement. These reforms, however, remain solely in the realm of theory and the letter of the law; they do not have any actual and practical effect.

An indisputable fact is that the achievement of e-procurement would reduce several times over the human element in the award process, and consequently the prevalence of subjectivity in evaluation, restriction of competition and corrupt efforts to manipulate procurement. This process, however, must be completely aligned with the legislative framework and with all other anticorruption measures and provisions introduced for that purpose.

A legal analysis is naturally not really able to determine conclusively whether the German e-model is the best, most expedient or efficient for Member States in similar situations as Bulgaria, but to conclude that the main tool to combat widespread corruption in this sector would be its removal from human hands is undeniable.

In connection with e-procurement, the development of whistle-blowing and software-based anticorruption systems is also of great importance. Despite severe criticism at the local level and the lack of official whistle-blower hotlines in the public sector, there is in Germany a well-developed whistle-blower protection system provided for public sector employees in law.[111] Civil servants are able to report cases of suspected corruption directly to law enforcement agencies.

Germany is criticised for the lack of specific protection with regard to private sector whistle-blowers.[112] According to the German institutions, however, existing laws provide sufficient safeguards for private sector employees, as they may use the so-called hotlines confidentially. A whistle-blowing system which has expressly been noted as good practice in Germany[113] is the Business Keeper Monitoring System (BKMS) used for processing anonymous reports and based on online portal software. The BKMS, which is used for instance by the authorities in Lower Saxony, is a tool providing anonymity for corruption reports made electronically and aims to facilitate the early and effective disclosure of risks within companies and public authorities. The BKMS is regarded as an especially effective system for the detection of high-level corruption because, as opposed to other systems, it is structured to guarantee absolute whistle-blower anonymity. Hensgen (2013) observes that the 'innovation of the certified BKMS System lies in the anonymous dialogue between whistle-blowers and an examiner directly at the customer's site (anticorruption officers, ombudsmen, audits and examinations with the company or administration), so that whistle-blowers can be notified about the processing status or can further be questioned about the matter of facts'.[114]

---

[111] The Act on Federal Civil Servants (*Bundesbeamtengesetz*) and the Act on the Status of Federal Civil Servants (*Beamtenstatusgesetz*).

[112] A draft of a Whistleblower Protection Act is a priority for the Bundestag for 2016.

[113] See above (n 10).

[114] Ibid, 37.

Furthermore, as a consequence of the development of whistle-blowing systems in Germany and in response to criticism by TI,[115] some initiatives for the implementation of a corruption register at federal level have been attempted, as well as in several federal states (eg Hamburg and Bremen, Berlin and North Rhine-Westphalia, and Schleswig-Holstein). The corruption register is to contain a list of unsound companies and/or persons (on the basis of convictions for bribery, illegal employment, competition law infringements and so on). Listed companies and persons must be excluded from the award of public contracts. So far, these federal initiatives have not been successful and currently, there are corruption registers only at the level of the *Länder*, although the legal basis varies from *Land* to *Land*. With the transposition of the new procurement legislation the creation of such register is increasingly on the agenda.

> Combating procurement law violations, corruption and similar economic offenses would be facilitated by the introduction of a nationwide central corruption register. Such a register, which makes centrally available to the contracting entities […] all established findings of federal, state and local authorities of corruption and other economic offenses of bidders and their representatives is […] urgent and overdue.[116]

However, there are some issues which need to be resolved even in Germany before launching such register, such as the type of offences to be registered, the rehabilitation of bidders, the reflection of the self-cleaning mechanism in it etc.

The situation in Bulgaria points to different conclusions. Over the last decade, the introduction of hotlines in Bulgaria has been decidedly encouraged in larger state institutions. Their existence has become something of a trend which has been picked up by various bodies (and contracting authorities) such as the Bulgarian Industrial Association, the Ministry of the Interior, the Ministry of Transport etc. The fact is, however, that the launch of hotlines (usually in the form of telephone services and not of a comprehensive software system similar to the German BKMS) has not resulted in the exposure of large cases of corruption, least of all in the public procurement field. Nor has it resulted in the 'emancipation' of Bulgarian civil servants, enabling them to develop a sense of trust and confidence in the anonymity guaranteed by hotlines.[117] The existence of such hotlines is still rather a formality which does not bring about the exposure or prevention of cases of corruption. Consequently, this reality would probably benefit from a comprehensive whistle-blowing system similar to the German one – or any other software-based system which would help in

---

[115] 'Policy document on Public Procurement and Anti-Corruption Strategies' (Berlin: Transparency International Deutschland, 2011).

[116] Motion for the third reading of the Federal Government Bill – Draft Law on the modernisation of public procurement law (Procurement Law Modernisation Act – VergRModG) (2015) German Bundestag.

[117] Germany is among the few Member States which publish comprehensive statistics on cases reported to the police and criminal investigations launched. In 2011 the Federal Criminal Police recorded 46,795 corruption reports to the police, and 1,528 ongoing investigations.

the detection of corruption loopholes[118] – and from the elimination of hotlines which again depend on the human factor as the main anticorruption model.

As for the so-called 'blacklisting' (eg the corruption register), in the earlier review of the Bulgarian legislation it was noted that the previously applicable PPA also contained a similar clause regulating the creation of blacklists for bad contractors (including corrupt ones). This provision failed to yield any significant results in Bulgaria, thus this weapon appears in practice not to be a reliably effective and appropriate measure in the fight against corruption in public procurement, even in the version provided in the New PPA.[119] The provision was drafted so that it provides for too broad a spectrum of interpretation as to how the blacklisted entities should be rehabilitated, registered and potentially excluded from further participation in procurement awards. This again demonstrates that the existence of provisions is one thing, but ensuring their effectiveness is quite another.

6.11.3   Centralised Procurement

In addition to everything discussed on the different anticorruption methods and policies employed by Germany, using CPBs should be highlighted as one of the pillars which appears to make a substantial contribution to the success of German policy in combating corruption in public procurement. The German government and the separate *Länder* use the option provided by the Procurement Directives for the creation of CPBs (Article 11 Directive 2004/18/EC) to its fullest extent.

The question arises why the award of public procurements by means of a central body should be seen as an efficient anticorruption measure. The simplest answer could be because such system would involve at least one more entity to be bribed in order to win a contract. On a more serious note, any method of separating the individuals requiring goods or services from those engaged in the implementation and control of the procedure for selecting the winning contractor constitutes a significant obstacle to the employment of the most common corrupt methods. CPBs take on the functions of a contracting entity which acquires goods and services designated for one or more contracting entities by organising public tenders for those goods and services. This authority may also conclude framework agreements for works, goods or services designated for one or more contracting entities. Contracting entities may depend on CPBs for all the steps from the publication of the competition notice through to the final implementation of the resulting procurement or procurements.

---

[118] The Bulgarian BORKOR project has attempted to introduce another widely-used German anticorruption model – the V-model. The V-model is a software product created in 1999 to be used mainly for government defence projects. It has already been adopted by several countries as it is regarded as both efficient and relatively easy to use.

[119] A similar provision for blacklisting with 'informative character' is also found in the new national procurement legislation (Art 57(4) New PPA). Practice will reveal whether it will yield any positive results against corrupt procurement participants.

Contracting entities may transfer their legal obligations to the CPB but only to the extent to which the CPB accepts obligations related to certain stages. Where, however, certain stages of the award process or actual contract implementation are undertaken by the contracting authority, the latter will continue to be responsible for those obligations. Regardless of the fact that CPBs are generally used for more standard goods and services and mostly for the conclusion of framework agreements: '[a] central purchasing body may very well offer both standardized products and services of non-strategic importance and products and services of significant strategic importance. In the latter case, the centralised arrangement is often driven by the owner's objectives to improve administrative efficiency and effectiveness within the public sector as a whole by ensuring interoperability and standardisation of the administrative systems used by contracting authorities'.[120]

In Germany almost every region[121] has its own CPB which assists in the activities of the separate contracting entities while at the same time ultimately severing any overly close contacts between the actual contracting entity and potential bidders. The choice falls entirely into the hands of the central authority which, in this case, acts as an independent intermediary.

For example, the functions of the Federal Ministry of the Interior (*Beschaffungsamt*) in its capacity as a CPB[122] are as follows: (i) procurement of goods and services, including preparation of all documents required under a specific public procurement exercise as well as the implementation of measures to guarantee the quality of goods designated for the proper functioning of the Federal Ministry of the Interior; (ii) provision and maintenance of an e-procurement system, management of framework agreements, coordination of the interaction of public procurement award offices differentiating between standard activities and products by means of framework agreements with the CPBs of the different areas within the remit of the Federal Government with a view to procurement optimisation; (iii) collection, aggregation and, where necessary, forwarding of data, including statistics, acquired in the course of the procurement procedures; and (iv) consultation with the Ministry of the Interior on all issues related to the procurement award etc.

As has already been noted in this book, Bulgaria has had one attempt at developing such a body, before transposition of the new EU legislation, which unfortunately was not particularly successful in terms of its operations and anticorruption effects. The CPCCOC proposed the expansion of such a centralised structure and the creation of one similar to the German model. As was observed in the analysis of the CPCCOC's activities in Chap. 4, the proposal is in itself positive (although the CPCCOC is burdened by the overweening and often contradictory functions of the centralised bodies and is subject to conformity with Bulgarian legislation), but is scarcely feasible under the current legislation regulating public procurement in Bulgaria. The new legal framework is of course formulated to provide an opportu-

---

[120] 'Central Purchasing Bodies' (2011) SIGMA Public Procurement Brief 20, 7.

[121] Logistik Zentrum Niedersachsen, Hessen Central Procurement Authority etc.

[122] See Bescha.bund.de, *Beschaffungsamt – Startseite* (2015) <www.bescha.bund.de/DE/Startseite/home_node.html> accessed 25 April 2016.

nity for new CPBs, especially given that the new legislative procurement package actually expands the functions of such bodies and the possibilities for their use, and even creates, in addition, the role of the procurement service provider. The option exists, if not for the entire procurement process and contractor selection to be carried out by an intermediary before the CPB, then at least for part of the process to be facilitated in this way.[123] Hopefully, forced by the now harmonised legislation, the state institutions will start to create more centralised procurement bodies and to shift at least part of the award process to them.

As discussed above, the differentiation and the resulting relative independence from the actual contracting entity is a good approach to combating corruption which is now underpinned in the new legislation in the public procurement field in all Member States and could serve to reduce subjectivity in the assessment of candidates. Naturally, such a legislative change should not and cannot remain just a theoretical aspiration, as has so far been the case in Bulgaria. The necessary legal leverage and sanctions need to be created to safeguard the interests of the actual contracting entity and to support the anticorruption aim. Analysing the various types of infringements, however, does not help define who the central entities should be for this much-needed cure, especially at the contractor selection stage, because in reality, the person currently bribed to get a preferred candidate selected would simply be replaced by another. Such a differentiation would, however, be especially efficient in counteracting corrupt schemes aimed at amending the parameters of concluded contracts. As noted above, this is currently the most obscure stage in a procurement procedure's development. Quite often the contract signed between the parties is only a framework which defines the price to be paid to the contractor and which serves to meet publicity and transparency expectations. Control at contract implementation level is weak and inefficient. The introduction of a CPB could resolve this problem as it would obviate the possibility of subsequent arrangements with the actual contracting authority. The agreement of certain conditions with the CPB body and their inclusion in the contract would make subsequent modification in negotiation with the actual contracting entity far more complicated, bearing in mind the division of responsibility between the central authority and the contracting entity and the distribution of their control functions. Moreover, following implementation of the New Procurement Directives, the selection of contractors based on the 'lowest price' criteria is now usually a thing of the past (in at least part of the Member States). In this case the objective selection of the bidder on the basis of the 'most economically advantageous tender' by the central authority and the subsequent corrupt arrangement at the Contract Implementation Phase (one which is beneficial to both parties) will be significantly obstructed.

---

[123] By means of: (a) technical infrastructure enabling contracting authorities to award public contracts or to conclude framework agreements for works, supplies or services; (b) advice on the conduct or design of public procurement procedures; (c) preparation and management of procurement procedures on behalf and for the account of the contracting authority concerned (Art 2(15) Directive 24/2014/EU).

6.12   Lessons to Be Learned from Germany

The analysis of the German legal system in the public procurement field and its good practice in curbing corruption definitely helps to the benchmarking part of this book. From the comparison with a quite opposite case as Bulgaria the essential conclusions about which anticorruption tools work and fail to work stand out more clearly. Of course the comparison captures the purely national characteristics of the two legal systems, but this helps further to identify the good practices which yield results in countries such as Germany but which remain inapplicable in less economically developed countries with greater socio-historical tendencies towards corruption, such as Bulgaria.

One of the material conclusions which crystallises in addition to the purely legal observations is that regardless the legislative changes needed in a certain country and regardless how public spending is regulated, a key factor is of course the actual implementation, control and sanctioning of these norms. The cycle of efficient and/or preventive measures against corruption in the award process can be defined as complete when combined with an efficient judicial system and a much larger number of anticorruption proceedings initiated and concluded with enforceable judgments. This means that the legislative changes which can be borrowed from Germany comprise only a small portion of the weapons needed in the fight against corruption in public procurement – undeniably the main part, but not the only one.

Germany, however, is an invaluable example which Member States can follow not only in view of its legislative framework – which (compared to Bulgaria's) is higher-level, mainly outlining essential terms, rights and obligations[124] – but also in view of its application in practice. Instead of imperatively promulgating a huge number of transparency rules as statutory norms while allowing corruption schemes to run unhindered, Germany has opted for methods which facilitate publicity but also for control over the activities of both contracting authorities and contractors. Just one of the examples in this direction are the e-procurement platforms which are constantly under development. Reducing the human element is of great significance to achieving a corruption-free environment and is definitely a good practice which should be borrowed at all costs; a practice for which it is high time that financial resources should be found in countries like Bulgaria, instead putting forward nonsensical criticism of investment in software and e-platforms.

---

[124] This comment mostly refers to the main German federal laws. Some of the acts enacted by the individual regions which regulate procurement (and are not part of the object of this work) can turn out to be more detailed or complicated, but the main parameters, rights and obligations of participants in public procurement procedures are set out in a very specific, clear and plain manner and are not subjected to quarterly bouts of supplementation and amendment, which creates an atmosphere of stability in the application of the provisions and confidence as regards the rules which need to be observed in order to ensure the lawful conduct of an award. These are all elements and features of an effective legal system which are painfully absent from the relevant Bulgarian legislation.

Another important point is the efficient institutional apparatus in Germany. The entire development of the award and implementation stages of a public procurement in Germany depends on the well-oiled administrative apparatus,[125] which exercises control over the activities of contracting authorities and quickly sanctions any irregularities. In addition, the efficient judicial system and the National Court of Auditors act as controlling and sanctioning bodies and also have a restraining and disciplining effect on all participants in the award and implementation process. The comment made in the International Comparative Legal Guides to Public Procurement 2014 is very indicative on this point: 'With regard to the roughly 2,000 rulings of the German award review bodies over the last 10 years, one may come to the conclusion that a 'culture of enforcement' has been well established in Germany for pan-European contract awards'.[126] According to the statistics of the Federal Ministry for Economic Affairs and Energy (*Bundesministerium für Wirtschaft und Energie*) for 2013, there have been 751 first instance appeals before the procurement tribunals, and 110 second instance appeals before the High Regional Courts.[127]

Last but not least are the CPBs, which can also be regarded as a viable option the functioning of which could commence simultaneously with the changes in the Member States legislation (where missing) required by transposition of the New Procurement Directives. This is obviously an effective mechanism which limits subjective contracting authority–candidate relationships. Separation of the functions of the actual user of the goods, works or services from those of the individual carrying out and controlling the procedure introduces a very active party to the procedure which, in addition to serving as a buffer to potential corrupt intent also constitutes an additional control body over the entire procedure. Furthermore, according to the new procurement package, CPBs will be the first to move onto complete e-procurement (by 2018), which will further serve to strengthen the anticorruption effect of their functions by not only mediating the award process on behalf of the contracting authority, but also by freeing participants from the interference of the human element in the selection process.

The option to create CPBs is not recent in the example of Bulgaria. Its application is still almost non-existent and is completely inadequate. This is why the German model is highly relevant and why its adoption would serve as a positive first step in the fight against corruption. The introduction of such authorities requires

---

[125] In 2014 the First EU Anti-Corruption Report (see above (n 9) 3) expressly highlighted that 'Detailed rules regulate the work of the public administration. Comprehensive codes of conduct aim to prevent corruption at federal level and in many *Länder*. According to the research, 99% of the authorities contacted apply the 'four eyes' principle, whereby two individuals must approve important decisions, 80% have internal anti-corruption guidelines, 74% randomly monitor decision making where the risk of corruption is more prevalent, 62% have identified areas with high corruption risks, and 57% have appointed an anti-corruption commissioner. [...]. Certain German municipalities, such as Hamburg, provide examples of local best practice for fostering integrity in the public sector'.

[126] See above (n 43) 76.

[127] As cited by M Brakalova in the German Chapter of *Public Procurement 2015* (2016) International Comparative Legal Guides <www.iclg.co.uk/practice-areas/public-procurement/public-procurement-2015/germany> accessed 25 April 2016, 119.

restructuring and reorganisation of the existing model. If however such a rupture in relations between contracting authorities and potentially bribing bidders could, as hoped, be accomplished according to the German model (as well as the implementation of the new EU rules), these efforts would be repaid fully many times over.

In addition to everything which has been discussed so far, the 'door' to this chapter should be closed with a comment which gives meaning to the comparative analysis between the Bulgarian and German award systems, two countries illustrating two opposite approaches towards the transparency principle. Ensuring transparency at every step and with regards to every action of the contracting authority is obviously not essential in the fight against corruption in the sector. Without downplaying the importance of adequate and proportional provision of information in the award process, procurement legislation needs to focus more closely on ensuring a wider competitive environment, on flawless and timely control and the creation of provisions with a clear disciplining effect if it truly aims to limit the handing out of procurements to pre-selected candidates. Perhaps this aspect should be explored in the annual monitoring report of Bulgaria also. The EU mantra 'increasing transparency in public procurement' needs to be replaced by more constructive advice and analyses of the actual state of public procurements at legislative, but also practical level. Indeed, even avowed champions of the transparency principle in public procurement admit that a '[c]areful balance would have to be drawn between the expectations of full transparency and other considerations [...] [T]ransparency is not an all cure remedy to corruption. Over-reliance on transparency may not be always appropriate as it may also have counterproductive tendencies under certain circumstances'.[128]

Bibliography

A Hantschel and A Schlange-Schöningen, 'Public Contracts in Germany' (2010) Executive Agency for Competitiveness and Innovation (Leaflet) <www.een-ireland.ie/eei/assets/documents/uploaded/general/Public%20Contracts%20in%20Germany.pdf> accessed 25 April 2016

A Pulito, 'Germany the anti-corruption laggard' (2012) Academia.edu <www.academia.edu/2225981/Germany_the_anti-corruption_laggard> accessed 25 April 2016

C Sesterhenn, 'Erfolg durch Präqualifikation in Deutschland und Europa?' (2009) Seminar paper: 11th Interdisciplinary Conference of Construction Economics and Building Law in Hanover (*Seminarunterlagen zur 11 Interdisziplinären Tagung für Baubetriebswirtschaft und Baurecht, Hannover*) <www.semina.de/verlag/pdf/11_praequalifikation.pdf> accessed 25 April 2016

F Raddatz, 'Modernisation of public procurement law – will this impact the healthcare industry?' (2015) Noerr.com <www.noerr.com/en/press-publications/News/modernisation-of-public-procurement-law.aspx> accessed on 25 April 2016

J Ellison and L Baudrihaye (eds) *International Comparative Legal Guides to Public Procurement 2014* (London: Global Legal Group Ltd, 2013)

---

[128] K Osei-Afoakwa, 'How Relevant is the Principle of Transparency in Public Procurement?' (2014) 4(6) *IISTE: Journal of Developing Country Studies* 145.

J Olaya, 'Case study: the implementation of an Integrity Pact in the Berlin Schönefeld Airport Project' (Transparency International, 2010)

K Osei-Afoakwa, 'How Relevant is the Principle of Transparency in Public Procurement?' (2014) 4(6) *IISTE: Journal of Developing Country Studies*

K Pashev and K Marinov (eds), *Reducing the risks of corruption and introducing good practices in public procurement management* (Sofia: Governance Monitoring Association and Economic Policy Institute, 2009)

K Pashev, 'Reducing Corruption Risks and Practices in Public Procurement: Evidence from Bulgaria' (2009) Paper presented at the First Global Dialogue on Ethical and Effective Governance Amsterdam

L Hensgen, *Fight against corruption in the Danube region: A study of regional best practices*, (Max Plank Foundation for International Peace and the Rule of Law, Sankt Augustin: Konrad Adenauer Stiftung, 2013)

M Brakalova, *Germany Chapter – Public Procurement 2015* (2016) International Comparative Legal Guides <www.iclg.co.uk/practice-areas/public-procurement/public-procurement-2015/germany> accessed 25 April 2016

M Burgi, 'Public Procurement Law in the Federal Republic of Germany: Annual Report' IUS Publicum <www.ius-publicum.com/repository/uploads/09_02_2012_9_43_Burgi.pdf> accessed 25 April 2016

R Caranta, 'The Comparatist's Lens on Remedies in Public Procurement' (2011) Istituto Universitario di Studi Europei ECLI Working Papers Series No 2011-1/2-ECLI <http://workingpapers.iuse.it/wp-content/uploads/2011/08/2011-02-ECLI.pdf> accessed 25 April 2016

T M Funk, 'Germany's Foreign Anti-Corruption Efforts – Second-Tier No More' (2014) 1 *ZDAR* 24.

Chapter 7
Public Procurement in Austria – Reforms Limiting Corruption

'Never neglect an opportunity;
Change at the right moment,
Sometimes be constant...'
('Cosi fan tutte' W.A.Mozart, Act 2, Scene 1, Despina)

7.1 Why Austria?

The choice of this particular country for the benchmarking analysis is again guided by several main motives underpinning the logic of this comparative study: corruption levels, procurement system efficiency, and historical, substantive and economic connections with Bulgaria. The main statutory rules regulating public procurement are examined, as well as the existing transparency and anticorruption rules. The comparison with current Bulgarian solutions again aims to draw a clear dividing line between the mandatory provision of a torrent of information and demonstrative publicity in the award process as an end in itself, and truly effective anti-bribery measures.

7.1.1 Legislative Similarities

As with Germany, the Austrian legal system is of continental type, but is even more similar to the Bulgarian one in terms of legislative structure. Further, being Member States, Austria and Bulgaria of course adhere to European values and harmonise their national legislation according to EU law.

In addition, Austria holds a historic place and has played a significant role in the creation of Bulgaria's post-liberation[1] legal system and in the process of the Europeanisation of its commercial and economic regulation from the nineteenth century onwards. Although not directly adopted, one of the masterpieces of Austrian legal thought, the Austrian Civil Code (*Das Allgemeine Bürgerliche*

---

[1] As was noted in the previous chapter, this term refers to the period of restoration of the Bulgarian state after being part of the Ottoman Empire for five centuries and runs between 1879 and 1920.

© Springer International Publishing AG 2017
I. Georgieva, *Using Transparency Against Corruption in Public Procurement*,
Studies in European Economic Law and Regulation 11,
DOI 10.1007/978-3-319-51304-1_7

Gesetzbuch),[2] which recently marked its 200th anniversary, has had a major impact on Bulgarian law, particularly in civil proceedings. Further, the Bulgarian Civil Procedure Code of 2007 was drawn up with extensive assistance from leading Austrian procedural experts.[3]

The legislative framework of acts regulating the award of public contracts is in many ways very similar to the Bulgarian one (the resemblance here is much greater than with the German framework). Despite its division into federal states, Austria has a single public procurement act,[4] as does Bulgaria, and there are also several similarities with the Bulgarian PPA and the New PPA. Given Austria's federal structure, each of the nine states has its own procurement legislation[5] (as is the case in Germany), but it is focused mainly on the regulation of appeal proceedings before the state court. Nevertheless, the Austrian legislator desired that the main act regulating public procurement in the country be as imperative as possible, setting out all fundamental elements in procurement awards, appeals and implementation. The text, however, follows the EU law as closely as possible to preclude any ambiguous interpretations,[6] which is a major difference from the current legislative basis in Bulgaria. Austrian secondary legislation supplements its primary legislation and facilitates the actions of contracting authorities in the separate districts but cannot derogate from the main rules which apply with equal force for all.[7]

An active procurement player in Austria is the Federal Public Procurement Agency (*Bundesbeschaffung GmbH*, BBG) which has similar functions to the Bulgarian PPAgency and regulates the award process. Quite separately from these

---

[2] Enacted 1881.

[3] Dr Peter Bauer, Dr Peter Joham, Dr Oscar Kolman.

[4] Regulating this subject matter only, separately from the laws regulating competition (as opposed to the German model).

[5] Which are beyond the scope of this book.

[6] In addition, Austria is one of the Member States which tends to codify preliminary reference judgments of the ECJ, again with the aim of achieving clarity and ensuring maximum focus of regulation into a single main legal text.

[7] In this context see also M Fruhmann in the chapter on Austria in U Neergaard, C Jacqueson and G Ølykke (eds), 'Public Procurement Law: Limitations, Opportunities and Paradoxes', in *The XXVI FIDE Congress in Copenhagen* (Copenhagen: Congress Publications, 2014), vol 3, 221 et seq. Fruhmann defines the close link to the New Procurement Directives as one of the specifics of Austrian legislation in the field of public procurement, but also comments that this is not always possible 'Furthermore, it must be said that (award) legal concepts of the Union legislature is often difficult to or cannot be classified in the historically evolved scheme of a national legal system' ('*Ferner ist zu konstatieren, dass (vergabe)rechtliche Konzepte des Unionsgesetzgebers oft nicht oder nur schwer in die historisch gewachsene Systematik des nationalen Rechtssystems eingeordnet werden können*').

functions, however, the BBG is also a CPB in Austria with its own Code of Conduct with respect to anticorruption measures, as will be discussed further below.

7.1.2 Corruption Level

In 2015, according to the Transparency International CPI, Austria was sixteenth of 168 countries with a score of 76 points, six points behind Germany and the United Kingdom.[8] There have been several significant corruption scandals in Austria over the last few years which have increased the public 'perception of corruption' and this has had an immediate effect on its CPI levels.[9] From this perspective, Austria is all the more interesting for analysis and comparison with Bulgaria because, following criticism at the European level and low evaluations from non-governmental organisations (something which also occurs on an annual basis in Bulgaria), Austria has focused on launching anticorruption measures in several spheres, some of which are already bearing fruit. The analysis below discusses precisely those measures and examines whether they could also have a positive effect in Bulgaria.

Regardless of the increased corruption levels, the situation in the country and its role as a major economic player make Austria a reliable benchmarking source, especially given the fact that Austria ranks corruption eleventh from a total of 16 factors hindering business, while for Bulgarians corruption comes first.[10]

The First EU Anti-Corruption Report of 2014[11] comments on problematic areas and the need to improve anticorruption measures but also acknowledges the seriousness demonstrated by Austria in its efforts to further minimise corruption.

---

[8] Austria has greatly improved its ranking since 2014, where it came 23th of 175 countries with a score of 72 points, which ranked the country 11th among all EU Member States and approximately ten points behind Germany.

[9] In the public procurement field, the most widely discussed scandal involved a former interior minister allegedly receiving kickbacks in return for awarding a contract for a new digital police radio network, totalling several millions of EUR; he was sentenced to four years in prison. Further, a deputy governor of the Austrian central bank was one of a group of nine people charged in connection with bribes allegedly paid to win contracts to supply banknotes to Azerbaijan and Syria. A former deputy chief executive of Telekom Austria was convicted of diverting funds to the Austrian party Freiheitliche Partei Österreichs – FPÖ and also received a prison sentence. In 2012 the Austrian Green Party released a report on a parliamentary corruption investigation, estimating that corruption reduced the nation's economic output by about 5 percent, or EUR 17 billion.

[10] K Schwab and X Sala-i-Martín, *The global competitiveness report 2014–2015.* (Geneva: World Economic Forum, 2014), 116 (Austria) and 136 (Bulgaria).

[11] Commission (EU), First EU Anti-Corruption Report COM(2014) 38 final, 3 February 2014.

With regards to corruption in the public procurement field, the results for Austria are as follows:

> According to the 2013 Eurobarometer Business Survey 38% of business representatives think that corruption is an obstacle to doing business, and 41% of them think nepotism and patronage is also problematic in this context. 18 % of those who participated in public procurement in the last three years reported that they were prevented from winning because of corruption. Respondents in Austria reported tailor-made specifications for particular companies in 66% of cases, which is above the EU average. Collusive bidding was reported as a widespread practice by 57%. In addition, 45% of respondents noted conflicts of interest in the evaluation of bids and 35% pointed to unclear selection or evaluation criteria. According to the World Economic Forum's Global Competitiveness Report 2013-14, Austria is ranked the 16th most competitive economy in the world, out of 152 countries.[12]

Again, to help compare Austria to the other benchmarking example – Bulgaria, below are figures, as produced by Globaleconomy.com,[13] which illustrate all the critical differences more straightforwardly (Figs. 7.1, 7.2 and 7.3):

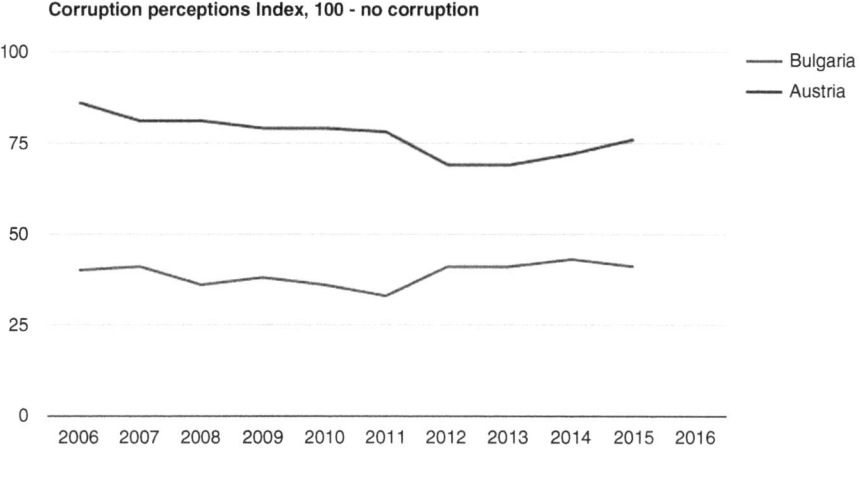

Corruption perceptions Index, 100 - no corruption

Source: The GlobalEconomy.com,World Bank

Fig. 7.1 Movement of the CPI (2006–2016)

---

[12] Ibid, Annex 20 – Austria, 3. See also table 5.1 in Chap. 5 which provides for a comparison between the three benchmarking countries as to matter of most common infringements detected in the procurement process.

[13] TheGlobalEconomy.com, 'Compare countries, compare economies, compare indicators' (2015) <www.theglobaleconomy.com/compare-countries/> accessed 26 April 2016.

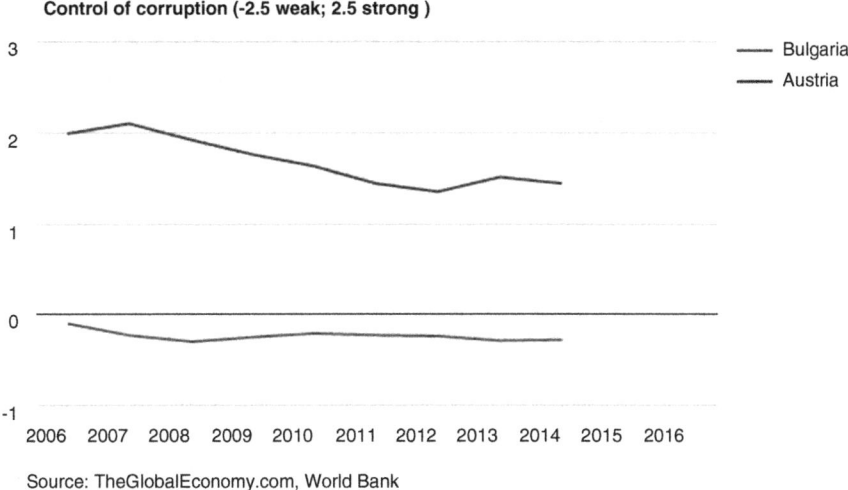

Fig. 7.2 Control over corruption (2006–2016)

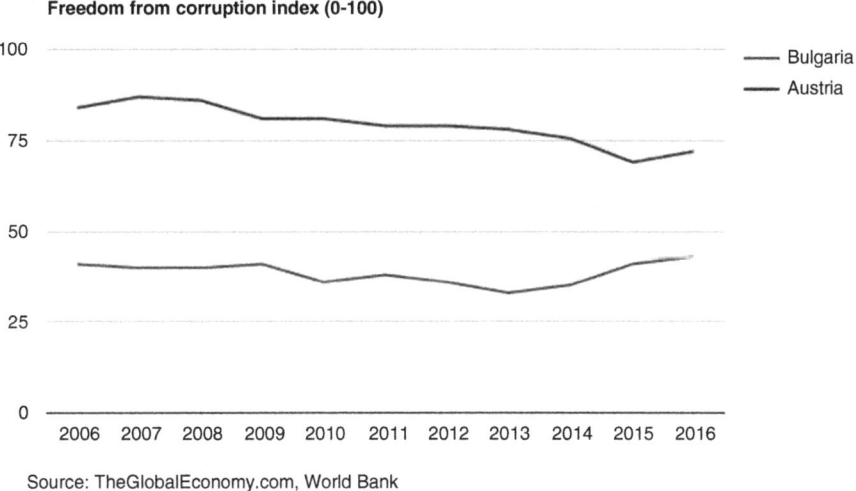

Fig. 7.3 Freedom from corruption (2006–2016)

7.1.3 Public Procurement System

There are many more similarities to be found between Austria and Bulgaria as regards how public procurement is organised than between Bulgaria and Germany. These similarities are distinctly highlighted and discussed in the comments below. It should, however, be noted that Austrian rules in the public procurement field do not tend to go further than the European rules. Regardless the similarities with the

Bulgarian system in terms of structure and organisation, there is no such abundance of transparency rules as in the Bulgarian procurement legislation, nor is there such a fixation on additional requirements creating unnecessary burdens on all participants in the award process. While there are specific regional rules, they are also free of the superfluous hyperbolisation of transparency rules or 'anticorruption measures' leading for example to overloading contracting authority officials with requirements for overly detailed documentation, which is exactly what is happening in Bulgaria, as seen in the previous chapters.

7.1.4   Socioeconomic Differences

Naturally, when comparing the legislation, good practices and effective methodologies of the two countries, account must be taken of their differences, which are not only of a legal but also of a socioeconomic, cultural and lifestyle nature. This was also done for Germany in the previous chapter.

Austria is a federation, divided administratively into nine federal states, and is a parliamentary democracy. Austria ranks twenty-first in the world in terms of gross domestic product *per capita*. It enjoys a high living standard and a socially-oriented market economy, which until the 1990s was to a large extent state-owned. Following accession to the EU, speedy privatisation took place. Today, the balance between the private and public sectors is comparable to the EU average level. With its well-developed market economy and qualified work force, Austria is strongly connected to other economies in the EU, particularly to that of Germany. The global financial crisis led to a severe but short-lived recession, the consequences of which were brought under control following the adoption of stabilisation measures.[14]

As for Bulgaria, there is not much to add to what has already been stated in the course of the comparison with Germany. Over the last decade, successive governments have demonstrated commitment to economic reforms and responsible fiscal planning. However, despite the favourable investment regime, including low, flat corporate income taxes, the standard of living is far from high and, against this background, trust in the political and judicial systems has collapsed completely. 'Corruption in public administration, a weak judiciary, and the presence of organised crime continue to hamper the country's investment climate and economic prospects'.[15]

For visualisation purposes and to graphically highlight the social and economic differences between Austria and Bulgaria, reference is made to information published by Globaleconomy.com again on economic growth, gross domestic product, government costs, administration efficiency and regulatory quality (Figs. 7.4, 7.5, 7.6, 7.7 and 7.8):

---

[14] Austrian GDP fell by 3.8% in 2009 but saw positive growth of about 2 percent in 2010 and 2.7% in 2011. Growth fell to 0.6% in 2012.

[15] *Analysis of Good European Practices in Quality Management of the Judiciary* (2013) <www.sac. government.bg/home.nsf/vPagesLookup/prj-3-research~bg/$FILE/13.12.16%20Analiz.pdf> accessed 26 April 2016, 7—8.

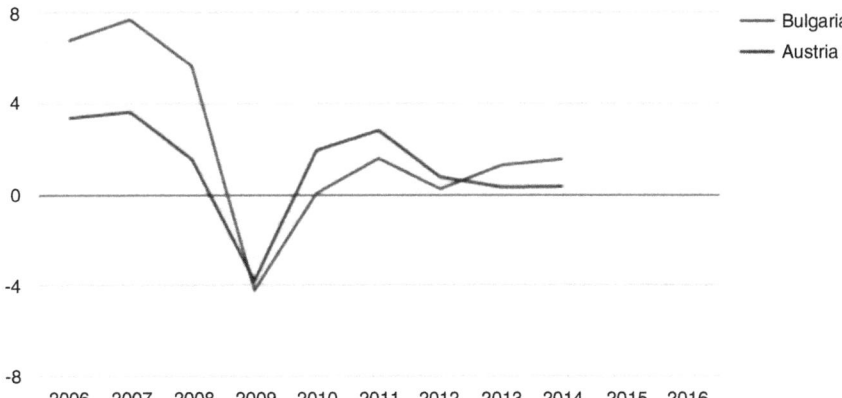

Fig. 7.4 Changes in economic growth (2006–2016)

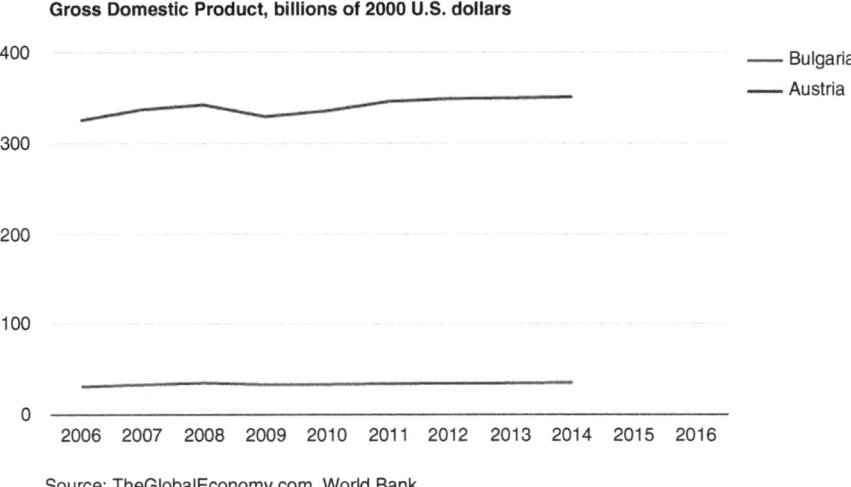

Fig. 7.5 Gross Domestic Product (2006–2016)

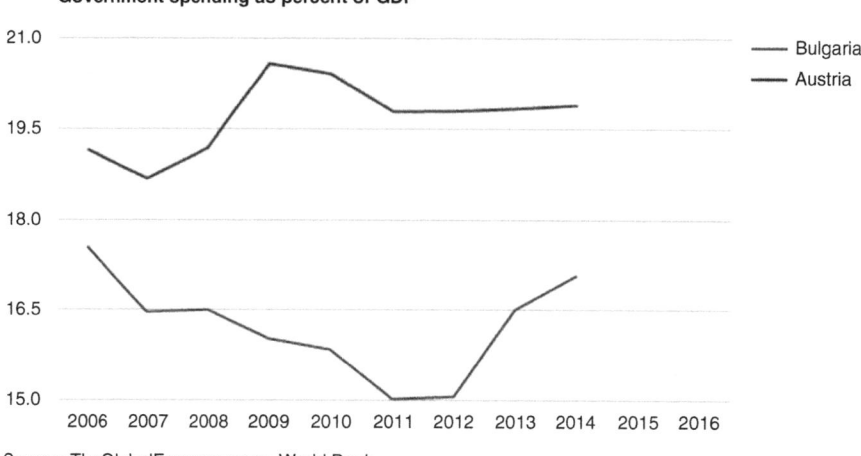

Government spending as percent of GDP

Source: TheGlobalEconomy.com, World Bank

Fig. 7.6 Government spending (2006–2016)

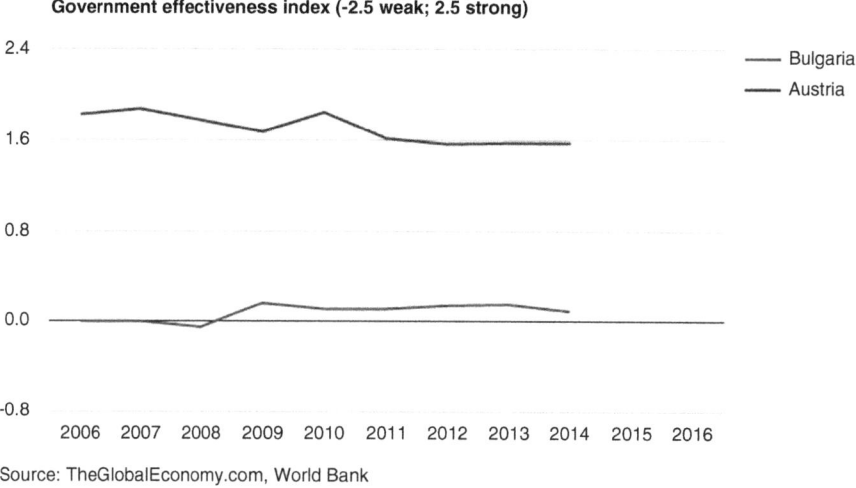

Government effectiveness index (-2.5 weak; 2.5 strong)

Source: TheGlobalEconomy.com, World Bank

Fig. 7.7 Administration efficiency (2006–2016)

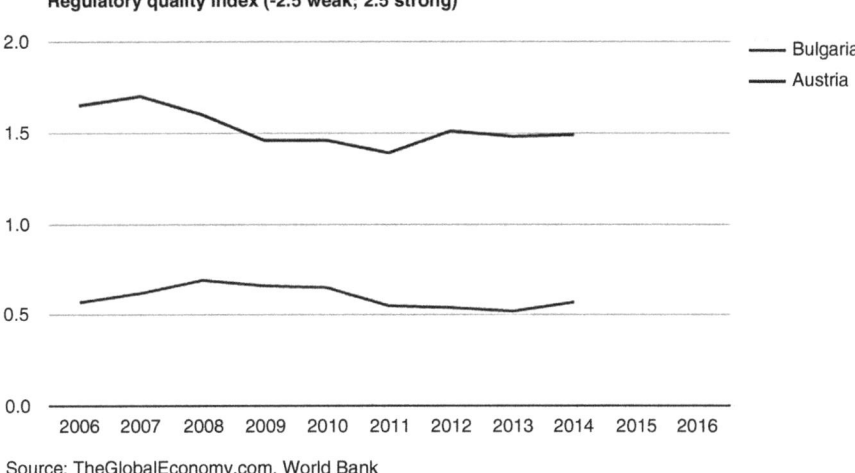

Regulatory quality index (-2.5 weak; 2.5 strong)

Source: TheGlobalEconomy.com, World Bank

Fig. 7.8 Regulatory quality (2006–2016)

7.2 Main Characteristics of the Austrian Public Procurement System – Applicable Legislation

The New Procurement Directives are in a process of transposition in Austria, but the deadline of April 2016 has not been met and there is still no piece of legislation covering the new procurement package entirely. However, Austria has already confirmed the advance effect of certain provisions of the New Procurement Directives[16] (as Germany has done as well) and acts in conformity with their main provisions. Further, in contrast to Bulgaria, some of the decisions provided for in the new procurement package (such as the self-cleaning mechanism and the ESPD) were already part of the Austrian national legislation in concept and they will not constitute novelties for the participants in the procurement process once transposition has occurred.

As in Bulgaria, the award of public contracts in Austria is regulated by a designated legal act which implements the EU rules and regulates the award process

---

[16] Decision of 14 May 2015 of the Administrative Court of Lower Austria LVwG-AV-194/002-2015, taken in view of the *effet utile* principle, which holds that during the transposition period, Member States must refrain from taking any measures liable to seriously compromise the result prescribed (Case C-129/06). The decision is in accordance with ECJ cases C-129/06 *Autosalone Ispra Snc v European Atomic Energy Community* [2006] ECR I-131; Joined cases C-397/01 to C-403/01 *Bernhard Pfeiffer and Others v Deutsches Rotes Kreuz, Kreisverband Waldshut eV* [2004] ECR I 8835; and C-221/04 *Konstantinos Adeneler and Others v Ellinikos Organismos Galaktos (ELOG)* [2006] ECR I 6057. See also J Stalzer, 'Austria: court confirms advance effects of the new procurement directives' (Blog post, 6 August 2015) < www.lexology.com/library/detail.aspx?g=4698e021-9af7-48bf-a223-edf3e8f3e442 > accessed 26 April 2016.

conducted by both 'standard' and 'utilities' contracting authorities. This is the Federal Procurement Act (*Bundesvergabegesetz*, BVergG).[17] A separate act regulates public procurement in the field of national security and defence.[18] As noted above, each of the nine states employs its own legal acts, applied in accordance with the specifics of the respective district and local appeal rules.[19]

The BVergG sets out the main award principles and rules and all the types of procedures, methods of control and appeal. A significant aspect of the Austrian system which resembles the Bulgarian solution (but differs from the German one) is that these strict rules apply both to procurement above the European thresholds and to those falling below them.[20] Austria has several mechanisms in place to facilitate procedures below the relevant threshold,[21,22] and as might be expected, the EU-wide notice of the tender invitation is not mandatory. Direct awards are thus possible in Austria if the expected value of the procurement is under EUR 100,000.[23,24] Bulgarian legislation also sets out additional national thresholds and simplified pro-

---

[17] BGBl. No 17/2006, as amended.

[18] The Federal Defence and Security Procurement Act (*Bundesvergabegesetz Verteidigung und Sicherheit*, BGBl. I Nr. 10/2012, as amended) which has transposed Directive 2009/81/EC [2009] OJ L216/76, as amended. This piece of legislation is not part of the present book.

[19] *Burgenländisches Vergabe-Nachprüfungsgesetz*, LGBl. Nr. 34/2003), as amended; *Kärntner Vergaberechtsschutzgesetz*, (LGBl. Nr. 17/2003, as amended; *NÖ Vergabe-Nachprüfungsgesetz*, LGBl. Nr. 7200-0, as amended; *Oö. Vergabenachprüfungsgesetz*, LGBl. Nr. 153/2002, as amended; *Salzburger Vergabekontrollgesetz*, LGBl. Nr. 103/2002, as amended; *Steiermärkisches Vergabe-Nachprüfungsgesetz*, LGBl. Nr. 43/2003, as amended; *Tiroler Vergabenachprüfungsgesetz*, LGBl. Nr. 123/2002, as amended; *(Vorarlberger) Vergabenachprüfungsgesetz*, LGBl. Nr. 1/2003, as amended; and *Wiener Vergaberechtsschutzgesetz*, LGBl. Nr. 25/2003, as amended.

[20] §12–18 BvergG.

[21] In this context see T Bianchi and V Guidi (eds), *The Comparative Survey on the National Public Procurement Systems Across the PPN* (Rome: Authority for the Supervision of Public Contracts 2010), 1–4; J Stalzer, 'Austria Chapter – Public Procurement 2015' (2014b) International Comparative Legal Guides <www.iclg.co.uk/practice-areas/public-procurement/public-procurement-2015/austria> accessed 26 April 2016 etc.

[22] BVergG 2012 introduced a few measures designed to simplify procurement procedures and reduce costs. For instance, the contracting authority is no longer obliged to demand any evidence from the candidates and tenderers in order to establish their suitability, not even from the successful tenderer. Another simplification concerns references in order to establish the required technical capacity. The candidates and tenderers may now present references obtained during the previous ten years, if the contracting authority so decides.

[23] This threshold will be valid until the end of 2018, in compliance with the latest extension from 13 September 2016; this is a positive step towards preserving the possibility for 'authorities to award small and medium-sized contracts unbureaucratically and efficiently' (see J Stalzer, *Austria: Extension of the threshold regulation until the year 2016* (Blog post, 30 September 2014) <www. schoenherr.eu/knowledge/knowledge-detail/austria-extension-of-the-threshold-regulation-until-the-year-2016> accessed 26 April 2016 and <https://www.iclg.co.uk/practice-areas/public-procurement/public-procurement-2017/austria> accessed 30 January 2017.

[24] Further, there are also specific exemptions and thresholds for certain procedures below the EU threshold, such as the direct award procedure with prior publication (below EUR 130,000 – §41a BVergG) or the negotiated procedure without prior publication for purchasing additional services (below EUR 103,000 – §38(3) BvergG).

cedures which apply only to procurements falling below these national thresholds. The main difference between the two legislative solutions, however, arises from the far more complicated regulatory system in Bulgaria, where the contracting authority must observe both European thresholds and national thresholds, which in turn differ depending on whether the procurement concerns services, works or supplies; there are also thresholds for low-value contracts envisaged.[25] Such a solution has its advantages and can also be observed in other European states.

> The following Member States have essentially the same regulations for below- and above-threshold contracts: Austria, Bulgaria, Cyprus, the Czech Republic, Denmark, Estonia, Hungary, Latvia, Lithuania, Luxembourg, the Netherlands, Poland, the Slovak Republic and Sweden. The main variation from the provisions of the above-threshold regime concerns the provision of proof of qualification requirements.[26]

The countries which have selected this approach aim to provide strict control even at the level of smaller procurements, and this approach tends to facilitate the procedure to some extent, as the regime is essentially the same for all procurements (with the relevant exceptions) regardless of the thresholds. Of course, there are procedures for which the award process has been considerably facilitated. This mechanism is in place in both countries and is subject to continuous improvement in the search for the most successful model.[27] A higher level of control is intricately linked to a higher level of operation and efficiency in the supervisory and law enforcement institutions. It is precisely for this reason that a comparison between the two countries is so interesting: most reports[28] note an increase in corruption levels in Austria over the last few years, but what is more peculiar is that the public is clearly aware of the corruption issue and acknowledges its increase as a phenomenon in itself, but this does not in any way undermine the prestige and authority of the legal system, supervisory and administrative authorities in which Austrians tend to place a great deal of trust.[29]

The above demonstrates a major difference from the Bulgarian situation, where corruption is indeed a serious problem in public procurement. Failure to cope with it, however, does not originate solely from legislative shortcomings but is caused to a much greater extent, by the inept control apparatus and the inefficient judicial system. This conclusion is supported by in the further analysis and comparison of the two countries. Like Germany, Austria has a high percentage of corruption-

---

[25] Art 20 New PPA.

[26] 'Public Procurement in EU Member States – The Regulation of Contract Below the EU Thresholds and in Areas not Covered by the Detailed Rules of the EU Directives' (2010) SIGMA Papers No 45, OECD Publishing; also 'Public Procurement in EU Member States – The Regulation of Contract Below the EU Thresholds and in Areas not Covered by the Detailed Rules of the EU Directives' (2010) SIGMA Papers No 17, OECD Publishing.

[27] 'For procurement procedures below the thresholds a 'lighter' and more flexible regime for the award of contracts has been established', see Bianchi and Guidi, *The Comparative Survey* (n 21) 1.

[28] See *First EU Anti-Corruption Report* (n 11); 'The Special Eurobarometer Report 374 Corruption' (2012) TNS Opinion & Social at the request of Directorate-General Home Affairs etc.

[29] 'The Special Eurobarometer Report 374 Corruption' (2012) TNS Opinion & Social at the request of Directorate-General Home Affairs, 102.

related proceedings as well as a high conviction rate. This has a huge hindering and preventive effect on future corruption. In Bulgaria legal proceedings in the field can be counted on the fingers of one hand while those which have resulted in an effective sentence are even fewer. This effectively encourages contracting authorities and contractors whose activities remain unsanctioned, while the overall perception of impunity aids the implementation of new and novel corruption schemes aimed at embezzling taxpayers' money.

In this connection the conflicting conclusion regarding the approach to regulating public procurement by means of an almost identical set of rules both above and below the relevant thresholds is especially intriguing. This model obviously works for Austria, although voices can always be heard in support of even further simplification of contracts below the thresholds. In Bulgaria, despite the rather more rigid rules, their application does not result in more efficient control and tends to obstruct the award process. Often, a simplified procedure is initiated without the legal prerequisites for this purpose being met, as is the case in negotiated procedures without notice, and, unsurprisingly, corruption thrives.[30] Bulgaria faces criticism for the excessively complicated manner in which individual thresholds are determined, which also impedes the effective fight against corruption. The clearer, less ambiguous and less interpretative the legislative framework is, the easier it would be to detect corrupt chicanery. Moreover, the law would not provide fertile ground for the justification of technical or deliberate errors in the determination of the proper regime. As a result, the current considerable loss of public funds is expected to diminish.

7.3 Main Principles. Transparency Obligations

Austria implements the mandatory EU principles in public spending – free and fair competition, equal treatment of bidders, non-discrimination and proportionality. Even the texts of § 19 and § 187 BVergG, which are analogous and list the principles of contract award governing contracting authority actions in the standard or utilities sector, explicitly highlight 'considering the Union-legal basic freedoms as well as the discrimination prohibition'.[31]

The two texts (targeting standard and utilities sector contracting authorities) list the different social principles primarily dealing with non-discrimination against foreign contracting entities or certain professions, the employment of women, the elderly, the disabled etc. In addition, the principles explicitly set out the rule that contracts should be awarded to qualified, efficient and reliable entrepreneurs only,

---

[30] This is expected to be overcome to some extent with the stricter rules for using light regimes according to the new procurement package, as already transposed in Bulgaria. It is however something which will only become apparent from practice.

[31] Part of the text of § 19 and § 187 BvergG.

and at adequate prices (this is also the case in Germany).[32] The texts also respond to the obviously growing trend for socially-oriented legislation, precisely of the type offered by the New Procurement Directives, which are currently being transposed by the Member States. There is no separate text or reference to the transparency principle in the BVergG. Furthermore, several of the specialist works on the public procurement award system in Austria do not explicitly list transparency as a fundamental principle.[33]

As explained by Steiner (2010), '[i]n Austria a general transparency principle in an act does not exist, but the whole administration is based on the Principle of Legality (*Legalitätsprinzip*) to ensure that every act of the administration is determined by law. [...] In any other case of public contracts no special method of transparency is necessary, because the administration is required by law to treat each case legally and like other, similar ones'.[34]

The transparency principle can be observed in a broader interpretation of the provisions of the BVergG and in the analysis of other stand-alone texts referring to the promulgation of procurements (*Bekanntmachungsbestimmungen*).[35] The BVergG does not set out any exceptional measures for the observation of publicity and transparency nor does it introduce any rules which differ significantly from those prescribed by the EU legislation.

The rules for the promulgation of procurements applicable to standard and utilities sector contracting authorities are almost identical, with one exception added by the legislator – namely the obligation for publication in a daily newspaper or electronic procurement platform for those procurements which fall below European thresholds.[36] The contracting authority announces the procurement, although there is also variation between districts as well.[37]

---

[32] §19(1) 2nd sentence &§187(1) 2nd sentence BvergG: '*The award shall be made to authorized, efficient and reliable contractors at reasonable prices*'.

[33] See eg J Stalzer, *Austria* (n 21); 'Lex Mundi 2009 Public Procurement Guide' (2009) Lexmundi. com <www.lexmundi.com/Document.asp?DocID=5953> accessed 26 April 2016, 3–7 etc.

[34] M Steiner, 'Comparative law on public contracts' in R Noguellou (ed), *Droit comparé des contracts publics / Comparative law on public contracts* (Brussels: Bruylant, 2010) 390.

[35] Promulgation in the OJEU, promulgation in Austria, promulgation in the media etc. (§50 *et seq* BVergG for conventional contracting authorities; BVergG, §207 *et seq* for utilities sector contracting authorities).

[36] § 55 *et seq* BvergG.

[37] Public procurement notifications are published at a national level, depending on the district in the: (a) Official Journal of the Viennese Newspaper (*Amtsblatt zur Wiener Zeitung – Amtlicher Lieferungsanzeiger*), online: www.wienerzeitung.at; www.lieferanzeiger.at; (b) Online platforms: www.auftrag.at; (c) the nine local publication media – the Official Journal of the city of Vienna (*Amtsblatt der Stadt Wien*); the Official News of the province of Lower Austria (*Amtliche Nachrichten Niederösterreich*), the Official Journal of the state of Burgenland (*Landesamtsblatt für das Burgenland*), Official Journal of the state of Upper Austria (*Amtsblatt für Oberösterreich, Linzer Zeitung*), the Official Journal of the Authorities, Departments and Courts of the state of Salzburg (*Amtsblatt der Behörden, Ämter und Gerichte Salzburgs, Salzburger Landeszeitung*), the Official Journal of the state of Styria (*Amtsblatt für die Steiermark, Grazer Zeitung*), the Official Journal of the Authorities, Departments and Courts of the state of Tyrol (*Amtsblatt der Behörden,*

In compliance with the New Procurement Directives,[38] the BVergG has also provided the option for contracting authorities to use the 'buyer's profile' (*Beschafferprofil*) to announce the main elements of the procurement. This, however, is neither mandatory for the contracting authority, nor is it bound by any time limits the non-adherence to which could lead to administrative sanctions.[39] It is expected that this legislative decision will remain as it is now and not to become more burdensome with the transposition of the new rules. According to the BVergG:

> Contracting authorities may publish a buyer profile on the Internet. The buyer profile may include notices, information on ongoing procurement procedures, scheduled purchases, contracts concluded, revoked procedures, and any other information concerning a procurement procedure or information of general interest such as point of contact, telephone or fax number, postal address and e-mail address.[40]

In addition, the BVergG also defines the minimal requirements for information to be published on the respective platform (if different from or supplementary to the OJEU) while allowing additional freedom to the separate *Länder* to set out more specific rules in this respect. The main publication requirements for procurements are set out by the Chancellor in a set of rules which are then promulgated in the 'Federal Journal' of Austria and are deemed mandatory.

The Bulgarian solution, as outlined in this book, of overloading the national legislation with publicity requirements differs significantly from the Austrian model. The Austrian legislator has judged that the normal operation and implementation of the award procedures requires a level of transparency which allows control and improves competition in the sector concerned, but not to such a level as to obstruct the entire award process and burden the contracting entity. The Austrian model does not render all publication and information options provided by the EU legislation mandatory, so that almost every document produced by a contracting authority[41] must be scanned and published in the buyer's profile at the very least – this to be done simultaneously with publications in other places, as is the case with the other Member State considered here. Only the minimum information package is published, in compliance with the requirement that no participant should be discriminated against through lack of information regarding a certain procedure, which would limit competition. On the whole, the Austrian legislator does not seem intent on turning the publication of all sorts of information on ongoing procurements into a 'mantra' against corruption in the sector, as seems to be the case with its Bulgarian peer.

As will demonstrated below, the measures which Austria finds useful to implement are aimed at changes in control authorities and improvement of their functions

---

Ämter und Gerichte Tirols, Bote für Tirol), the Official Journal of the state of Carinthia (*Amtsblatt des Landes Kärnten, Kärntner Landeszeitung*) and the Official Journal of the state of Vorarlberg (*Amtsblatt für das Land Vorarlberg*).

[38] Art 48 Directive 2014/24/EU.

[39] §48 for conventional and §209 BvergG for utilities sector contracting authorities.

[40] §48(1) and (2) BvergG.

[41] Sometimes regardless of its significance.

and efficiency, and at the simplification of some of the award rules, but not at stretching publicity and transparency rules beyond recognition.

There are voices in Austria urging for increased publicity – this however is normal in any efficient democracy, and in some cases there are even certain legislative changes which might be desirable in this direction, but these are not viewed as an aim to be achieved for its own sake, nor are they directed steadfastly towards the fight against corruption in the public procurement sector.[42] The drive to enact such changes is not solely based on the desire to achieve greater transparency for the purposes of anticorruption policies but is rather aimed at ensuring the bidders other rights, eg that in the event of an appeal, the bidders involved will have sufficient information to obtain adequate legal protection.[43]

7.4 Contracting Authorities Under BVergG

According to §3 BVergG, *first tier contracting authorities* are the State, each separate region, the municipalities and the municipalities associations. *Second tier contracting authorities* are entities which have been established (a) for the specific purpose of meeting needs in the general interest, which do not have an industrial or commercial character; (b) which have the legal capacity, at least in part;[44] and (c) whose business is for the most part financed by public agencies from the first tier or other bodies in the second tier, or whose operations are subject to supervision by the latter, or whose management is made up of members of the latter. *Third tier contracting authorities* are any possible associations between the first and the second tiers. In addition, the BVergG also applies to entities engaged in *utilities sector activities* (energy, water, transport).

The constant expansion of the set of companies and their associations which fall within the scope of the definition 'body governed by public law' must not be ignored. All sorts of combinations of associations, including private companies owned by the state can be deemed contracting authorities and obliged to apply the BVergG.

The award system in Austria is characterised as decentralised and the use of CPBs is not as widespread as it is in Germany. The *Länder* usually carry out most

---

[42] eg in 2011 'the Federal Public Procurement Office held that even award decisions with respect to non-priority services must now contain the same information as all other such communications [...] [T]he contracting authority must inform unsuccessful bidders of the characteristics and relative advantages of the winning tender, the name of the successful tenderer and the award sum, regardless of the fact that Section 131 of the act (which provides that the award decision must contain this information) does not apply to non-priority services': B Müller, 'Court requests greater transparency for award decisions' (2011) International Law Office <www.internationallawoffice.com/newsletters/detail.aspx?g=63a0a8da-bcb0-4723-9687-4873c1c5985b> accessed 26 April 2016.

[43] The applicable BVergG now sets out the specific obligations in terms of the minimum content of the award decision to apply to non-priority services – see §141 BVergG.

[44] Hospitals, universities, Austrian national television etc.

of their procurement through the administrative organisations of the regional governments. There is however, a trend for CPBs to act in the regions, as well as for procurements to be organised by cross-regional-border CPBs,[45] which is expected to grow further with the transposition of the New Procurement Directives.

In 2001, precisely with a view to streamlining the procedures and in connection with some budgetary restrictions, the Austrian procurement agency BBG was established. The BBG is a limited liability company to handle the procurement of services and supplies for the federal state and its companies. The BBG's functions are similar to those of the Bulgarian PPAgency but it also acts as the CPB for the Federal Government of Austria. The BBG provides central procurement services, 'in particular to negotiate framework contracts and make them available to the agencies. Its primary tasks are to bundle requirements to obtain better prices and terms from suppliers and to standardise public purchasing to reduce processing costs and legal risks'.[46] As a contracting entity, the BBG observes BvergG's requirements for exclusion of corrupt participants from all award procedures. Its operational goals mainly centre on conserving award resources, which in practice means that BBG monitors the efficient spending of these resources. The BBG is a non-profit organisation providing free services to their mandatory clients, ie the federal institutions, which are obliged to procure through the BBG unless they are able to obtain the same product under better conditions elsewhere.

The main tasks of the BBG are the organisation of public tenders[47] and establishing framework contracts for federal authorities or for public entities (on special request); catalogue management regarding concluded contracts, goods and services; the definition of purchasing strategies and purchasing marketing strategies; implementation of standards and specifications, and control. The BBG is focused on rationalisation of purchasing decisions by standardising and consolidating requests, promotion of e-commerce; using e-procurement-tools, and simplification of internal procurement procedures. The activities of the BBG are public activities, and it is funded by the Ministry of Finance. It purchases more than twenty groups of goods mainly to meet the needs of the federal administration. The agency's purchases result in approximately 15 percent economies for the state. The volume of public contracts is around EUR 1 billion per annum, where usually 70 percent of the orders arise from the federal system and the remaining 30 percent from public organisations (federal provinces). 'In 2014 the [BBG] executed 150 tendering procedures, of which only one was set as invalid'.[48]

As the largest CPB, over the last few years the BBG has developed its own compliance mechanism: an anticorruption strategy, aimed at combating corruption in

---

[45] See Commission (EU), 'Final Report Cross-Border Procurement Above EU Thresholds' (2011) DG Internal Market and Services, 70 et seq.

[46] 'Bundesbeschaffung GmbH: About the Federal Procurement Agency' (2015) Bbg.gv.at <www.bbg.gv.at/english-information/about-the-fpa/> accessed 26 April 2016.

[47] Examples of products procured by the BBG: energy, fuels, transport, IT, newspapers, books, insurance and cleaning.

[48] Information published by BBG <www.bbg.gv.at/english/facts-figures/> accessed 26 April 2016.

the award system. It has adopted a code of conduct, to be signed and observed by each BBG employee. In fact this is perhaps the only specific anticorruption tool created distinctly with regard to the award process and not as a general measure, as will be discussed further below.

In one of its recent reports, the OECD[49] highlighted the BBG's mechanisms as reflecting good practice in the efforts against attempts to taint public procurement in Austria.

> [BBG's] [a]nti-corruption Strategy has been developed mainly as a tool for preventing corruption. In order to achieve this, BBG defined actions which have to be taken into consideration: (a) Precise organisational procedures (clear definition of roles and structures); (b) Anti-corruption measures need to be integrated in the workday life; (c) The strategy needs constant reassessment and improvement; (d) Raising awareness of staff is done constantly; (e) Sharpening the focus on the consequences of corruption. The Strategy is based on three main pillars: the obligation of conducting transparent procurement procedures, the active commitment against corruption and the anti-corruption directive.[50]

As opposed to legislation and the relevant by-laws regulating the award and implementation of public procurement, the strategy adopted by the BBG attaches due importance to transparency but relegates it solely to practical mechanisms providing internal control over the activities of employees engaged in the award process. 'The four eyes principle' is strictly observed, as well as the division of functions, rotation of staff and other mechanisms which protect competition in the choice of contractor. In addition, the BBG introduces several internal obligations through its code of conduct, which are mandatory for its employees. Employees are not permitted to accept any gifts and any attempted bribery of an official will be promptly exposed. Moreover, like other institutions combating corruption (the Federal Bureau of Anti-Corruption and the Prosecution Service), the BBG organises regular training and seminars for its staff to ensure appropriate knowledge of all corruption risks and the measures applicable to each type.[51]

The practice of combining a 'public procurement institution' with the CPB, as in Austria, is especially advantageous – while performing support functions across the process, it is at once a participant in procurement procedures in its capacity as a CPB; it is thus well placed to observe actual problems in practice. This approach unites two fundamental functions of BBG, as the main organisational structure for

---

[49] *Compendium of Good Practices for Integrity in Public Procurement.* (2015) OECD GOV/PGC/ETH(2014)/REV1.

[50] Ibid, 20 *et seq.* Further, the survey sets out that '[t]he anti-corruption directive is a compliance management tool for the prevention of corruption. It contains an explicit regulation of the main values and strategies regarding prevention of corruption, clear definition of grey areas (eg the difference between customer care and corruption; what is permitted, what not), clear rules on accepting gifts as well as rules on additional occupation. It also offers the employees a clear view on the emergency management'.

[51] The reports of the Austrian Audit Office on BBG activities also differentiate between anticorruption policies and the strategies they impose. For example, see, 'Bericht des Rechnungshofes – Bundesbeschaffung GmbH, Follow-up-Überprüfung' (2011) Bund 2011/8 <www.rechnungshof.gv.at/fileadmin/downloads/2011/berichte/teilberichte/bund/bund_2011_08/Bund_2011_08_3.pdf> accessed 26 April 2016.

the entire procurement award and implementation process. It can serve as an example to other contracting authorities of how to conduct procurement in the most expedient manner. In this respect the comparison with Bulgaria serves to stress the differences between two similar institutions and outline a good practice which could in any case have a major impact if implemented in other Member States suffering corruption such as Bulgaria. Unlike the BBG, the PPAgency in Bulgaria has mainly organisational and analytical functions but does not act as a CPB. Of course, the PPAgency is a public procurement contracting authority and does indeed award contracts itself, but not as a CPB. The BBG's efforts to be an example and a model for anticorruption behaviour are also not such a priority for the PPAgency as well.

As was noted in the chapter dedicated to Germany, the overall trend in Europe is for increasing the use of CPBs, which can support the process and act as a barrier against attempts to 'fix' procurement procedures; the New Procurement Directives expand the functions of CPBs and encourage their creation and use. According to the Comparative Survey on the Transposition of the New EU Public Procurement Package,[52] Austria, like most other Member States, finds that the use of CPBs (as a form of aggregated procurement) is definitely beneficial and intends to continue to use them.[53] Additional benefits of the adopted approach arise from the anticorruption model elaborated by BBG. Concentrating all these functions into a single institution allows it to place itself, by means of its employees, 'on both sides of the barricade' and to acquire significant practical experience as to how procurement award and implementation is actually carried out. This helps highlight the actual transparency rules which need to be created and observed. It is on this basis that BBG created its code of conduct – by using its own experience in the award process. Thus it defines its employees' obligations, restricts them from certain activities with the purpose of bribery prevention, and places them under strict internal control in order to make their actions transparent, but takes further care not to turn control into a stumbling block for the administrative apparatus.

As opposed to the BBG's functions, the PPAgency (through its Executive Director, as commented in Chap. 4) focuses mainly on (a) the issuance of methodological guidance with a view to ensuring a unified national policy in the public procurement field; (b) the timely transposition of European legislation; (c) monitoring of the public procurement market; and (d) maintenance of a public procurement portal and register. The latter activity ensures implementation of publicity and transparency principles: all European procurement procedures are entered into the register (even those whose value is lower than European thresholds but higher than national ones). The most important role of the PPAgency from the perspective of the national anticorruption strategies is related to its control functions, which have been expanded in recent years and further with the transposition of the New Procurement Directives, as noted in previous chapters. This control has a preventive function and

---

[52] 'Comparative Survey on the Transposition of the New EU Public Procurement Package' (2014) Department for European Union Policies, Italian National Anti-Corruption Authority, Presidency of the Council of Ministers.

[53] Ibid, 14 and 42 et seq.

could be viewed as a form of methodological assistance also. It does not aim to administer punishment, but aims to prevent the contracting authorities of wrongs. Its main task is to minimise the risks which can arise upon conclusion of contracts under which payments may subsequently need to be refunded due to violations in the rules for application of public funds.

In reality, the functions of the PPAgency serve as a corrective force on the actions of actual participants in the procedures, or rather, mainly those of contracting authorities. The PPAgency, however, lacks the resources (financial, for the time being, and human) to undertake wider functions – even as it is, the PPAgency is struggling due to having to exercise *ex ante* control as well as to provide guidance on compliance with the law. The PPAgency is therefore sometimes slow to act and is unable to respond to all inquiries regarding the application of the highly complicated legal framework. Questions entered by participants are often urgent as they concern a specific procedure, but the PPAgency could not always provide a timely and/or adequate answer.

In searching for good anticorruption practices, suitable for Member States with issues similar Bulgaria's, the BBG approach stands out as a decidedly positive and appropriate solution. In particular, since for the time being the PPAgency does not have the necessary experience also to act as a CPB, this Member State could at least strengthen the role of the other CPBs, allowing a greater number of procurement procedures to pass through them, and to urge them to create their own operationally implemented anticorruption strategies.[54] Because of the impetus given by the New Procurement Directives, the New PPA presents a completely new piece of legislation in Bulgaria. Accordingly, the trend towards the use of CPBs is expected to increase. A problem which may curb the initial enthusiasm is, however, that as already observed in previous chapters, Bulgaria had only one central authority before transposition of the new EU legislation which cannot boast of having achieved any particular success in the course of its existence. Unlike Austria, Germany and other Member States, Bulgaria has yet to take its first steps towards introducing CPBs.

As can be seen in the comparative analysis, which highlighted the general functions of both procurement institutions in Austria and Bulgaria, the PPAgency is mainly an advisory body as regards to proper implementation of public procurement procedures. It may well be that this function will remain a leading one even after the presented legislative novelties, which would be justified given that the institution lacks the resources to take on further obligations. This does not undermine the conclusion drawn here that the way that Austria has chosen for the BBG to function could turn out to be a very positive influence on the efforts of Bulgaria and other Member States to tackle corruption. Moreover, in view of the habit of the Bulgarian legislator to revise its legislation at least annually, or even semi-annually, this change could be reflected at a later stage.

---

[54] Such anticorruption strategies/policies should not to remain 'on paper' only, as is currently the case in some Bulgarian institutions.

It is clear that the use of the BBG as a CPB is important not so much in terms of its role as an intermediary between businesses and contracting authorities – as is the case in Germany – but in terms of its role as a 'guiding light'. The good example which this public procurement body provides while blending the two activities – advisory and practical – is a very positive approach for countries such as Bulgaria. The analysis of Austria in this respect is invaluable – from genuine practice towards strategy and elaboration of anticorruption measures and not *vice versa* – from theory to a complex and cumbersome bureaucratic apparatus created by contracting authorities.

7.5 Procedures

In compliance with the Directives, the BvergG permits public procurement contracts in Austria to be awarded through (i) open procedure, (ii) restricted procedure (with and without prior notice), (iii) negotiated procedure (with and without prior notice), (iv) direct award, (v) direct award with prior notice, (vi) competitive dialogue, (vii) dynamic purchasing system, (viii) electronic auction, (ix) design and realisation contests, or (x) a framework agreement. The new EU procedures (eg e-catalogue and innovation partnership) would also be available after the transposition of the New Procurement Directives.

As in the case of Bulgaria, contracting authorities are free to choose between the open procedure and the restricted procedure. The other procedures require certain conditions and imperative provisions to be met. The distinguishing features of these individual procedures are set out in the BVergG.[55]

The German legislative decision before the transposition of the new procurement package, ie to give priority to the open procedure over other procedures is much more suitable for Member States which seek to strengthen the disciplining element in the conduct of procurement procedures (as discussed in detail in Chap. 6). This is because of the anticorruption efforts required (even accepting that some business representatives would perceive such measure as burdensome). In this case, the similarity between the Austrian and Bulgarian models cannot be regarded as positive. The wider freedom of choice works well for Austria, but leaves too many openings for corruption in the Bulgarian climate. However, this is again an example of one (EU) legislative decision which yields results in developed Member States which value the freedom of choice. Nonetheless, for countries such as Bulgaria, freedom of choice can sometimes prove to be counterproductive. I definitely support the argument that the restrictive approach has a far more organising effect in countries where freedom is often distorted and used for perverse purposes. It can be concluded that in cases such as Bulgaria the restrictions on the freedom of action and judgment of the contracting authority inversely increased competition in the sector.

---

[55] §25 BvergG.

In the desire to simplify some of the award procedures, an additional procedure was introduced into the BVergG in 2012: direct award with prior notice.[56] This promotes a 'relaxed' regime and restricted remedies, provided again that economic operators are qualified, capable and reliable. The contracting authority is enabled to conduct the award procedure at its discretion, to decide whether to negotiate or not, to collect offers or not, or to award the contract directly. It is only obliged to publish a contract notice with minimum information for the benefit of those economic operators which will participate in the direct award. Marboe and Franzmayr (2016) observe that:

> As to remedies, economic operators may merely challenge the choice of the award procedure and the contract notice. In contrast, the selection criteria, the selection of the successful tenderer, the withdrawal of the award or the award decision cannot be contested.[57]

The lighter regime in Austria is actually rarely used since the threshold (EUR 130,000) is only slightly different from the direct award threshold (EUR 100,000). Bidders enjoy a reduced level of legal protection under this procedure, because they may only challenge the choice of procedure, but not other decisions during the procedure.

In contrast, the Bulgarian equivalent to this more flexible procedure before transposition was called 'public procurement award via public invitation'. The weakness of the Bulgarian legislation, however, did not miss this form of 'relief' which was actually characterised by a higher level of formality than the previous system. Candidates selected as contractors have to submit a package of documents and declarations comprising the minimum set required by the PPA prior to contract conclusion. In practice, contracting authorities require both these and also other declarations and documents from the participants, as early as the application phase. Accordingly, instead of achieving the goal of simplification, the contracting authority needlessly complicates the process. In addition, the deadlines for tender submission are unrealistically short, and it turns out that within this specific regime, the options granted for eg contractual amendment and/or appeal are precluded. This was contrary to the European case-law,[58] and although it underwent several modifications in 2014, the problems in essence remained almost the same until the New PPA came into force in April 2016. The lighter regimes introduced in the New PPA are still too new to be analysed, although at a first glance they also do not leave the impression that they will be less burdensome in practice.

This comparison does not help in choosing the better option on this point much, also bearing in mind the restrictive policy of the new procurement package in that respect. Nevertheless, it still serves as a good reference point to conclude that the

---

[56] Admissible for supply and service contracts not exceeding the threshold of EUR 130,000, and for works contracts below EUR 500,000. See (§41a and §201a BvergG).

[57] P Marboe and P Franzmayr, 'Austria: Recent Public Procurement Law Introduces a New Award Procedure while a Last-Minute Regulation Dispels Confusion on Threshold Values' <http://www.mondaq.com/Austria/x/174552/Government+Contracts+Procurement+PPP/Recent+Public+Procurement+Law+Introduces+A+New+Award+Procedure+While+A+LastMinute+Regulation+Dispels+Confusion+On+Threshold+Values> accessed 26 April 2016.

[58] Ibid. See Case T-258/06 *Germany. v. European Commission* [2010] ECR II-2027; Case C-6/05 *Medipac-Kazantzidis AE v Veniseleio-Pananeio* [2007] ECR I-04557, para 33.

Austrian model is far too 'lenient' for the Bulgarian reality, while Bulgarian legislation often demonstrates excessive complexity and the inability to safeguard the main principles of public procurement. In any event, however, the options for use of a simplified award procedure for certain types of procurement (defined by the Member States themselves) and for those falling below the thresholds are significantly restricted following transposition of the New Procurement Directives, which are mindful of the unwarranted application of the lighter regime and circumvention of the law. Further research will thus be necessary to analyse the situation after the transposed New Procurement Directives have built up some practice under the national legislation in both Member States.

7.6 Award Criteria

The two countries again display some similarities with respect to their legislative decisions before the transposition of the new EU rules regarding award criteria. Until recently, they used both of the criteria considered above – 'most economically advantageous offer' and 'the lowest price'; one did not predominate over the other, unlike in the legislative solution adopted by Germany. Hence both Austria and Bulgaria will need to adapt to the application of only the 'most economically advantageous offer' following the transposition of the New Procurement Directives.

What was done in the New PPA is that Bulgaria took advantage of the option for the price remaining a decisive factor and in practice being an available sub-criteria for awarding, along with and separately from (a) the level of expenditures (taking into account cost-effectiveness, including the cost of the life cycle) and (b) the optimum quality/price ratio, which is assessed on the basis of price or cost level and performance, including quality, environmental and/or social aspects related to the subject matter of the contract.[59] Given that the 'most economically advantageous offer' as a criteria is endlessly fertile ground for the imagination of the procurement participants in terms of corruption opportunities, the decision of the Bulgarian legislator not to abandon its ability to use of 'the lowest price' criteria completely is gathering some praise, as commented below as well.

The situation in Austria demonstrates quite a different approach. The amendments to the BVergG with respect to the changes in the award criteria[60] entered into force on 1 March 2016, before full transposition took place. This preliminary amendment aimed to combat social and labour dumping and focus on quality when awarding public contracts. Therefore the amendments to the BVergG established the general priority of the 'most economically advantageous offer' criteria. The 'lowest price' criteria should only be applied under certain (exceptional) circumstances (such as standardised off-the-shelf works, services and goods). Furthermore, the amendments suggest that the quality criteria needs a sufficient weight to ensure

---

[59] Art 70(2) items 2 and 3 New PPA.
[60] §79(3) and §236(3) BvergG.

its realistic impact on the evaluation of the best bid. Other adjustments refer to the mandatory transparency of the complete subcontractor chain, the necessary reasoning when deciding not to award contracts in lots and to certain obligations in relation to social dumping.[61]

What happens in Austria and Bulgaria on this point is of great interest. Elimination of the 'lowest price' criteria, as it has been known so far, is regarded by the EU as a step towards a more complex and more expedient contract award process. While this is not a radical change,[62] and Member States remain free to select the contractor on the basis of price as the main factor, the effect on corruption in the field cannot as yet be determined. Only analysis of the situation in individual Member States will provide an answer to this question in due course. The change was introduced to promote more efficient spending of public funds, because in the race towards the lowest price, stakeholders often missed the truth that the cheapest service or product does not necessarily mean 'the best' offer. According to some authors '[t]he relationship between best value and anti-corruption provisions is that where contracts are awarded as a result of corrupt activity, this will have adverse implications for the best value, since corruption stifles competition and the costs of corruption may be passed onto the government'.[63] This however is only one side of the coin.

As already observed, there can be no certainty that the adoption of this change will have a positive effect in all Member States. The analysis of the infringements in the award of procurements performed in Chap. 5 reveals that the 'lowest price' criteria presents fewer opportunities for circumventing the law due to it being much more specific in how the criteria should be applied: it also takes into account the market values of the respective services, goods or works. A corrupt practice typical of this criteria is the offer of a low price in the tender and renegotiation of certain conditions only after the contract has been concluded in the absence of any publicity whatsoever. Another form of infringement which has also been highlighted as typical, is related to prior coordination between participants/candidates: the candidate who offered the lowest price is selected as contractor but declines the contract and the contract is then awarded to the next participant in line, who had offered a higher price.

As to the 'most economically advantageous tender', as Bovis (2007) notes, '[t]he meaning of the most economically advantageous offer includes a series of factors chosen by the contracting authority, including price, delivery or completion date, running costs, cost-effectiveness, profitability, technical merit, product or work quality, aesthetic and functional characteristics, after-sales service and technical

---

[61] More with this respect also by J Stalzer, 'Austria: 'Fair procurement' – initiative requires MEAT as sole award criterion for construction contracts' (17 February 2015) <www.thelawyer.com/knowledge-bank/white-paper/austria-fair-procurement-initiative-requires-meat-as-sole-award-criterion-for-construction-contracts/> accessed 26 April 2016.

[62] As noted in S Arrowsmith, *The law of public and utilities procurement. Vol. 1.* (London: Sweet & Maxwell, 2014) 737.

[63] S Williams-Elegbe, *Fighting Corruption in Public Procurement: A Comparative Analysis of Disqualification or Debarment Measures* (Oxford: Hart Publishing Ltd, 2012) 30.

assistance, commitments with regard to spare parts and components and maintenance costs, security of supplies. The above is not exhaustive'.[64] In other words, the
imaginations of contracting authorities and bidders with corrupt intentions will be
able to stretch much further when using the 'most economically advantageous tender'. This criteria provides an opportunity for technical parameters and/or requirements to bidders to assume rather exotic proportions and to point towards a certain
desirable bidder who can often remain undetectable and invisible for supervisory
bodies regardless of the full transparency provided. For this reason, corruption in
this type of contract award is much more widespread and varied.

The Bulgarian experience so far confirms that conclusion, as reviewed in the
preceding chapters. In this respect, the decision of the Bulgarian legislator not to
exclude the opportunity for contracting authorities to continue using the 'pure version' of the 'lowest price' criteria should be positively evaluated. Prioritising the
'most economically advantageous offer' criteria and requiring minimum weighting
of the quality criteria might increase potential corruption, given that price criteria
are in generally clear, transparent and most of all, objective. Quality criteria often
contain certain subjective criteria or weightings. Thus both 'tailor made' quality
criteria and 'tailor made evaluations' might be more likely to be subject to corruption than price criteria. Accordingly, for countries with high corruption profiles, the
general idea of the EU legislator to focus on quality is for the moment not optimal.

Given the above analysis of the two criterias from the perspective of the corruption opportunities they provide, the legislative decision of the EU in the New
Procurement Directives will indeed pose a serious challenge to states suffering from
corruption in the procurement sector, including Austria, which contrary to Bulgaria,
has chosen the opposite response to the imperative.

7.7   Appeal

Appealing public procurement decisions in Austria is affected by a significant
change in the organisation of the judicial system and more particularly of administrative control bodies. As of 1 January 2014, the former specialised appeal agencies
no longer exist.

Prior to 2014, the Austrian Administrative Court acted as the first and ultimate
appellate authority against acts of the executive power. Control of administrative
acts was conducted within the administration itself by means of challenging the
decisions through administrative channels. In accordance with the Austrian
Constitution of 1991, however, there were also independent administrative tribunals
operating in the various districts (*Unabhängige Verwaltungssenate in den Ländern*).
These are jurisdictions with quasi-judicial functions which ruled at first instance on
the merits of appeals against administrative violations. In addition to those tribunals, there were also other independent quasi-judicial institutions or administrative

---

[64] C Bovis, *EU Public Procurement Law* (Cheltenham: Edward Elgar, 2007) 466.

bodies with the status of special jurisdictions which also resolved issues related to contract award.

After almost two decades of discussions on the issues of administrative enforcement and legislative changes at the constitutional level, 2012 saw the adoption of the legislative basis for a fundamental and thorough reform of the Austrian system of administrative enforcement and administrative control.[65] This reform aims to build a comprehensive system of administrative enforcement, the model of which is similar to that applied in Germany. Appeals against administrative acts pursuant to administrative rules are restricted and a unified system of courts of general competence is created for each district, with a Federal Administrative Court (*Bundesverwaltungsgericht*) and Federal Fiscal Court (*Bundesfinanzgericht*) competent to review administrative disputes as courts of first instance. Independent tribunals and special jurisdictions are discontinued and their functions are transferred to these administrative courts. This is called the '9 + 2' model because it comprises nine administrative courts (one for each district) and two separate ones.[66] In reality the administrative instance is single, but two-tier.[67] The functions of the court on issues related to public procurement are undertaken by the Federal Administrative Court.[68]

> The distribution of competencies between the provincial administrative courts and the Federal Administrative Court accords with a constitutional general clause, which regulates these competencies in favour of the provinces. Accordingly, among its other duties, the Federal Administrative Court will review and decide on challenged decisions of the federal public procurement authorities.[69]

---

[65] The amendment adopted, *Verwaltungsgerichtsbarkeits-Novelle 2012*, entered into force on 1 January 2014. A legislative package was then promulgated on 14 February 2013, to regulate the activity of all administrative courts with the exception of the Federal Fiscal Court. The package regulates the transition to a two-instance administrative process in the period 2013 to 2014. The legislative package also amends several administrative laws in compliance with the reform in administrative jurisdictions commenced in 2012.

[66] eg G Grassl, 'Austria: Major reform of administrative jurisdiction system takes effect as from 1 January 2014' (Blog post 2013) <www.schoenherr.eu/knowledge/knowledge-detail/austria-major-reform-of-administrative-jurisdiction-system-takes-effect-as-from-1-january-2014/> accessed 26 April 2016.

[67] In addition to reducing the excessive fragmentation of competences between the different special and judicial instances which existed, among other reasons, because Austria is a federal state, Austria in practice is evolving towards an appeal model (similar to that employed by Germany), which Bulgaria has rejected. With the transposition of the Procurement Directives into the PPA in 2006, administrative courts ceased to have competence as a first instance of appeal in public procurement and the CPC undertook these functions in the capacity of a special jurisdiction. It has already been observed in Chap. 4 that this led to serious disputes over whether this change (although in conformity with the Remedies Directive) is unconstitutional, but ultimately the CPC has remained the first instance of appeal pursuant to the New PPA as well.

[68] The Federal Fiscal Court has jurisdiction where taxes and duties are enforced by the federal fiscal authorities; the Federal Administrative Court is competent for the law enforced directly by the respective federal authorities; all other competences are referred to the Administrative Courts in the *Länder*.

[69] B Müller and I Mayr, 'Amendment introduces new public procurement review bodies' (2013) <www.internationallawoffice.com/newsletters/detail.aspx?g=ddc59a8e-4514-49ea-a137-7580657fc81c> accessed 26 April 2016.

In accordance with the new organisation, almost all decisions issued by the administrative courts of first instance may be appealed to the Supreme Administrative Court (which is in fact the administrative court in operation until 2014). The court of first instance reviews the eligibility of the appeal and its decision may be appealed to the Supreme Administrative Court, which may carry out a wider check on the case and is not restricted by the conclusions contained in the lower court's decision.[70] Despite this, however, such cassation is possible only if the issue is of exceptional legal importance.

The new procedural rules for the administrative courts are based on the existing procedural law applied before the authorities reviewing administrative decisions. Nevertheless, the competence of the first instance authority to issue a preliminary decision on the complaint was extended (ie *Beschwerdevorentscheidung*).

Decisions of the administrative courts as public procurement review bodies can be challenged before the Supreme Administrative Court. However, this court is not limited to upholding or reversing the challenged decision; with the jurisdiction reform the Supreme Administrative Court has also been empowered to issue a new decision in lieu of the challenged decision. It will be difficult for bidders in tender proceedings to request a decision from the Supreme Administrative Court – under the new regulation, an appeal to the court is admissible only if the subject of the appeal is an important point of law.

In reality, the main change is that today control authorities have the status of courts and are more unified as institutions. The previous system included the Federal Review Authority (*Bundesvergabeamt*) as the main tribunal for control over public procurements, seven autonomous tribunals in seven of the Austrian districts and two more control senates in Vienna and Salzburg.

The appeal itself does not have an automatic suspensive effect over the procurement, but on request by the appellant and at the discretion of the court, an interim 'suspension' measure may be implemented. This is also the current solution adopted in Bulgaria. The BVergG[71] provides that the court may on request adopt interim measures and prohibit contract conclusion until it reaches a judgement. In addition, the Austrian legislation has set the standstill period for conclusion of contracts above the threshold at 10/15 days (depending on the use of e-communication or not) and for those below the threshold at 7 days.[72]

If any shortcomings within the appeal system for public procurement in Austria need to be highlighted (with a view to identifying good practices which can be applied in other Member States), these arise from the lack of automatic suspensive effect of the appeal, as is also the case in Bulgaria. In the latter, in order to comply with the Remedies Directive, appeal against the final decision of the contracting authority relating to the choice of contractor has an automatic suspensive effect. Upon conclusion of the public contract, the mandatory fourteen-day standstill period must be observed to make sure that the decision will not be appealed. In all

---

[70] The cassation instance is competent to repeal the appealed decision of the court of first instance or to reject the appeal.

[71] §328 BVergG.

[72] §132 BVergG.

other cases of appeal against the actions or omission of the contracting authority, the PPA has not envisaged an automatic suspensive effect. The New PPA has not changed this situation.

§328 BVergG makes it plain that the view of Austrian legislator is similar to the Bulgarian: the appellate authority implements the necessary and suitable interim measures only upon the appellant's request. However, Austrian appellate authorities generally act on such requests and may only refuse an application where the relevant requirements for the application have not been fulfilled. More than 90 percent of applications are accepted.[73] This approach is dramatically different from the Bulgarian situation where not only is there no automatic suspensive effect, but the court allows suspension of the procedure only on very rare occasions.

As already observed, justifications for the completion of a tainted (or allegedly tainted) public procurement procedure quoting economic interest are fundamentally flawed. Legislative solutions in which the appeal suspends performance of the contract (in combination with a speedy and efficient process) are much more sensible and serve as better motivation for contracting authorities to avoid the corrupt practices leading to wrongful contract awards. As was seen in Chap. 6, the German legal system in the public procurement sector is a better option for countries with severe corruption problems such as Bulgaria than the Austrian system. Under German law, an appeal has a suspensive effect as a general rule. Of course, such a legislative decision would be denounced as causing delays in dynamic market relationships and running counter to the needs of contracting authorities, but if some other, much more burdensome imperative rules are removed, as exist in abundance in Bulgaria, the award process could well afford to wait for the result of an appeal against decisions of the contracting authority at each phase of the procedure where suspicions of infringements exist. Such an approach would definitely have a disciplining and preventive effect on the contracting authority itself, which would inevitably be forced to increase the quality of its internal *ex ante* and ongoing control exercised during the preparation of the document package for each procurement procedure. Where there is a reciprocal and adequate legislative reaction to each action or omission, then a large portion of the attempts to bribe the contracting authority as early as the choice of procedure and object selection stages would inevitably be thwarted. Nevertheless, the Austrian model does demonstrate positive effects because the court practically always allows suspension of the procedures, once requested. However, in the case of Bulgaria this approach would require more far-reaching legislative and case law changes in order to achieve the necessary disciplining influence on participants in the procurement process.

When commenting on the appeal process in Austria, the scope of appeal should also be taken into account. The Bulgarian model is more similar to the German one here, allowing in practice appeal against each action or omission of the contracting

---

[73] See eg *Report of the Bundesvergabeamt* [*Bundesvergabeamt Tätigkeitsbericht*] (2012) <www.parlament.gv.at/PAKT/VHG/XXIV/III/III_00417/imfname_306182.pdf> accessed 26 April 2016, 17 et seq.

authority.[74] The Austrian solution is somewhat different[75] – the BVergG explicitly lists[76] those decisions which can be appealed independently and those which can only be appealed along with ones listed for independent appeal. On a similar note, with a view to preventing corruption in public procurement in Bulgaria, the Bulgarian award system must rest on much more rigorous restrictions and active administration of the law, which would 'dampen' the desire to manipulate public procurements: thus the Austrian model cannot be recommended as a good example for Bulgaria. With regard to the scope of appeal, the Bulgarian legislator has definitely provided wider opportunities for protection of participants,[77] having explicitly set out in the New PPA that:

> Any decision by the contracting authorities […] shall be subject to appeal in procedure for:
>
> 1. procurement, including through the conclusion of a framework agreement, dynamic purchasing system or qualification systems;
> 2. conclusion of a framework agreement;
> 3. creating a dynamic purchasing system or qualification systems;
> 4. design contest.[78]

The observation that these wide legal opportunities need to be supported by a fast-acting judicial apparatus, timely decisions of both instances and reliable expert capacity, is an altogether different issue. Precisely these elements of an effective appeal and control system regarding decisions of contracting authorities are in place in Austria, as will be discussed below. In the presence of these elements, the detection of corrupt schemes concealed behind discriminatory criteria or tailor-made notices will be much more reliable and the anticorruption policy becomes meaningful. Currently, the exact opposite situation can be observed in Bulgaria – the law is liberal with regards to the scope of appeal, but the first and second (first judicial) instances have the capacity only to detect infringements which are strictly legal (and procedural) in nature, with not much left over for in-depth control of the factual context of the procurement to detect whether these infringements are deliberate.

Despite the administrative legal system in Bulgaria being generally different from the Austrian one, there are certain similarities which in turn give rise to similar problems. In both countries there is a large number of different (including special) jurisdictions, the decisions of which are subject to control by a single supreme administrative court. This concentration of competence generates a huge load on the supreme administrative jurisdictions in both countries. Connected to this, the *technical and organisational measures* to regulate the workload of the administrative court in Austria could usefully be applied in Bulgaria as well.

---

[74] Art 196 New PPA,.

[75] See inter alia G Gast, *Das Österreichische Vergaberecht* (Vienna:WUV Universitätsverlag, 2002) 120 et seq.

[76] §2Z(16)(a) BvergG.

[77] See M Krivachka, 'Certain Specifics in the Appeal of Decisions of Contracting Authorities pursuant to the Public Procurement Act' (2006) 10 *Pazar i Pravo*.

[78] Art 196(1) New PPA.

The reform in administrative enforcement in Austria by transforming the special jurisdictions into a Federal Financial Court and Federal Administrative Court helps redistribute the load, differentiate competences and set apart the Supreme Administrative Court as a court of second instance in administrative disputes. A *better organised court structure* (first and second instance) could have a significant effect on the speed and efficiency of operation. This could restore the motivation of bidders and contractors in public procurements to appeal the acts of contracting authorities. More particularly, if such improved organisation of the appellate bodies could result in more definitive protection of the rights of participants in the procedures and more frequent interaction between appeal instances and the prosecutor's office, corruption prevention would also take on an entirely new meaning in countries such as Bulgaria. Currently, regardless of the efforts in this direction in Bulgaria, public procurement is identified as 'an important risk area for corruption [...] [T]he limited administrative capacity in many parts of the public administration due to a lack of sufficient qualified staff and experts, high staff turnover and a lack of supporting structures for smaller contracting authorities [*can be highlighted as a serious problem in the country*].[79] Important delays in the treatment of appeals related to public procurement also appear to follow from limited capacity in the judicial system.'[80]

Another important point of the judicial control system of Austria is the relative (financial) *independence* of the courts following the reforms. If this could be achieved in most Member States (and especially in those suffering corruption like Bulgaria), then the impartiality and transparency in the monitoring of bodies entrusted with control of the legality of actions of the executive power would be questioned much less often; their effectiveness, once again, would be decisive for the elimination of corruption in public spending. As for the independence of the judicial system and of administrative and government bodies in Bulgaria, any positive comparisons remain in the realm of wishful thinking, because even the most well-meaning legislative imagination, eager to incorporate the good practices of other countries could not overcome the status quo in the absence of conscious and purposeful political will. In this context, it is well known that '[a] judiciary that is not independent can easily be corrupted or co-opted by interests other than those of applying the law in a fair and impartial manner'.[81] As has also been shown in the preceding chapters, Bulgaria requires much more rigorous restrictive and sanctioning rules for the award of public contracts in order to combat the widespread corruption and improper spending of public funds in a not particularly economically stable

---

[79] The note has been added to the quote.

[80] Commission (EU), Bulgaria: Technical Report (2014), accompanying the document *Report from the Commission to the European Parliament and the Council on Progress in Bulgaria under the Co-operation and Verification mechanism*, Commission Staff Working Document Brussels, SWD(2014) 36 final.

[81] As stated by G Knaul, the United Nations Special Rapporteur on the independence of judges and lawyers, in the presentation of her annual report to the UN General Assembly, New York (24 October 2012) ohchr.org <www.ohchr.org/EN/NewsEvents/Pages/DisplayNews.aspx?NewsID=12692&LangID=E> accessed 26 April 2016.

country. These rules need to be supported by frequent and timely implementation, particularly on behalf of instances which are independent of politics and business circles. Only when these elements operate simultaneously can the good examples identified in the course of this book or other similar works achieve positive results.

The introduction of an *electronic document exchange system* in the administrative procurement process and the introduction of computerised finance and human resource management systems as in Austria may be expected to improve matters. The introduction of 'e-justice' in Bulgaria requires a massive amount of funds but is beyond doubt yet another cornerstone in the streamlining of the public procurement appeal process which could ensure speed, impartiality and publicity.

As is evident from Austria's example, the use of different types of software would be decisively useful not only for faster allocation and review of administrative proceedings against ongoing or finalised procurement procedures, but also for the creation of control, internal monitoring and activity assessment systems for the courts (eg delayed cases; statistics for the number of cases reviewed and finalised by means of an effective sentence; detected corruption cases etc). At present this is highly necessary for the Bulgarian judiciary in general, not just with regards to procurement. The expected effect from the implementation of these practices would be optimisation of time limits for case review by administrative courts, improved efficiency and increased transparency of court activity.

7.8   Corruption Prevention

As mentioned above, in recent years Austria has been frequently mentioned as a state with problems with corruption control, while some overly zealous critics describe the country as a 'corruption paradise'.[82] Several serious scandals exploded in the field of public procurement and public private partnership in Austria,[83] which ultimately had an effect on social perceptions of corruption and consequently resulted in a lowered CPI ranking for Austria, which lags behind other large economically developed countries (including Germany).

In its recent efforts to restore its image as a country in which business is not characterised by corruption, Austria has proposed and already implemented several anticorruption measures. Most of these are not specifically or purposefully related to public procurement, but where the anticorruption policy is relevant for the purposes of this work, it is discussed below.

---

[82] A Pulito, 'Austria: The Alpine corruption paradise' (2013) Academia.edu <www.academia.edu/2432598/Austria_-_the_Alpine_corruption_paradise> accessed 26 April 2016.
[83] Above (n 9).

7.8.1 Corruption Prevention Legislation

Austria has ratified most existing international agreements and conventions regulating the fight against corruption, including the Council of Europe's Criminal Law Convention on Corruption[84] and the Additional protocol[85] thereto. Austria is also a State Party to the OECD Anti-Bribery Convention (with a reservation for facilitation payments). Austria is a member of the GRECO of the Council of Europe and has a leading role in IACA.

In recent years, Austria has introduced several amendments in its national legislation and in particular the Criminal Code (*Strafgesetzbuch*, SGB)[86] under pressure from the EU, precisely with the purpose of covering almost all possible types of corrupt behaviour. These changes, however, refer mainly to the 'providing of advantages' to employees and not specifically to public procurement. Measures against money laundering, lobbying and limiting funding of political parties were expanded in 2012 and 2013.[87] The SGB criminalises in general, attempted corruption, bribery (active, passive, of foreign officials etc), extortion, fraud, embezzlement and money laundering.[88] Of course, in accordance with European legislation, all manifestations of active and passive corruption and the offering of gifts to officials are explicitly listed in the BVergG as grounds for exclusion of participants from a public procurement procedure[89] (a final court judgement is not necessary for exclusion). These exclusion grounds are mandatory and the affected companies are excluded from taking part in procurement, irrespective of whether they intend to participate as bidders, subcontractors, or jointly with other bidders (even if the latter are reliable). They will be duly supplemented with the new exclusion grounds following transposition.

At a purely legislative level, no other measures aimed specifically against corruption in contract awards (except for exclusion and possible blacklisting) can readily be pinpointed. As reported in the Phase 3 Report on Implementing the OECD Anti-Bribery Convention in Austria,[90] blacklisted companies are not necessarily excluded from participating in future bids.

The Bulgarian solution, as set out in the PPA, and now somehow reformed in the New PPA, regards that lists of 'informative character'[91] of unreliable (excluded in a procurement) contractors do not help the choice of contractor, nor is there any clear

---

[84] Strasbourg, 27 January 1999, CETS 173.

[85] Strasbourg, 15 May 2003, CETS 191.

[86] Promulgated 13 November 1998, BGBl. I S. 3322, as amended.

[87] The US Department of State 2012 notes that the law provides access to government information and these laws have generally been respected in practice.

[88] eg §133, §146, §147, §148, §153 and §165 SGB etc.

[89] In particular, §153, §153a, §1536, §302 and §307 SGB are among the exclusion criteria in §68 and §229 BvergG.

[90] *Phase 3 Report on Implementing the OECD Anti-bribery Convention in Austria* (2012) <www.oecd.org/daf/anti-bribery/Austriaphase3reportEN.pdf> accessed 26 April 2016, 47 and 48.

[91] Art 57(4) New PPA.

option for rehabilitation of a bidder.[92] It is impossible to say which approach is better because there is no practical evidence that would indicate positive results or a reduction in corruption. This demonstrates again the ineffectiveness of the overrated transparency rule. In the case of 'blacklists' it serves merely to expose and condemn but does not actually prevent corruption in Bulgaria. In the Austrian model, where blacklisting is applied, this has a profoundly negative effect on the business of the affected undertakings and has its logic, but in Bulgaria the effect is almost zero for the moment. The importance of the cultural perceptions of corruption should not be underestimated either.

Furthermore, the new Directive 24/2014/EU expands on one hand, the grounds for exclusion of participants[93] (as already transposed in Bulgaria), but creates, on the other hand, a rather liberal solution – the 'self-cleaning' mechanism where the bidder is allowed to provide the contracting authorities with sufficient evidence to rehabilitate itself and permit its continued participation in the procedure.[94] Unlike in Bulgaria, the 'self-cleaning' mechanism was familiar to and used in Austria and in Germany long before the new procurement package was implemented, as discussed in Chap. 6 as well. Both of the latter Member States have managed to demonstrate the logic behind this mechanism, as it does not pose an obstacle to the fight against corruption and does not detract from the main aim of the preconditions for exclusion of participants under Article 45(1) Directive 2004/18/EC; it has, at the same time, assisted in increasing competition.[95] As Arrowsmith, Prieß and Friton (2009) maintain in their observation of the Austrian and German experience in self-cleaning:

> Although exclusions are suitable means for achieving the objectives of the mandatory exclusions in the procurement directives[96] it is submitted, however, that exclusion is not *always necessary* to achieve these objectives. A less severe method, short of an absolute exclusion, is to take into account, in certain individual cases, self-cleaning measures which the affected company has taken. Further, [...] the accomplishment of a complete self-cleaning can often, in fact, *positively support* the objectives of the mandatory exclusions provisions.[97]

Whether this mechanism will have a positive effect in combating corruption in procurement in Bulgaria it is still too early and too debatable to judge, bearing in mind that the provisions of the New Procurement Directives with this respect were copied verbatim into the New PPA without any consideration of their actual

---

[92] Except for the expiry of the limitation period for offenses, for example – Art 57(3) New PPA.

[93] eg offering the option for blacklisting and exclusion of economic operators which have demonstrate persistent failings in performing procurement contracts in the past.

[94] Art 57(6) Directive 24/2014/EU.

[95] When a participant is able to prove that there are no longer any grounds for its exclusion, the participant again is deemed equal to other participants and acts to increase the number of competitors for the relevant procurement.

[96] ie The Procurement Directive.

[97] S Arrowsmith, H Prieß and P Friton, 'Self-cleaning as a Defence to Exclusions for Misconduct: An Emerging Concept in EC Procurement Law?' (2009) 6 *Public Procurement Law Review* 276.

applicability in this Member State.[98] Years of practice in the award of public procurement in Bulgaria reveal that when a certain element of the procedure is left to the discretion of the contracting authority (or the members of the tender assessment committee), and when a way to circumvent the main and more severe rule exists, the door to corruption remains wide open. Given that the contracting authority may be convinced, by means of sufficient evidence, that a certain bidder need not be excluded (in the absence of a clear definition of the term 'sufficient evidence'), scepticism as to the motives of the contracting authority to accept the evidence provided as sufficient is perfectly justified. It has been repeatedly noted in the course of this work that given the characteristics of the Bulgarian model, restrictive measures are a much more appropriate to combat poorly detected and sanctioned corruption effectively. Only practice, however, will tell whether the 'self-cleaning' mechanism will contribute to an increase or decrease in corruption in Bulgarian awards. However, if I may offer one speculation about the future of this provision in Bulgaria, it is rather to be expected that it will be seriously amended (since in its current draft it is still-born), or remain only to be applied in cases where no other corrupt method will serve to keep a desired candidate in a procedure.

Back to Austria, up to a little over a decade ago the issue of corruption and its manifestation was virtually offensive to Austrian legal writers and lawyers. Fabrizy (2001)[99] states that:

> Corruption is not an issue of policy in Austria today and had not been in the years before [...] Corruption is not mentioned in the latest report of national security [...] even not in connection with organised crime [...] There is also no public discussion about corruption going on [...] Corruption is really a minor problem in Austria [...] corruption rather happens in the field of public procurement, especially in construction.[100]

Obviously, however, corruption in public contracts did exist even then, but the fact that comments on corruption in Austria have swung from one extreme to the other (from 'not an issue in Austria' to 'a corruption paradise in EU') within a relatively brief period cannot be ignored. Probably due to the corruption cases revealed at high political levels over the last few years and the sharp drop in the CPI ranking, Austria has focused on the development of strategies, policies and legislative changes (including being one of the initiators of IACA). The distinct features of the problem in the field of public procurement seem to have become diluted in the general picture and anything specific is in most cases hard to identify.

Despite the above, the absence of specific anticorruption measures aimed at public procurement does not mean the absence of measures in the case of proven corruption in the award process. In addition to the mandatory exclusion from further participation in public procurement, corruption detected in the procedures may be

---

[98] See comments made in Chap. 5 in this context.

[99] EF Fabrizy, in T Beken, B Ruyver and N Siron (eds), *The organisation of the fight against corruption in the Member States and candidate countries in the EU* (Antwerp/Apeldoorn: Maklu, 2001) 35–48. Fabrizy was then the Deputy Chief Advocate General at the Supreme Court in Vienna, later becoming Chief.

[100] Ibid, 35.

deemed a constituent element of an infringement under SGB and may result in significant sanctions (including deprivation of liberty). As noted below in connection with the functions of the various bodies investigating corruption in public procurement, if a specific contract is deemed to restrict competition (which also covers certain types of bid rigging) in the sector concerned, or if fraud or bribery have been detected, then these offences automatically entail a breach of criminal law.[101]

Of course, criminal provisions differentiate between corruption in the public and the private sectors in terms of the punishment imposed, but nevertheless, the SGB sanctions *inter alia* the acceptance by or the offer of benefits to contracting authority employees for the purpose of winning a contract or obtaining data from a competitor's bid (subject to monitoring by control bodies), when the act restricts competition in the award process.[102]

Jaros and Stalzer (2014)[103] note the presence of a 'legal chain reaction' of corrupt behaviour in public procurement procedures, which may result not only in restrictions of a penal nature, but also means that '[a]ny such legally binding judgment or substantial evidence for a respective offence constitutes a very high risk for the company being – at least temporary – 'blacklisted' in public procurement procedures. [T]he potential risk of being temporally excluded from public procurement procedures may have a substantial negative effect on the company's future business and turnover (depending on the company's business sector and clients)'.[104]

7.8.2 *Responsible Bodies*

Action against corruption in Austria is undertaken primarily by the centralised body – the Federal Bureau of Anti-Corruption (*Bundesamt zur Korruptionsprävention und Korruptionsbekämpfung*, BAK), an institution of the Federal Ministry of the Interior. Between 2001 and 2010, the Federal Bureau for Internal Security was active in Austria in the capacity as the main anticorruption body exerting police oversight, but following changes in legislation (dictated in part precisely by the corruption scandals during the same period), the BAK took over these functions, concentrating specifically on corruption and enjoying significantly wider powers. The BAK has nationwide jurisdiction in preventing and combating, and investigating and fighting corruption and any related economic offences perpetrated by state administration officials and employees in undertakings with state participation, and

---

[101] Particularly §168b and §146 SGB. Offences under §168b can be penalised with a maximum imprisonment of three years, and bribery under §146 with up to ten years imprisonment.

[102] See §331 *et seq* SGB.

[103] K Jaros and J Stalzer, 'Austria: Corruptive behaviour in public procurement procedures as a deal breaker for mergers and acquisitions transactions?' (Blog post 2014) <www.schoenherr.eu/knowledge/knowledge-detail/austria-corruptive-behavior-in-public-procurement-procedures-as-a-deal-breaker-for-mergers-and-acqu/> accessed 26 April 2016.

[104] Ibid.

in the private sector as well. The BAK cooperates closely with the second main anticorruption body in Austria – the Central Prosecutor's Office for Economic Crimes and Corruption Cases (*Zentralen Staatsanwaltschaft zur Verfolgung von Wirtschaftsstrafsachen und Korruption*) and with different international anticorruption institutions.

BAK's activities are concentrated in four main areas:[105] (i) prevention, through analysis of corruption models and elaboration of preventive measures in cooperation with criminal police and other institutions; (ii) law enforcement, through police investigations into corruption and related criminal offences in the public and private sector; (iii) education, through information exchange and development of training programmes aimed at increasing the competences of employees throughout the state administration; (iv) cooperation with other national, European and international institutions in the field of anticorruption, as well as the exchange of good practices.

One of the main instruments employed by the BAK in developing prevention projects is the analysis of previous cases and investigations. The focus of analysis is not only on statistical data and initiated/completed investigations, but also on an in-depth review of individual cases of complex or specific acts of corruption, and organised and systematic behaviour of individuals and undertakings.

> The aim is to identify the different structures and mechanisms which support the manifestation of corruption. This approach investigates certain details related to the circumstances which have led to detection of the crime, specific operational aspects, as well as the outcome of any subsequent legal or disciplinary proceedings. [...] This data is then assessed against selected parameters in order to detect similar models and specific features in the profiles of suspects and the models of corruption exhibited.[106]

One of the main reasons for the overhaul of the former Federal Bureau of Internal Affairs, in addition to the acts of bribery established among high-ranking officials in the Austrian police and other institutions, was the desire of the state to create a body which would enjoy a significantly higher level of independence from politics, and which would be able to perform its duties in the detection and prevention of corruption free of any external pressure.[107] The BAK was created on the basis of a Federal Law on the Establishment and Organisation of the Federal Bureau of Anti-Corruption (*Bundesgesetz über die Einrichtung und Organisation des Bundesamts zur Korruptionsprävention und Korruptionsbekämpfung*, BAKG)[108] which expressly provides that the BAK will be an independent institution outside the scope of the

---

[105] See Bak.gv.at, *Federal Bureau of Anti-Corruption – General Information* (2015) <www.bak.gv.at/cms/BAK_en/general/start.aspx> accessed 26 April 2016. Further information also in L Hensgen, 'Fight against corruption in the Danube region: A study of regional best practices' (2013) Max Planck Foundation for International Peace and the Rule of Law, Sankt Augustin: Konrad Adenauer Stiftung, 57.

[106] R Dzhekova, F Gunev and T Bezlov, *European Experience in the Fight against Police Corruption* (Sofia: Center for the Study of Democracy, 2013) 93.

[107] Which is connected to certain criticisms of Austria by GRECO.

[108] BGBl I No. 72/2009

Directorate General for Public Security, although subordinate to the Austrian Ministry of the Interior.

In addition, the BAK's functions and tasks are clearly set out. It has full authority to perform police investigations of criminal offences under the Criminal Code (among other instruments) relating to agreements restricting competition in procurement procedures and (commercial) fraud on the basis of such agreements. It enjoys extensive rights and employs numerous methods for investigation of corruption cases involving all state administration officials, employees of undertakings with state participation and, in specific cases, entities from the private sector. The BAK is in close and constant cooperation with the Prosecutor's Office, acting explicitly on the basis of alerts provided by the latter, while on the other hand, the police authorities are obliged to report to the BAK any cases of suspected corruption. This creates an excellent interaction between law enforcement bodies and the judiciary, while the fight against corruption remains at the same time a separate and independent action unit (over which oversight is exercised separately by a special committee). Last but not least, the BAK is the body for cooperation with international institutions performing corruption investigations, such as OLAF and INTERPOL.

A comparison with the benchmark Member State in this book – the Bulgarian model – reveals several differences.

Firstly, similar centralised, anticorruption activities in Bulgaria are conducted by the CPCCOC,[109] but its initial institutional characteristics and projects in the field of public procurement have been unable to evolve fully, due to the unstable situation in this Member State and the rapid succession of governments over the last couple of years. The fate of CPCCOC (and BORKOR) remains unclear for the time being due to the project's links with the political aspirations of Bulgarian politicians and the significant resources required for its implementation. There is an evident lack of political will, and perhaps of the requisite public support for the CPCCOC to continue adequately its role as a centralised anticorruption body and for comprehensive implementation of the BORKOR project.

Secondly, even if the CPCCOC were to commence proper operation, its functions, at least for now, only cursorily cover the four-pillar approach to work adopted by the Austrian BAK. The analysis of corruption models is indeed strongly expressed in the BORKOR project Solution Model, simply because the project itself has been successfully borrowed from Germany's experience in this area. Under the remaining three pillars, however, Bulgaria has done almost no work whatsoever. Police investigations of corruption are a rare occurrence, and in the field of public procurement it would be difficult to identify even a handful of such investigations.[110]

Another important difference which cannot be ignored is the principle and actual independence of the institutions investigating corruption which applies in Austria.

---

[109] See Chap. 4.

[110] No claims are made as to comprehensiveness of the examination of the frequency of this type of investigation and its results because police investigations remain outside the context and objectives of this work.

This underlies the legislative changes and the expanded powers of institutions such as the BAK and the Central Prosecutor's Office, which will be discussed further below. In reality, the exact opposite is evident in Bulgaria – the NAO is a relatively independent body, albeit with rather limited powers due to the many recent legislative changes, which controls public procurement in Bulgaria. Yet given the enormous political interests concentrated around the NAO, its fate has been largely uncertain in recent years, with each new government attempting to lay its hands on and influence the choice of its members and mandates, thus limiting its independence (as discussed in Chap. 4).

Finally, the training of the Bulgarian administration in the timely recognition of corruption, responses in cases of attempted bribery etc is insufficient, or where in place, is definitely not a priority. Particularly in the field of public procurement, such training, along with effective whistle-blowing systems with guaranteed anonymity could have a decided effect on the detection of corruption involving public procurement participants.

As discussed, the judicial body working in closest cooperation with the Austrian BAK is the Public Prosecutor's Office for White-Collar Crime and Corruption (*Zentrale Staatsanwaltschaft zur Verfolgung von Wirtschaftsstrafsachen und Korruption*, the WKStA). The functions of the WKStA are similar to those of the BAK, with the two bodies working in close cooperation and complementing each other. The WKStA is part of the Public Prosecutor's Office and investigates corruption, bribery, financial crimes, fraud, as well as anti-competition agreements. Prosecutors have the power to initiate and terminate investigations and proceedings. The offences are generally of a high public and/or material interest, as well as financial crimes. Public procurements also fall in this scope as a separate control and prevention item. The WKStA proposes to increase the number of experts employed and allocated by the state, both to the WKStA and to the BAK, with significant resources in support of their functions.

As previously mentioned, the BAK does not conduct own-initiative investigations, but acts on information lodged by the WKStA or another prosecutor's office or court. Following receipt of an alert and its preliminary assessment, the BAK, in cooperation with the WKStA determines whether the case should be investigated by the BAK or another qualified body (usually the Federal police) if the BAK has no available capacity to carry out the investigation at the relevant time. Thus the BAK acts as an intermediary between the prosecution and the police in launching anticorruption measures.

In addition to these two bodies, acting as the main anticorruption units with general and more specific functions in the field of public procurement, there are also several other relevant organisations such as (i) the Coordinating Body on Combating Corruption (whose role is to coordinate anticorruption measures and whose members include Members of Parliament, BAK, the Chamber of Commerce and other governmental authorities and private sector representatives); (ii) the Department for Economic and Financial Crime; (iii) the Austrian Financial Intelligence Unit –

A-FIU (focused on suspicious transactions within the banking sector); (iv) the Audit Office (*Rechnungshof*, AO)[111]; and (v) the Austrian Ombudsman Board.

With respect to the AO, despite the fact that its primary function is to control the financial conduct of procedures 'it is possible in this context to compare, whether the conclusion of public contracts that replace rulings (and hence avoid the costs of possible objections against these rulings) is financially advantageous'.[112] The AO is also a good example of an audit office which carries out external audits and is empowered to make recommendations for the improvement of the procurement process.[113] Again, as in Germany, the opportunity emerges for the AO to act by exerting control over the proper spending of public funds. In addition, the AO, like the BAK and the WKStA, is also independent and able to provide objective and impartial monitoring of the financial part of the procedure – an element which the Bulgarian NAO most certainly lacks, as already noted. The functions and authority of the AO serve as additional proof of the absolutely imperative synergy which must exist between the legal framework and the control and administrative apparatus. In the absence thereof, all existing rules (even those aimed at achieving transparency and/ or strengthening anticorruption policies) lose their meaning. The AO in Austria does not suffer constant legal changes and its stability and clear functions leave no doubt as to the importance of an active, independent body exercising control over public spending. However, the AO has no sanctioning tools, but is only an advisory body, which, as already observed, would certainly not suit for the Bulgarian model, which urgently needs more active sanctioning mechanisms if it is to deal with corruption in the sector.

A review of the functions, actions and tasks of the main bodies engaged in tackling corruption in Austria leads to several important conclusions when these are compared to a Member State suffering much more prevalent corruption in public procurement:

1. The good practices which could be adopted in view of the organisational structure of the Austrian authorities are related mainly to the strong tendency for these bodies to be relatively independent of government as well as the adequate coordination between police forces and the prosecution, united both in the investigation and in the prevention of corruption;
2. The functions of all bodies are strictly defined and focus on timely and proper control over procurement implementation – from both a legal and a financial standpoint, with these bodies also being actively involved in the improvement of the awarding process. There is no room for interpretation, misinterpretation or duplicated effort, as observed in Bulgaria (eg in the functions of NAO and the PFIA or the strict procedural control maintained by the CPC and the SAC).
3. Specifically to public procurement, the approach of criminalising the restriction of competition in the sector is very interesting, as is the focus on cases of bid

---

[111] Along with the respective regional audit offices.

[112] Above (n 34) 398.

[113] See *Integrity in Public Procurement: Good Practices from A to Z* (OECD Publishing, 2007) 95.

rigging. This is in complete compliance with the ideas in the New Procurement Directives. Bid rigging is an issue which has been highlighted in recent years in most Member States, due to the clear conclusion that such practices not only distort or restrict competition, but also create avenues for corruption (on a horizontal line between the participants in a procurement process). The Austrian experience could thus be a valuable example of positive practice against this phenomenon.

Given the new rules set out by Directive 24/2014/EU, the functions of the BAK and the WKStA are expected to increase, along with criminalisation of the other grounds contained in the Directive requiring the exclusion of a bidder.[114] However, making allowance for the fact that the organisational and structural changes made to these anticorruption bodies are rather new, what is also important is that their activities show 'a serious will to effectively fight against corruption'.[115]

7.8.3   Other Anticorruption Efforts in Public Procurement

Some of the private and non-governmental initiatives in combating corruption in the field of public spending are briefly analysed below, especially those which demonstrate good practice and which could also be adopted in other Member States. Again, these do not differ significantly from the conclusions drawn from the review of the German system.

(i) The *development of the whistle-blowing mechanisms* available in Austria and the encouragement of citizens to make use of them are both very important. Whistleblowing Austria is the local branch of the Whistleblowing International Network (WIN). It provides whistle-blowers with assistance and advice. According to its website, it works on promoting the idea of whistle-blowing within Austrian society.

(ii) *Developing e-Governance* is also a priority for Austria, as is the case in Germany and most Member States. The main portals in Austria are Digital Austria and USP.gv.at, which offer online administrative services to citizens and companies. This results in significant reduction in the time necessary for obtaining all sorts of permits and certificates required in the course of participation in public tenders. 'Across Europe, Austria is the leading country regarding the implementation of eGovernment'.[116]

---

[114] According to Art 57 Directive 24/2014/EU, the main exclusion grounds are: participation in a criminal organisation, corruption, fraud, terrorist offences, money laundering, child labour and trafficking.

[115] Hensgen (2013) above (n 105), 63. This can also be recognised in the number of the WKStA's recent procedures and activities in relation to bid rigging and public procurement procedures.

[116] P Humann, *'eTendering in Austria'* <www.ippa.org/IPPC4/Proceedings/05e-Procurement/Paper5-6.pdf> accessed 26 April 2016.

(iii) Austrians also definitely recognise *the development of e-procurement* as an 'effective tool to fight corruption', which ensures 'reliable audit trial for the process of promoting, issuing, clarifying, evaluating, and awarding tenders'[117] and anticipate the transposition of the New Procurement Directives, which will provide an additional stimulus in this direction. E-procurement is getting increasingly popular in Austria. Many contracting authorities have already implemented e-procurement systems.[118] Yet there are no clear standards as to the software requirements and there are a number of different providers of e-procurement systems and tools. Most of the small and medium sized purchasers, however, do not yet have the necessary resources and there will be a huge demand as a result of the transposition of the New Procurement Directives.

As is by now well-known, the development and broad use of all types of electronic systems and portals aimed to facilitate the award process and to reduce bureaucracy is one of the main instruments in the fight against corruption in the procurement field. Given the historical background and corruption traditions in countries like Bulgaria, reviewed in the first few chapters of this work, all attempts to limit the human element in the award process can be regarded as extremely well-targeted. The practice of Austria is a positive example. The expected introduction of e-Certis, in accordance with the New Procurement Directives, and the strengthening of the role of e-procurement as promoted by these acts are additional positive steps.

In Bulgaria the introduction of e-procurement would be a real challenge, as discussed in the previous chapter as well. E-government is not expected to be a reality in practice earlier than 2020; e-procurement requirements need to be enforced by 2018. Nevertheless, the operation and use in practice of all e-platforms require much more investment in training and purely technical revisions before these e-platforms can be truly operative.

(iv) One element in the New Procurement Directives is *the introduction of the ESPD*, which involves self-declaration as means of proof that the economic operator fulfils the relevant selection criteria; this already exists in Austria, having been introduced in law.[119] In addition to ensuring considerable savings,[120] this instrument significantly reduces the administrative burden in the award procedure. This should also play a role in anticorruption policies by providing not only a lighter regime of proof which does not leave any opportunities for getting round the selection criteria, but also by distributing the responsibility

---

[117] J Stalzer, 'Challenges and opportunities of e-Procurement' (2014a) Roadmap 15 <http://roadmap2015.schoenherr.eu/challenges-opportunities-e-procurement/> accessed 26 April 2016.

[118] Such as the ÖBB, Asfinag, BBG etc.

[119] See Federal Law BGBl. I Nr. 15/2010.

[120] 'The savings following the introduction of the system of self-declaration were estimated at 12.3 Million Euros. Further savings of 3.2 Million Euros were estimated due to an extension of the system of self-declaration in 2012 (see Federal Law BGBl. I Nr. 10/2012)': High Level Group on Administrative Burdens, 'Case Study on ABR plus Item No. 5 Public Procurement' <http://ec.europa.eu/smart-regulation/refit/admin_burden/docs/141007_abrplus_case_study_no_5_public_procurement_final_en.pdf> accessed 26 April 2016, 15.

for contractor selection between the participant and the contracting authority, with the participant bearing the risk of any incorrect data. As already commented above, this document has been introduced in Bulgaria but without there being any practice in its implementation for firm conclusions to be drawn. However, it already opens some questions as to the real simplification it achieves, bearing in mind that the Bulgarian legislator has found it necessary to require enough other declarative documents from the bidders in addition to the ESPD, and this may not be felt as much support to the participants in the procedures.

7.9 What Can Be Borrowed from Austria?

The parallel drawn in the field of procurement awards and implementation in Austria is of great significance for the present work because it is a Member State which also faces some difficulties in managing corruption models and their prevention.

Although in a very different social and economic context, and with a different CPI (unsatisfactory when compared to other Member States but significantly better than that of Bulgarian example), Austria appears to have problems in limiting corruption both among high-ranking officials and more specifically in public spending (these two aspects are often inextricably linked). The corruption scandals of the last few years have toppled Austria from its pedestal as a remarkably stable and upright business partner, and the criticism in the EU reports sometimes sound close to that contained in the reports addressed to Bulgaria.

This is the central point for the comparison of these two Member States which face similar issues: how does Austria react to the attack that it has become a 'corruption paradise'? What statutory and structural changes has it introduced in order to escape this status quo?

The analysis of the legislation and procurement award systems of the two Member States distinctly reveals the differences in their approach and also the attitude towards transparency rules as an anticorruption instrument, which is the primary objective of this book. Evidently, and in contrast to the Bulgarian model, Austria has embraced in its desire to change its current situation, yet stricter legislative bodies and a yet better-oiled policing–prosecution apparatus, resulting in a large number of detected and prosecuted cases and effective sentences ('Austria is among the best-rated countries for the deterrent effects of successful prosecutions in corruption cases, according to the 2013 Eurobarometer').[121]

Even though there are similarities in terms of legislation, between the two example Member States, the reforms launched by Austria differ significantly from the Bulgarian ones. While the Bulgarian PPA has suffered countless transformations and unfortunately the New PPA (as drafted) is expected to fare the same way, the designated Austrian law has undergone only a few small-scale amendments in the last five

---

[121] *First EU Anti-Corruption Report* (n 11) 5.

years[122] (expectedly, it would also change as a result of the transposition of the new EU rules), but has reorganised its bodies to meet the needs of the contracting authorities and contractors for independent control bodies: a two-instance fast-acting, independent judicial system and a public procurement agency – the BBG – acting as a central purchaser and as a role-model against corruption practices.

The practical experience of the above bodies is not yet sufficiently extensive (considering the period after their reform and reorganisation) and their functions and responsibilities are expected to be further expanded to give effect to the New Procurement Directives. But even in their current modus operandi, they demonstrate a positive change and a focused fight against corruption – in practice, and not only on paper.

The legislative framework in the field of public procurement in Austria is not overly specific in terms of anticorruption instruments created specifically for this sector, but the increased control and broadened powers of the institutions are evidently able to achieve the desired effect. The BVergG provides the main instruments to fight corruption as presented in the Procurement Directives. Some rules do also mirror the Bulgarian approach, but this is again due to the harmonised EU legislation and/or the historical similarities, as discussed above, and not due to a specific approach being adopted by the domestic legislators.

As a summary of the main findings, the investigation into Austria's award system shows two main differences with the Bulgarian approach towards resolution of an equally grave problem – corruption in public resource allocation:

(i) Transparency rules are *not* an endless bibliographic list reproduced into Austrian legislation – on the contrary, transparency is achieved by means of an effective administrative machine, strengthening of e-procurement and working control and appellate apparatus.

(ii) Trust in Austria's law enforcement system and its constant refinement and efficient actions with the aim of speedy exposure of corruption cases puts a wide berth between where the two countries start in the fight against corruption in public contracts.

Again, as with the comparison with Germany, it is clear that effective control bodies along with a strong trend of limiting the human element in procurement award are the right path to restricting and curbing corruption in the procurement sector. This conclusion will inevitably remain valid following implementation of the New Procurement Directives' rules in Austria as well.

---

[122] Most of the legislative amendments in Austria were made with the aim of increasing flexibility and decreasing the burden of the procedure. However, Austrian procurement legislation was not as burdensome and complicated as the legal framework in Bulgaria, even before the amendments in BVergG were adopted.

Bibliography

A Pulito, 'Austria: The Alpine corruption paradise' (2013) Academia.edu <www.academia. edu/2432598/Austria_-_the_Alpine_corruption_paradise> accessed 26 April 2016

B Müller, 'Court requests greater transparency for award decisions' (2011) International Law Office <www.internationallawoffice.com/newsletters/detail.aspx?g=63a0a8da-bcb0-4723-9687-4873c1c5985b> accessed 26 April 2016

B Müller and I Mayr, 'Amendment introduces new public procurement review bodies' (2013) <www.internationallawoffice.com/newsletters/detail.aspx?g=ddc59a8e-4514-49ea-a137-7580657fc81c> accessed 26 April 2016

C Bovis, *EU Public Procurement Law* (Cheltenham: Edward Elgar, 2007)

EF Fabrizy, in T Beken, B Ruyver and N Siron (eds), *The organisation of the fight against corruption in the Member States and candidate countries in the EU* (Antwerp/Apeldoorn: Maklu, 2001)

G Grassl, 'Austria: Major reform of administrative jurisdiction system takes effect as from 1 January 2014' (Blog post 2013) <www.schoenherr.eu/knowledge/knowledge-detail/austria-major-reform-of-administrative-jurisdiction-system-takes-effect-as-from-1-january-2014/> accessed 26 April 2016.

G Knaul, the United Nations Special Rapporteur on the independence of judges and lawyers, in the presentation of her annual report to the UN General Assembly, New York (24 October 2012) ohchr.org <www.ohchr.org/EN/NewsEvents/Pages/DisplayNews. aspx?NewsID=12692&LangID=E> accessed 26 April 2016

J Stalzer, 'Challenges and opportunities of e-Procurement' (2014a) Roadmap 15 <http://roadmap2015.schoenherr.eu/challenges-opportunities-e-procurement/> accessed 26 April 2016

J Stalzer, 'Austria: court confirms advance effects of the new procurement directives' (Blog post, 6 August 2015) <www.lexology.com/library/detail. aspx?g=4698e021-9af7-48bf-a223-edf3e8f3e442>

J Stalzer, 'Austria Chapter – Public Procurement 2015' (2014b) International Comparative Legal Guides <www.iclg.co.uk/practice-areas/public-procurement/public-procurement-2015/austria> accessed 26 April 2016

K Jaros and J Stalzer, 'Austria: Corruptive behaviour in public procurement procedures as a deal breaker for mergers and acquisitions transactions?' (Blog post 2014) <www.schoenherr.eu/knowledge/knowledge-detail/austria-corruptive-behavior-in-public-procurement-procedures-as-a-deal-breaker-for-mergers-and-acqu/> accessed 26 April 2016

K Schwab and X Sala-i-Martín, *The global competitiveness report 2014–2015.* (Geneva: World Economic Forum, 2014)

L Hensgen, 'Fight against corruption in the Danube region: A study of regional best practices' (2013) Max Planck Foundation for International Peace and the Rule of Law, Sankt Augustin: Konrad Adenauer Stiftung

M Fruhmann in the chapter on Austria in U Neergaard, C Jacqueson and G Ølykke (eds), 'Public Procurement Law: Limitations, Opportunities and Paradoxes', in *The XXVI FIDE Congress in Copenhagen* (Copenhagen: Congress Publications, 2014), vol 3

M Krivachka, 'Certain Specifics in the Appeal of Decisions of Contracting Authorities pursuant to the Public Procurement Act' (2006) 10 *Pazar i Pravo*

M Steiner, 'Comparative law on public contracts' in R Noguellou (ed), *Droit comparé des contracts publics / Comparative law on public contracts* (Brussels: Bruylant, 2010)

P Humann, *'eTendering in Austria'* <www.ippa.org/IPPC4/Proceedings/05e-Procurement/Paper5-6.pdf> accessed 26 April 2016

P Marboe, P Franzmayr, 'Austria: Recent Public Procurement Law Introduces a New Award Procedure while a Last-Minute Regulation Dispels Confusion on Threshold Values' <http://www.mondaq.com/Austria/x/174552/Government+Contracts+Procurement+PPP/Recent+Public+Procurement+Law+Introduces+A+New+Award+Procedure+While+A+LastMinute+Regulation+Dispels+Confusion+On+Threshold+Values> accessed 26 April 2016

R Dzhekova, F Gunev and T Bezlov, *European Experience in the Fight against Police Corruption* (Sofia: Center for the Study of Democracy, 2013)

S Arrowsmith, *The law of public and utilities procurement. Vol. 1.* (London: Sweet & Maxwell, 2014)

S Arrowsmith, H Prieß and P Friton, 'Self-cleaning as a Defence to Exclusions for Misconduct: An Emerging Concept in EC Procurement Law?' (2009) 6 *Public Procurement Law Review*

S Williams-Elegbe, *Fighting Corruption in Public Procurement: A Comparative Analysis of Disqualification or Debarment Measures* (Oxford: Hart Publishing Ltd, 2012)

T Bianchi and V Guidi (eds), *The Comparative Survey on the National Public Procurement Systems Across the PPN* (Rome: Authority for the Supervision of Public Contracts 2010)

Chapter 8
Conclusions

'For the one who sows to his own flesh
will from the flesh reap corruption,
but the one who sows to the Spirit
will from the Spirit reap eternal life.'
(Galatians 6:8)

8.1 Groups of Conclusions

The conclusions drawn on the basis of this work can be organised in the following categories:

(a) Relevance and efficiency of the transparency principle as an anticorruption measure in public procurement;
(b) The role of control and appellate authorities in the prevention of corruption;
(c) Good practices which could be adopted and the most effective trends in handling the problem of corruption in public contracts.

These are now considered in turn.

8.1.1 Transparency Principle Efficiency Against Corruption

The work clearly demonstrates the inability of one of the example Member States (Bulgaria) to handle corruption in the public procurement sector by means of excessive reliance on publicity and transparency as pillars of lawful and efficient award.

Transparency emerged in response to society's need to fight corruption. It reflects the public's right to have access to a certain level of information on norms, rules, procedures and regimes and the actions of participants, presented in an understandable and clear manner; the information provided should at all times be sufficient for monitoring, verification and assessment. The transparency principle is strongly present in the public procurement regime, where it has taken on certain specific characteristics. EU legislation sets out certain requirements and restrictions on the parties involved in procurement procedures, with the aim of ensuring that the pro-

© Springer International Publishing AG 2017

I. Georgieva, *Using Transparency Against Corruption in Public Procurement*,
Studies in European Economic Law and Regulation 11,
DOI 10.1007/978-3-319-51304-1_8

cedures are conducted in openly and fairly. Some national legislative frameworks supplement these rules and develop an entire system aimed at ensuring transparent procedures (as is the case with Bulgaria), while other Member States keep to the level determined by the EU legislation.

An unresolved issue remains the lack of a common definition of transparency and the widely varying positions of the various states regarding the value of this principle. In particular, the Bulgarian approach to the transposition of transparency rules reveal a failure of understanding as well as a failure of the numerous attempts to put this principle in action. The continuous increase in transparency rules and the ever more complicated legislative basis has been examined and analysed in the course of this work. It has become patently clear that the example legislation of Bulgaria abounds in rules imposing 'absolute transparency' of award procedures, which sadly often overlap in both meaning and application, requiring that almost the entire public procurement file should be published on. Yet the EU claims that corruption in that Member State is increasing and the transparency obligations imposed on contracting authorities act purely as a burden on the award process. The outcome ultimately differs considerably from the desired result – the contractor selection process is greatly obstructed, the administrative apparatus labours under the numerous transparency rules, while corruption itself remains undisturbed. Hence, where the process does indeed require clarity and direct monitoring, the legislation turns out to be impotent.

Further, the overview of the origin and development of corruption worldwide and the focus on the individual historical and socioeconomic specificities of this phenomenon in Bulgaria outlines the main characteristics of corruption in public procurement. This description of corruption in Bulgaria is of value in the benchmarking part of this book, aiding the drawing of logical and objective conclusions as to which elements of the German and Austrian award systems have proved effective as anticorruption practices, but which remain inapplicable and unlikely to yield the desired results in Member States similar Bulgaria. Examples are provided of completely imprudent legislative decisions, ostensibly introduced for the purpose of combating corruption, but existing only pro forma, without achieving any success in that direction.

The conclusions regarding the unrealistic expectations of transparency as the main principle in public procurement are supported by an examination of theoretical developments and the work of certain institutions in their attempts to identify a successful method for preventing corruption in the award process.

TIBG's pilot project, the Pact, demonstrates tolerance towards publicity as a method for combating corruption in Bulgaria. The Pact is a voluntary act for additional monitoring and openness to the public in the award process. The sanctioning aspect for failure to fulfil the commitments undertaken under the Pact, however, is minimised and shifted to the background at the expense of the incentive aspect. The pilot implementation of the Pact shows that the model is a far cry from being a pillar against the severe corruption problems in the implementation of public procurement procedures. The comparison with the Integrity Pact, as applied in Germany, reveals that increasing the punitive element in the implementation of such a monitoring instrument is of utmost importance to provide the missing disciplining effect and for the latter to serve as a rod in the wheel of corruption.

In addition, particularly relevant to this first conclusion is the comparison between the work of the TIBG and the work of another anticorruption organisation in Bulgaria – the CPCCOC – which have certain similarities (both projects claim to offer an effective solution to reducing corruption in public procurement in Bulgaria and they basically use some of the best anticorruption practices of Germany). The approach of the two institutions, however, is completely antipodal, with the TIBG clearly championing increased trust between participants in the procedure and sufficient transparency, while the CPCCOC model offers measures which are far more radical and practical. A large part of the CPCCOC proposals are definitely applicable and also conform to the requirements of the New Procurement Directives. They highlight the European trend of focusing on other methods against corruption (eg promoting e-procurement, strengthening the role of CPBs etc). Although somewhat weak in certain points, the CPCCOC proposals are indeed constructive and demonstrate the trend for anticorruption policies which do not rely on stretching the transparency principle beyond recognition.

A significant part of this work, which demonstrates the broken link between transparency and corruption and illustrates where the gravest corruption 'ulcers' in the public procurement process award occur, is the infringements analysis (presented in Chap. 5). The list of infringements occurring in the course of the four phases of public procurement procedures (ie the Choice of Objects Phase, the Announcement Phase, the Procedure Conduct Phase and the Contract Implementation Phase, as defined in Chap. 3) can always be supplemented with other types of corrupt practices and specific infringements of the law or combinations thereof, depending on the type of procedure selected or the exact phase in which they occur.

On analysing the different types of infringements and their occurrence in the four phases, the following conclusions are underscored:

Most of the infringements which open up corruption loopholes are carried out in strict observance of publicity and transparency principles, even against a background of overly complicated and heavily bureaucratised procedures, with numerous additional transparency obligations imposed (as is the case of Bulgaria). In this context, *a large portion of professedly impeccable procedures turn out to be precisely those in which 'grand corruption' is perpetrated, with the subsequent loss of significant financial resources.* Some of the infringements (especially those occurring at the Choice of Object Phase), such as contractor selection in the absence of a procurement procedure, or splitting procurements in the absence of legal prerequisites, are relatively easy to detect. This is largely due to the fact that they are linked to a complete lack of publicity and occur directly outside legal rules. These infringements, however, are usually forms of 'petty corruption' and can be observed in smaller organisational units/contracting authorities (e.g. the patrons of municipalities).

In the remaining three phases transparency rules are either strictly observed or are altogether absent (e.g. in contract implementation infringements). The procedure runs as advertised, e.g. in the public procurement register, the OJEU, the buyer's profile, national daily newspaper etc. Despite all of this overt compliance, the procedure contains discriminatory requirements or provides a loophole for the selection of the only possible candidate, or the contract is implemented in complete disregard of the contract parameters. The methodology for the infringement analysis adopted for the purposes of the book (i.e. (i) description of infringed provisions; (ii) description of the infringement itself; (iii) violation of transparency rules, if any; and (iv) description of the types of corruption loopholes opened) clearly highlights *the prevalence of those infringements which open up significant corruption loopholes and which have, professedly, complied with all procedural and transparency rules*. This strongly supports the conclusion that publicity is not a cure for bribery and the selection of a 'favoured candidate' to the disadvantage of competitors.

8.1.2 Control and Appellate Authorities Effectiveness

This work reveals that where the administrative part of the procedure is deemed to have greater significance than its subject matter, it strongly influences how control over public procurement award and execution is carried out.

The example of the Bulgarian procurement model tends to show that in this Member State the control and appellate authorities monitor the strict observance of the law alone and the presentation of the specific set of documents required by contracting authorities. The control bodies' lack of human resources and financial capacity hinders the detection of intricate corruption schemes including deliberately convoluted technical requirements or evaluation methodologies. Infringements with corrupt intent often remain undisclosed. Yet even when detected, many of these infringements are penalised by means of fines which are disproportionately lower than the actual loss for society. Verdicts are far too rare to have a preventive effect on corrupt schemes. In reality, fiscal damage, restriction of competition, market distortion and the disillusionment of a large portion of candidates who no longer wish to participate in public procurement procedures cause damage to the state which cannot be compensated through sanctions, unless these sanctions can ensure reduced corruption in the sector.

It is apparent from this work that *the relationship between the various authorities in Bulgaria and their functions is extremely complex*, partly because of the EU legislative base, but partly because of the choices of the national legislator.

As stated, *most of the institutions monitoring and sanctioning the procurement process basically exercise legality control of contracting authority actions*, which is insufficient if the goal sought is that these institutions should somehow help in combating corruption. Furthermore, the structure of the control and appellate authorities is too burdensome and multi-instanced in comparison to the two other Member States reviewed. Some of the institutions have poorly defined powers to intervene in, or to improve the procurement process. *Ex ante* control is concentrated mainly in the powers of the Executive Director of the PPAgency and is restricted in scope. Ongoing control is implemented internally, is insufficiently independent and manages to prevent corruption at the lower and middle level of administration only. *Ex post* control is organised in a highly fragmented manner between the different authorities and is unable to achieve serious results in exposing corruption and infringements: (i) the financial inspection agency – PFIA – has greater responsibilities but is limited to the implementation of legality control only (monitoring mainly conformity with procedural rules); (ii) the audit office – the NAO – has the authority to analyse the efficiency and effectiveness of the awards but not to respond to alerts and complaints. Unfortunately, the actual operation of this auditing authority so far has been negligible due to constant restructuring and changes in its functions, and due to its being an object of political manipulation. Finally, the appellate authorities – the CPC and the SAC – also focus only on compliance with the letter of law and have neither the competence nor the expertise to detect corruption schemes hidden, for instance, in the requirements of seemingly procedurally-sound and transparent procurements.

Last but not least, it is important to underline *the lack of independence of the control and appellate authorities from the executive power* in Bulgaria. This factor definitely affects the efficiency and the meaningfulness of control which is expected to have a preventive and disciplining effect on participants in the award process and to dissuade them from using corrupt schemes. Lack of independence has a demotivating effect on eliminated or losing candidates, reflected in the reduced number of appeals which is in any event quite low. From this perspective, and although this conclusion goes beyond the scope of a purely analytical look at the regulation of public procurement in Bulgaria, it is evident that so long as there is no political will to ensure that the control apparatus functions effectively so that faith in it can be restored, corruption will not be curbed; on the contrary, the corruption will continue to take advantage of their current impunity.

It is furthermore evident from the analysis of the participants in the award process, of the control and appellate authorities and of the most common infringements revealing corrupt intent, *that against the background of strictly observed procedural rules, public administration in Bulgaria is not effective*. It is inadequate and insufficiently familiar with European standards. The level of technical and professional qualification of individual contracting authorities is in most cases also completely inadequate to address the proposed modern measures, and the legislative framework in public procurement cannot be made fit for the purpose by further 'experiments'.

8.1.3 Outline of Good Practices

Against the obviously unsuccessful attempts of the Bulgarian legislator to create a system of flexible and simple rules, interlinked with a functioning public spending control system and to fight corruption in the sector, the German and the Austrian models tend to demonstrate how this can be done more successfully. Not all the solutions used by these two Member States are applicable and/or acceptable for Member States with higher corruption and lower socioeconomic levels such as Bulgaria, but some of them are completely conventional and objectively successful methods for improving the procurement process and dealing with the manifestations of corruption.

The benchmarking process and the review of the control and appellate authorities of the two other discussed Member States, as well as their different approaches towards corruption in public procurement strongly support the conclusion made in p. 8.1.2 above.

The analysis of the public procurement award system in Germany and its comparison with the current state in the counter-example in this book – the Bulgarian system – in terms of corruption and the measures tackling it, has resulted not only in highlighting good German practices which could be borrowed by other Member States but also in a more comprehensive outline of the elements absent from procurement models such as the Bulgarian one.

An age-old conclusion drawn from this benchmarking process is that regardless the legislative changes needed and regardless how public spending is regulated, a key factor is the actual implementation, control and sanctioning effect of these norms. Efficient and preventive measures tackling corruption in the award process can be defined as comprehensive only when combined with an efficient judicial system and only where there is a much larger number of anticorruption proceedings initiated and concluded with an enforceable judgment. This inevitably demonstrates that the legislative changes which can be borrowed from Germany comprise only a small portion of the weapons needed in the fight against corruption in public procurement – undeniably an important portion, but not the only one.

Germany, however, is an invaluable example which Member States suffering from corruption in the award process can follow not only in view of its legislative framework, which is rather more schematic – mainly outlining essential terms, rights and obligations – but also with view to its application in practice. Instead of translating a huge number of transparency rules into statutory norms which fail to limit corruption, *Germany has opted for methods which facilitate publicity but also allow control over the activities of both contracting authorities and contractors*. A good example in this direction is the use of electronic platforms for e-procurement. Restricting the human factor is hugely important for a corruption-free environment and is definitely a good practice which should be borrowed at all costs, and the financial resources should be allocated as soon as possible instead of churning out nonsensical criticism against investment in software and e-platforms.

Another important element is the *efficient institutional apparatus in Germany*. The entire award and implementation stage of public procurement in Germany depends on a well-oiled and independent administrative apparatus, which exercises control over the activities of contracting authorities and sanctions any irregularities in good time. In addition, the efficient judicial system and the National Court of Auditors act as controlling and sanctioning bodies; they have a restraining and disciplining effect on all participants in the award and implementation process. In contrast with Bulgaria, the German Court of Auditors can actually intervene in the procurement process and suggest practical amendments to help the process result in the choice of a quality and cost effective service or work.

The experience in Germany further shows that *an effective central purchasing system could greatly limit subjective 'contracting authority-tenderers relations'*. Separation of the functions of the actual user of the goods, services or supplies from those of the entity carrying out and controlling the procedure introduces a very active element into the procedure which, in addition to serving as a safeguard against potential corrupt intent, is also an additional control body with regards to the entire procedure. What is more, according to the new procurement package, CPBs will be the first to move onto complete e-procurement (by 2018); this will further strengthen the anticorruption element of their functions by not only mediating the award process on behalf of the contracting authority, but also by limiting the human factor in the selection process.

In contrast, the application of the concept of CPBs in Bulgaria is at present almost non-existent and completely inadequate where it exists. This is why the German model is indeed relevant and why adoption of this model would serve as a positive start in the fight against corruption. The introduction of such a scheme requires substantial restructuring and reorganisation of the existing model at national level. If however such a separation between contracting authorities and potentially bribing bidders could be accomplished in the Member States, following transposition of the new EU rules, these efforts would be fully justified.

In addition to this analysis and the good practices outlined, the example of the German award system and the implementation and control over public spending also serves to support the conclusion that *ensuring transparency at every step and for every action of the contracting authority is clearly not the key element in combating corruption in the sector*. Indeed, while an adequate level of information in the award process is a must, Member States with severe corruption problems need to focus on ensuring a wider competitive environment, on flawless and timely control, and on the introduction of provisions with a clear disciplining effect if they truly wish to limit the handing out of public contracts to pre-selected candidates.

Moreover, some of the significant achievements of Germany in the fight against corruption in procurement underlie the New Procurement Directives. The current German practice could thus speed the adaptation of other Member States, like Bulgaria, to some of the rules which will be completely novel to them. *The analysis, however, also provides objective criticism of some of the new elements in the new procurement package, which, although effective for some countries (as evidently for Germany), may prove supportive of corruption in others* (e.g. the self-cleaning mechanism, using the most economically advantageous tender as the sole award criteria etc).

In summary, the legal review of the procurement system in Germany leads to the conclusion that a not so burdensome legal framework (additionally enlightened by the transposition of the new EU rules) combined with an efficient and independent control apparatus which monitors the effectiveness of the procedures and demonstrates a strong sanctioning mechanism could be a working recipe for the limitation of corruption in countries at different economic levels of development to Germany and with poor histories in fighting corruption. On the contrary – where the German system (overlapping some EU solutions as well) provides for a more discretionary approach and gives the contracting authorities a freedom of choice, this legislative direction cannot be followed by Member States with issues like Bulgaria's, without risking exacerbating their problems.

The parallel drawn in the field of public procurement award and implementation in Austria was of further significance for the present work, because like Bulgaria, Austria has also faced difficulties in managing corruption and its prevention in recent years. This helps identify several different aspects and to draw different conclusions from those outlined in the review of the German model. Austria is also much more similar in terms of legal system and regulation of public procurement to Bulgaria: this was regarded as a good basis on which positive Austrian practices could be introduced.

Although Austria has a very different social and economic context and a different CPI, it appears to have serious issues with corruption both among high-ranking officials and more specifically in public spending (as these two aspects are often inextricably linked). Corruption scandals over the last few years have toppled Austria from its position as a stable and upright business partner, while EU criticism on this issue now ringing similar to that in the reports addressed to Bulgaria. Despite the similar legislative framework for public procurement in the two countries, the analysis of the legislation and procurement award systems of Austria and Bulgaria reveals differences in their approaches and also in their attitudes towards transparency rules as anticorruption instruments.

As opposed to the Bulgarian model, in its desire to improve its status, *Austria has embraced stricter legislative bodies and improved policing–prosecution apparatus*, which has resulted in a large number of cases being detected and prosecuted and effective sentences being handed down. The reforms launched by Austria differ significantly from those adopted by Bulgaria. While the Bulgarian procurement legislation has suffered countless transformations, the corresponding Austrian law has undergone only a few small-scale amendments in the last years, and though Austria has seriously reorganised its control bodies in order to meet the needs of contracting authorities and contractors for independent control and a swift-acting judicial system. The practical experience of the reorganised Austrian bodies is still not sufficiently long-standing for complete conclusions to be drawn, and their functions and responsibilities are expected to be further expanded with view of the new EU legislative base. Yet even in their current format they demonstrate a positive change and a focus on the fight against corruption – in actual practice and not only 'on paper'.

The Austrian public procurement agency – *the BBG – acts as the main central purchaser and serves as a positive example, with its tailor-made strategy for combating corruption* and its code of conduct applicable to all employees. The use of the BBG as a CPB is important in terms of its role as an intermediary between businesses and contracting authorities, as is the case in Germany, but much more in terms of being a role model in the fight against corruption. The good example which this public procurement body provides while blending the two activities – advisory and practical – is a very positive approach. The analysis of Austria in this respect is invaluable – from genuine practice towards strategy and elaboration of anticorruption measures and not vice versa.

The legislative framework in the field of public procurement in Austria is not overly specific in terms of the anticorruption instruments created for this sector, but *the increased control and broadened powers of the institutions are evidently able to achieve the desired effect.* The Austrian law sets out the main instruments for combating corruption, as required by EU law. In some respects there are national solutions which overlap with the requirements of the New Procurement Directives, although they are not as common as is the case with Germany. Some rules do mirror the Bulgarian approach as well, but this is again due to the harmonised EU legislation and/or historical similarities and not due to a specific approach of the domestic legislator.

The investigation into Austria's award system shows two main differences from Bulgaria's approach toward resolution of an equally grave problem – corruption in public resource allocation. On the one hand, transparency rules are not an endless list of specific requirements in Austrian legislation, as has been the case in Bulgaria in the last few years; on the contrary, transparency is achieved by means of an effective administrative system, functioning e-procurement and a working control and appellate apparatus. On the other hand, *the trust in Austria's law enforcement system and its constant refinement and efficient action* is what has the greatest impact in combating corruption in public contracts, and distinguishes these two countries.

Again, it is clear that effective control bodies along with a considerable effort in limiting the human element in procurement award are the best approach to preventing and combating corruption in the sector. This conclusion is equally valid both for the current legal systems and for the situation following transposition of the new legislation package.

8.2 Recommendations

The analysis of the anticorruption policies, transparency rules and procurement award systems of the three Member States which are so close yet so far apart, as well as the highlighting of positive solutions, serves to set out the main recommendations for legislative and institutional measures which should be undertaken in EU countries needing to tackle corruption in procurement. They outline not only the weaknesses in national legislation, but also point out legal solutions incorporated in the EU base legislation which are inadequate for countries where corruption remains a serious problem. The work succeeded in questioning why 'the mantra' for transparency is constantly being repeated in the EU when commenting on the progress of the process of awarding contracts, where there are enough other effective methods which contribute to limiting corruption to manageable levels:

– The legislative framework for procurement at national level needs to present a significantly light, flexible (as to matter of administrative burden) and streamlined system of rules. From this perspective, transposition of the new procurement package needs to further take into account the general anticorruption policy and must carefully assess those rules which permit discretion to the national legislator in order to ensure that they do not open up additional loopholes for corruption. Apart from this, the legislative framework must contain a greater number of imperative rules and give less discretion to the contracting authority with regards to the main decisions related to contractor selection;

- Decrease of corruption depends directly on the presence of disciplining sanctions, which need to be applied in a timely manner in order to create the perception of proper law enforcement and stability in the legislative and judicial systems. Such sanctioning norms should predominate over incentive norms. The number of proceedings initiated and corruption schemes detected must be greatly increased;
- Efficient and independent control of the appellate authorities needs to be established, designed specifically to prevent and detect corruption (exercising effective *ex ante*, ongoing and *ex post* control), as well as a designated body to drive the fight against corruption. The control system must exercise control both with regards to the legality of procedures and the regularity of their implementation. In addition, control needs to focus both on the contracting authority and on the other process participants;
- Appeal must automatically suspend contract implementation and this suspensive effect must also be supported by speedy proceedings so as not to delay the supply of goods and services required by the contracting authority;
- An increase in the role of the centralised procurement is expedient. The CPBs serve as mediators in the award of standard procedures and increase the distance between the contracting authorities and the bidders-cum-contractors;
- Reducing the human factor in the award process is a priority. This can be achieved by boosting the use of e-procurement implemented in compliance with the provisions of the New Procurement Directives;
- The responsibility for the presence/absence of corruption in a given public contract should be proportionally distributed among all participants (generally the bribed contracting authority and bribing bidder), and rules need to be introduced concerning the actions of the individual candidates, with a strong disciplining effect;
- The audit office or auditing body must be a completely independent authority with broad competence in the implementation of public procurement procedures. Such an auditing authority needs to have significant expert capacity able to detect corruption schemes by means of audit analyses, and to act as a sanctioning body which may, in addition to administrative penalties, issue recommendations regarding contracting authority actions;
- The public procurement authority/agency needs to take on wider functions, including corrective anticorruption ones, and not only be responsible for methodological guidelines;
- Political will for adequate, functioning anticorruption measures must be evident, while the actions of the executive need to be consistent and efficient.

In the light of the above, the present work ultimately demonstrates that the fight against corruption in the procurement sector and the curbing of misuse of considerable public funds needs to be a national strategic objective in all Member States, focused on efficient policies to combat this phenomenon and not on the promotion of numerous palliative measures which cannot on their own achieve the desired result.

Printed by Printforce, the Netherlands